Study Guide & Skills Performance
Checklists to accompany

POTTER · PERRY

FUNDAMENTALS OF NURSING

fifth edition

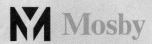

Mosby

A Harcourt Health Sciences Company

St. Louis   London   Philadelphia   Sydney   Toronto

Study Guide & Skills Performance Checklists to accompany

POTTER · PERRY

FUNDAMENTALS OF NURSING

fifth edition

Study Guide by

GERALYN OCHS, RN, MSN, CS-ANP
Assistant Professor in Adult Nursing
St. Louis University School of Nursing

Skills Performance Checklists by

PATRICIA A. CASTALDI, BSN, MSN
Associate Dean
Trinitas School of Nursing
Elizabeth, New Jersey
A Cooperative Program with Union County College
Cranford, New Jersey

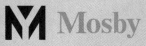 Mosby

A Harcourt Health Sciences Company

St. Louis London Philadelphia Sydney Toronto

Vice President, Nursing Editorial Director: Sally Schrefer
Senior Editor: Susan R. Epstein
Developmental Editor: Sharon Malchow
Project Manager: Gayle Morris
Production Editor: Jeanne Genz
Book Designer: Kathi Gosche

Mosby, Inc.
A Harcourt Health Sciences Company
11830 Westline Industrial Drive
St. Louis, Missouri 63146

Printed in the United States of America

International Standard Book Number: 0-323-01210-8

00 01 02 03 04   BD / EB   9 8 7 6 5 4 3 2 1

To my parents, George and Carolyn, for all your sacrifices, patience, love, and support. I am who I am because of this. Thank you.

CONGRATULATIONS

You now have access to Mosby's Fundamentals of Nursing Website!

Here's how to get there and what you'll find:

n on at:

www.mosby.com/MERLIN/Potter/Fundamentals/

A Website just for you as you learn fundamental nursing principles, concepts, and skills with the new 5th edition of *Fundamentals of Nursing*

t you will find:

- Content Updates
- Author Information • Information Exchange . . . and more

s:

WebLinks (only by using your personal passcode)

An exciting new program that allows you to directly access hundreds of websites keyed specifically to the content of this book. The WebLinks are continually updated and new ones added as they develop. **Simply peel off the sticker in the front cover of your textbook and register with the listed passcode. You cannot access the WebLinks without a passcode.**

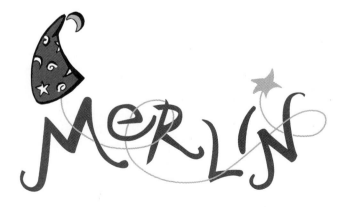

Mosby's **E**lectronic **R**esource **L**inks & **I**nformation **N**etwork

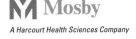

Introduction

The *Study Guide to accompany Fundamentals of Nursing,* fifth edition, has been developed to encourage independent learning for beginning nursing students. As you begin to read the text, you may note a difference in style or format from other books you've used in the past; the terms are new, and the focus of the content is different. You may be wondering, "How will I possibly learn all of the material in this chapter?" The essential objective of this study guide is to assist you in this endeavor—to help you learn *what* you need to know and then self-test with hundreds of review questions.

This study guide follows the text chapter for chapter. Whatever chapter your instructor assigns, you will use the same chapter number in this study guide. The outline format was designed to help you learn to read nursing content more effectively and with greater understanding. Each chapter of this study guide has the following sections to assist you to comprehend and recall.

The *Preliminary Reading* section is designed to teach prereading strategies. You need to become familiar with the chapter by first reading the chapter title, the key concepts and key terms (found at the end of each chapter), and all headings, as well as reviewing all photographs, drawings, tables, and boxes. This can be done rather quickly and will give you an overall idea of the content of the chapter.

The *Comprehensive Understanding* section is next and is in outline format. This will prove to be a very valuable tool not only as you first read the chapter but also as you review for tests. This outline identifies the topics and main ideas of each chapter as an aid to concentration, comprehension, and retaining textbook information. By completing this outline you will learn to "pull-out" key information in the chapter. As you write the answers in the study guide, you will be reinforcing that content. Once completed, this outline will serve as a review tool for exams.

The *Review Questions* in each chapter provide a valuable means of testing and reinforcing your knowledge of the material read and the answers written in the outline. Each question is multiple-choice and written in the NCLEX format. As a further aid for independent learning, each answer requires a rationale (the reason *why* the option you selected is correct). After you have completed the review questions, you can check the answers in the back of the study guide.

The clinical chapters, Chapters 26 to 30 and 36 to 49, include exercises based on the care plans found in the text. These exercises provide practice in synthesizing nursing process and critical thinking as you, the nurse, care for clients. Taking one aspect of the nursing process, you will be asked to imagine you are the nurse in the case study and to think about what knowledge, experiences, standards, and attitudes might be used in caring for the client. Write your answers in the appropriate boxes and check them against the answer key.

When you finish answering the review questions and synthesis exercises, take a few minutes for self-evaluation. If you answered a question incorrectly, begin to analyze the thoughts that led you to the wrong answer:

- Did you miss the key word or key phrase?

- Did you read into the question something that wasn't stated?

- Did you not understand the subject matter?

- Did you use an incorrect rationale for selecting your response?

Each incorrect response is an opportunity to learn. Go back to the text and reread any content that is still unclear. In the long run, it will be a time-saving activity.

A performance checklist is provided for each of the skills presented in the text. These checklists may be used by instructors to evaluate your competence in performing the techniques. The checklists represent generally accepted nursing principles and practice. You may need to adapt these skills in order to meet a client's special needs or follow the particular policy of an institution.

The learning activities presented in this study guide will assist you in completing the semester with a firm understanding of nursing concepts and process that you can rely on all of your professional career.

Contents

Study Guide & Skills Performance
Checklists to accompany

POTTER • PERRY

FUNDAMENTALS
OF NURSING

fifth edition

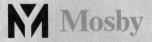
Mosby

A Harcourt Health Sciences Company

St. Louis   London   Philadelphia   Sydney   Toronto

Health and Wellness

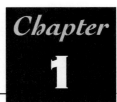

Chapter 1

Viewing health as an either-or situation ignores the health-illness continuum. In the approaching twenty-first century, health will be viewed from a broader perspective.

PRELIMINARY READING
Chapter 1, pp. 1-20

COMPREHENSIVE UNDERSTANDING
• Define the concept of *health*: _____
_____

• Define *illness behavior*: _____

HEALTHY PEOPLE DOCUMENTS
• *Healthy People 2000* focuses on three broad public health goals for Americans. List them.

  a. _____
  b. _____
  c. _____

• Goals for *Healthy People 2010* include:

  a. _____
  b. _____

• The four focus areas of *Healthy People 2010* are:

  a. _____
  b. _____
  c. _____
  d. _____

DEFINITION OF HEALTH
• Define *health:* _____
_____

• The WHO definition of health promotes a positive concept of health. Identify these characteristics.

  a. _____
  b. _____
  c. _____

- Life conditions have positive and/or negative effects on health. List some examples of life conditions.

  a. _____
  _____

  b. _____

  c. _____
  _____

  d. _____
  _____

MODELS OF HEALTH AND ILLNESS

- Health and illness are complex concepts. Models are used to understand the relationships between these concepts and the client's attitudes toward health and health practices.

- Health beliefs are a person's _____, _____, and _____ about health and illness.

- Health beliefs can impact health behavior, and they can positively or negatively affect a person's health. Identify some practices of each *health behavior*.
  a. Positive health behavior: _____
  _____
  _____

  b. Negative health behavior: _____
  _____
  _____

- Models represent different ways of approaching complex issues and helps us to understand a client's attitudes and values about health and illness.

HEALTH-ILLNESS CONTINUUM MODEL

- Describe the *health-illness continuum model*.
  _____
  _____

- Central to the health-illness continuum model are *risk factors*. Identify some common risk factors.

  a. _____
  _____

  b. _____
  _____

  c. _____
  _____

- Identify the advantages and disadvantages of this model.
  a. Advantages: _____
  _____

  b. Disadvantages: _____
  _____

HEALTH BELIEF MODEL

- The *health belief model* demonstrates the relationship between a person's belief and their behavior.

- Identify the three components of the *health belief model*.
  a. _____
  b. _____
  c. _____

HEALTH PROMOTION MODEL

- The focus of this model is to explain why individuals engage in health promotion activities.

- Identify the three functions on which the health promotion model focuses.
  a. _____
  b. _____
  c. _____

BASIC HUMAN NEEDS MODEL

- List in order the five levels of Maslow's hierarchy of needs.
  a. _____
  b. _____
  c. _____
  d. _____
  e. _____

HOLISTIC HEALTH MODELS

- Define the main concepts of the *holistic health model*: _____
  _____

- Clients use alternative therapies because: _____
  _____
  _____

THE WELLNESS-ILLNESS MODEL

- The wellness-illness model describes the relationship between *health, disease, wellness* _____, and _illness_ _____ as distinct parts of a process involving the person in the changing world.

- In this model, health is viewed as: _objective process characterized by stability balance & integrity of functioning._

- In this model, disease is viewed as: _____ a _dysfunction or alteration in functioning._

- In this model, wellness-illness is affected by the following factors. Give examples of each.
  a. Intrapersonal: _personality, past experience and emotional state_
  b. Interpersonal: _Social support & relationships_
  c. Health-disease related: _health promotion orientation, functional status_
  d. Extrapersonal: _____ _Sociocultural & economics_

THE HEALTH-HEALING/DISORDERING MODEL

- Define health and illness in this model.
  health is a dynamic process conceptualized as a functional state. Illness is deviation from normal state in which disordering processes occur.

- The health-healing/disordering model is a conceptual map. The model denotes a concept of health, which incorporates both healing and disordering processes as aspects of health.

- Briefly explain the following processes of the model.
  a. Health process: _____
  _____
  b. Disordering process: _____
  _____
  c. Healing process: _____
  _____

A MODEL WITHIN A MODEL

- A "model within a model" addresses the determinants of health from an individual and community level.

- List the five "environments" of health determinants for the individual.
  a. _Psychosocial environment_
  b. _Work_ "
  c. _Microphysical_ "
  d. _Behavioral_ "
  e. _Race/class/gender_ "

- List the four categories of social determinants of health for the community.
  a. _political & economic environment_
  b. _Local control & cohesiveness_
  c. _Macrophysical environment_
  d. _Social justice equity_

VARIABLES INFLUENCING HEALTH BELIEFS AND PRACTICES

- Internal and external variables can influence how a person thinks and acts. Understanding the way in which these variables affect a client allows the nurse to plan and deliver individualized care.

INTERNAL VARIABLES

- Internal variables include a person's developmental stage, intellectual background, perception of personal functioning, and emotional and spiritual factors. Identify and cite a personal example of how each of the following internal variables affects the client's health belief and practices.

  a. Developmental stage: _The concept of illness to a child_

  b. Intellectual background: _body functions & illness_

  c. Perception of functioning: _____

  d. Emotional factors: _____

  e. Spiritual factors: _____

EXTERNAL VARIABLES

- External variables influence a person's health beliefs and practices, including family practices, socioeconomic factors, and cultural variables. Identify and cite a personal example of how each of the following external variables affects the client's health belief and practices.

  a. *Family practices:* _____

  b. *Socioeconomic factors:* _____

  c. *Cultural background:* _____

HEALTH PROMOTION, WELLNESS, AND ILLNESS PREVENTION

- The concepts of health promotion, wellness, and illness prevention are closely related, and in practice overlap to some extent. All are focused on the future; the difference between them involves motivations and goals. Briefly explain each one.

  a. *Health promotion:* _activities such as routine exercise & nutrition maintain_

  b. *Wellness:* _Education teaches people how to take care of themselves in a healthy level_

  c. *Illness prevention:* _Such as immunization protects people from actual or potential threat to health_

- Nurses emphasize the following. Explain each one.

  a. *Health promotion activities:* _motivate people to act positively to reach style_

  b. *Wellness strategies:* _help people to understand & control their lives_

  c. *Illness prevention:* _motivate people to avoid decline or function level in health_

- The goal of a total health program is to _improve client's well being in all dimensions, not just physical_

- Give examples of the following practices or factors that affect health status.

  a. Individual practices: _poor eating habits no exercise_

  b. Physical stressors: _poor living environment exposure to air pollutants & unsafe_

  c. Psychological stressors: _emotional, intellectual, social, developmental spiritual_

- There are passive and active strategies for health promotion. Give two examples of each.

  a. *Passive strategies:* _The fluoridation of drinking water, fortification of_

  b. *Active strategies:* _weight reduction, smoking cessation_

4   Chapter 1: Health and Wellness

physically & emotionally health

LEVELS OF PREVENTIVE CARE

- Identify the health activities of each of the following levels of preventive care.
  - a. *Primary:* It precedes disease or dysfunction & applied to clients considered
  - b. *Secondary:* focuses on individuals who are experiencing health problems
  - c. *Tertiary:* occurs when a defect or disability is permanent & irreversible

RISK FACTORS

- Define *risk factor:* habit, social, environmental, physiological, psychological, developmental or spiritual variable that increases the vulnerability to an illness
- Identify at least two risk factors for each of the following categories.
  - a. Genetic and physiological factors: family history of disease, pregnancy, overweight.
  - b. *Age:* bearing children after 35 The risk of heart disease & cancer
  - c. *Environment:* industrial workers exposed to certain chemicals, poor housing unclear
  - d. *Lifestyle:* poor nutrition, overeating, poor healed etc insufficient sleep, tobacco use, alcohol & drug use

RISK FACTOR MODIFICATION AND CHANGING HEALTH BEHAVIORS

- Risk factor modification, health promotion, illness prevention activities, or any program that attempts to change unhealthy lifestyle behaviors can be considered a wellness strategy.

- Briefly explain the five stages of *health behavior change.*
  - a. *Precontemplation:* Not intending changes within the next 6 months.
  - b. *Contemplation:* Considered change within 6 months
  - c. *Preparation:* Make small changes in preparation for a change in the next month
  - d. *Action:* Actively engaged in strategies to change behavior. This stage may last upto 6 months
  - e. *Maintenance:* sustain change over time. This stage begins 6 months after action has started & continues indefinitely.

ILLNESS

- Define *illness:* is a state in which a person physical, emotional, intellectual, social, developmental or spiritual functing is diminishing or impaired
- Briefly explain the difference between disease and illness. does not have effect on functioning & well being in all dimention

ACUTE ILLNESS AND CHRONIC ILLNESS

- Explain the two general classifications of illness.
  - a. *Acute illness:* short duration & severe
  - b. *Chronic illness:* usually longer than 6 months & can affect functioning in all dimention.

ILLNESS BEHAVIOR

- _____,
  _____,
  _____, and
  _____ can
  all affect behavior.

- Illness behavior may become abnormal when it is disproportionate to the present pathology and the patient persists in the sick role.

VARIABLES INFLUENCING ILLNESS BEHAVIOR

- Give examples of the following:
  - a. *Internal variables:* _____
    _____
    _____
  - b. *External variables:* _____
    _____
    _____

IMPACT OF ILLNESS ON THE CLIENT AND FAMILY

- Illness is never an isolated event. The client and family commonly experience the following. Briefly explain each one.
  - a. *Behavioral and emotional changes:* _____
    _____
    _____
  - b. *Impact on body image:* _____
    _____
    _____

Chapter 1: Health and Wellness   5

c. *Impact on self-concept:* _____

_____

_____

d. *Impact on family roles:* _____

_____

_____

REVIEW QUESTIONS

The student should select the appropriate answer and cite the rationale for choosing that particular answer.

1. Internal variables influencing health beliefs and practices include:
   a. Family practices and cultural background
   b. Socioeconomic factors and intellectual background
   c. Spiritual factors and developmental stage
   d. Cultural background and perception of functioning

   Answer:_____   Rationale: _____

   _____

   _____

2. Any variable increasing the vulnerability of an individual or a group to an illness or accident is a (an):
   a. Illness behavior
   b. Risk factor
   c. Negative health behavior
   d. Lifestyle determinant

   Answer:_____   Rationale: _____

   _____

   _____

3. All of the following characterize illness behavior *except:*
   a. Calling a physician
   b. Ignoring a physical symptom
   c. Interpreting physical symptoms
   d. Withdrawing from work activities

   Answer:_____   Rationale: _____

   _____

   _____

4. The term *high-level wellness* is best defined as:
   a. Being free of chronic disease
   b. Surviving beyond one's life expectancy
   c. Fluctuating on a wellness-illness continuum within the health spectrum
   d. Functioning at one's best biophysical level

   Answer:_____   Rationale: _____

   _____

   _____

5. Marsha states, "My chubby size runs in our family. It's a glandular condition. Exercise and diet won't change things much." The nurse determines that this is an example of Marsha's:
   a. Acute situation
   b. Active strategy
   c. Positive health behavior
   d. Health beliefs

   Answer:_____   Rationale: _____

   _____

   _____

The Health Care Delivery System

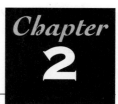

Chapter 2

With the costs of health care spiraling and no end in sight, employers, third-party payers, and the government search for new approaches that would reduce health care costs.

PRELIMINARY READING
Chapter 2, pp. 21-47

COMPREHENSIVE UNDERSTANDING

HEALTH CARE REGULATION COMPETION

* Total health expenditures have grown significantly from 1965 to 1985. Identify the reasons for rising costs.

  _____

  _____

  _____

* Briefly explain the following regulatory or government interventions that attempt to control health care spending.

  a. *Professional standards of review (PSRO):* _____

  _____

  _____

  b. *Prospective payment systems (PPS):* _____

  _____

  _____

* Competitive approaches to contain health care costs have supplemented and in some cases replaced regulatory approaches. Two common competitive approaches have been the following. Briefly summarize each one.

  a. *Managed care and health maintenance organizations (HMOs):* _____

  _____

  b. *Preferred provider organizations (PPOs):* _____

  _____

  _____

NURSING IMPLICATIONS

* Briefly explain how these regulatory and competitive approaches affect the nursing profession and the quality of care. _____

  _____

FINANCING HEALTH CARE

- Briefly explain the following common health plans.

  a. *Managed care:* _____

  _____

  b. *Preferred provider organization:* _____

  _____

  _____

  c. *Medicare:* _____

  _____

  d. *Medicaid:* _____

  _____

  e. *Private insurance:* _____

  _____

  f. *Long-term care insurance:* _____

  _____

PAYMENT MECHANISMS

- Capitation, fee-for-diagnosis, fixed payment, and direct contracting are payment mechanisms that an organization relies on and that affect its cost control approaches.

- Briefly define the following payment mechanisms.

  a. *Capitation:* _____

  _____

  b. *Fee-for-diagnosis framework:* _____

  _____

  c. *Fixed payment:* _____

  _____

  d. *Direct contracting:* _____

  _____

LEVELS OF HEALTH CARE

- The health care industry is moving toward health care practices that emphasize managing health rather than managing illness.

- A wellness perspective places focus on the health of populations rather than that of individuals. With this perspective, health care systems are moving toward *integrated delivery systems* (IDNs). Briefly explain this system.

  _____

  _____

  _____

PREVENTIVE AND PRIMARY CARE SERVICES

- Define *primary care*: _____

  _____

- Explain the focus of the following levels of care and the nurse's role in each.

  a. Health promotion services: _____

  _____

  b. Preventive care: _____

  _____

  c. School health services: _____

  _____

  d. Occupational health services: _____

  _____

  e. Physician's offices: _____

  _____

  f. Clinics: _____

  _____

  g. Nursing centers: _____

  _____

  h. Block and parish nursing: _____

  _____

  i. Volunteer agencies: _____

  _____

  _____

- *Primary health care* is an approach for:

  _____.

- The primary health care model focuses on collaboration of: _____

  _____

  _____

SECONDARY AND TERTIARY CARE

• Hospital emergency departments, urgent care centers, critical care units, and in-patient medical-surgical units are sites where secondary and tertiary levels of care are provided. In these settings, nurses work closely with all members of the health care team to _____, _____, and _____ for clients who are seriously ill.

• With the arrival of prospective payment and managed care, emphasis is placed on efficiency and the use of only those resources that are necessary to adequately care for the client until discharge. Identify some approaches that hospitals are using.

_____
_____
_____
_____
_____

• Explain the services provided by rural and urban hospitals.

_____
_____

• Explain the following sites where secondary and tertiary levels of care are provided.
  a. Public hospital: _____
  _____
  _____

  b. Private hospital: _____
  _____
  _____

  c. For-profit hospital: _____
  _____

  d. Not-for-profit hospital: _____
  _____
  _____

  e. Intensive care: _____
  _____
  _____

  f. Subacute care: _____
  _____
  _____

  g. Psychiatric facilities: _____
  _____
  _____

  h. Rural hospitals: _____
  _____
  _____

• Rural primary care hospitals (RPCH) are a new health care entity. Briefly explain the services they provide. _____
_____

RESTORATIVE CARE

• The goal of restorative care is: _____
_____.

• Explain the function of the restorative care team. _____
_____

• Briefly define *home health care*. _____
_____

• Home health nursing is a synthesis of community health nursing and selected technical skills from other nursing specialities.

• Home health care agencies provide: _____
_____.

• *Rehabilitation* is: _____
_____

• Drug rehabilitation centers help: _____.

• Rehabilitation services include the following. Briefly explain each.
  a. Physical therapy: _____
  _____

  b. Occupational therapy: _____
  _____

  c. Speech therapy: _____
  _____

• An *extended care facility* is: _____

CONTINUING CARE

- Continuing care/long-term care offer services for: _____
_____

- List the reasons why the need for continuing health care services is growing. _____
_____
_____
_____

- With the Omnibus Budget Reconciliation Act of 1987, the term 'nursing facility' became the term for nursing homes and other skilled nursing facilities where long-term care was provided.

- Briefly explain the services provided in a nursing facilities. _____
_____
_____

- Interdisciplinary functional assessment of residents is the cornerstone of clinical practice within nursing facilities. The focus is:
_____
_____
_____

- The Resident Assessment Instrument (RAI) consists of _____,
_____, and _____.

- Briefly define *assisted living* and described the services provided _____
_____
_____

- Define *respite care*: _____

- Identify the services provided by *adult day-care centers.* _____
_____

- *Hospice* is a system designed to: _____
_____

- The focus of hospice care is: _____
_____.

CANADIAN HEALTH CARE SYSTEM

- The Canadian medicare health care plan provides _____, _____, and _____.

- Identify some of the limitations in this health plan. _____
_____

ISSUES IN HEALTH CARE DELIVERY

- Consumers of health care want to access appropriate, cost-effective, quality health care.

- Access to care refers to: _____
_____.

- The success of any health care business depends on nursing's participation in _____
_____
_____

COMPETENCY OF HEALTH CARE PROVIDERS

- Identify the two principal mechanisms designed to ensure competent professional nursing practice.
  a. _____
  b. _____

- The Pew Health Professions Commission (1991) identified six critical competencies needed for health professions. Identify them.
  a. _____
  b. _____
  c. _____
  d. _____
  e. _____
  f. _____

POPULATION-BASED CARE

- To improve the health of the population there is a need to refocus health care in ways that better inform the public and to redistribute resources for health promotion and disease prevention efforts.

10   Chapter 2: The Health Care Delivery System

- Provide examples of ways that nurses can make a significant contribution in educating the public about their health.

  _____
  _____
  _____

REDESIGNING ACUTE CARE DELIVERY

- Explain each of the following.
  a. *Work redesign:* _____
  _____

  b. *Assistive personnel:* _____
  _____

  c. *Delegation:* _____
  _____

QUALITY HEALTH CARE

- Quality health care is difficult to define. Health care providers are trying to define and measure quality in terms of outcomes.

- Examples of outcomes are: _____
  _____
  _____.

- Health Plan Employer Data and Information Set (HEDIS) is a database of: _____.

- The Picker/Commonwealth Program for Patient-Centered Care identified seven dimensions of care that affect a client's experiences with health care. Name them.
  a. _____
  b. _____
  c. _____
  d. _____
  e. _____
  f. _____
  g. _____

THE CONTINUUM OF HEALTH CARE

- When an individual presents with a health problem, there is the potential of requiring a variety of services to enable the patient to regain or maintain his or her health.

- An integrated health care system has as its aim the delivery of care across the continuum. Most settings do not function as an integrated system but as independent levels.

- Define *discharge planning:* _____
  _____

- Discharge planning begins: _____
  _____

- List five tips that make the referral process successful.
  a. _____
  b. _____
  c. _____
  d. _____
  e. _____

- The Joint Commission on Accreditation of Health Care Organizations requires the following instructions on discharge from a health care facility._____
  _____
  _____
  _____
  _____
  _____
  _____

- Define *care delivery models:* _____
  _____

- Briefly explain the following care delivery models.
  a. *Care management:* _____
  _____

  b. *Care map/critical pathways:* _____
  _____

  c. *Case management:* _____
  _____

  d. *Patient-focused care:* _____
  _____

THE FUTURE OF HEALTH CARE

- Briefly summarize Nursing's Agenda for Health Care Reform from the American Nurses Association (1991). _____
  _____
  _____

REVIEW QUESTIONS

The student should select the appropriate answer and cite the rationale for choosing that particular answer.

1. The federal law allowing nurse practitioners to deliver primary health care in underserved areas is the:
   a. Rural Health Clinics Act
   b. Hill-Burton Act
   c. National Health Planning and Resources Development Act
   d. Social Security Amendment Act of 1972

   Answer:_____ Rationale: _____
   _____
   _____

2. Health promotion activities are designed to help clients:
   a. Reduce the risk of illness
   b. Maintain maximal function
   c. Promote habits related to health care
   d. All of the above

   Answer:_____ Rationale: _____
   _____
   _____

3. Rehabilitation services begin:
   a. When the client enters the health care system
   b. After the client requests rehabilitation services
   c. After the client's physical condition stabilizes
   d. When the client is discharged from the hospital

   Answer:_____ Rationale: _____
   _____
   _____

4. An example of an extended care facility is a:
   a. Home health agency
   b. Suicide prevention center
   c. State-owned psychiatric hospital
   d. Nursing facility

   Answer:_____ Rationale: _____
   _____
   _____

5. A client and his or her family facing the end stages of a terminal illness might best be served by a:
   a. Rehabilitation center
   b. Extended care facility
   c. Hospice
   d. Crisis intervention center

   Answer:_____ Rationale: _____
   _____
   _____

Community-Based Nursing Practice

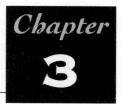

Chapter 3

The health care climate is changing, with a gradual transition from acute care delivered in hospital set-tings to care that is provided in the community.

PRELIMINARY READING
Chapter 3, pp. 48-63

COMPREHENSIVE UNDERSTANDING

ACHIEVING HEALTHY POPULATIONS AND COMMUNITIES

- Define *public health*: _____

    _____

- Identify the major public health problems of today.

    _____

    _____

- There are three essential services that constitute the core function. Identify them and give an example of each.

    a. _____
    b. _____
    c. _____

- Identify the five levels of health services.

    a. _____
    b. _____
    c. _____
    d. _____
    e. _____

- The principles of public health services aim at: _____

    _____.

COMMUNITY HEALTH NURSING

- Briefly identify the focus and educational requirements of the following.
    a. *Public health nursing:* _____

    _____

    _____

b. *Community health nursing:* _____
_____
_____

NURSING PRACTICE IN COMMUNITY HEALTH

- Population focused nursing practice requires a unique set of skills and knowledge.

- Briefly describe the practice of a community health nurse.
_____
_____
_____

COMMUNITY-BASED NURSING

- Community-based nursing involves: _____
_____

- Explain the human ecological model, which is the philosophical foundation for community-based nursing. _____
_____
_____

- The context of community-based nursing is family-centered care within the community.

VULNERABLE POPULATIONS

- *Vulnerable populations* are: _____
_____ .

- Explain how a nurse becomes culturally competent.
_____
_____
_____

- List some of the reasons why vulnerable populations typically experience poorer outcomes.
_____
_____
_____

- Briefly describe the following vulnerable groups and identify their risk factors.

a. Poor and homeless: _____
_____
_____

b. Abused clients: _____
_____

c. Substance abusers: _____
_____

d. Severely mentally ill: _____
_____

e. Older adults: _____
_____
_____

COMPETENCY IN COMMUNITY-BASED NURSING

- A nurse in a community-based practice must have a variety of skills and talents in assisting clients within the community.

- Briefly explain the competencies the nurse needs in the following roles.
a. Case manager: _____
_____
_____

b. Collaborator: _____
_____

c. Educator: _____
_____

d. Counselor: _____
_____

e. Client advocate: _____
_____
_____

f. Change agent: _____
_____
_____

COMMUNITY ASSESSMENT

- The community is viewed as having three components. Briefly explain each one.
a. Structure: _____
_____
_____

b. Population: _____

_____

_____

c. Social system: _____

_____

_____

- Once the nurse has a good understanding of the community, any individual client assessment is then performed against that background.

CHANGING CLIENTS' HEALTH

- The challenge is how to promote and protect a client's health within the context of the community.

- The most important theme to consider in order to be an effective community-based nurse is to:_____

_____.

- Identify some factors that nurses must consider in community-based practice.

_____

_____

_____

_____

REVIEW QUESTIONS

The student should select the appropriate answer and cite the rationale for choosing that particular answer.

1. Which of the following is *not* an example of a primary care setting?
   a. Elementary school
   b. Hospital
   c. Business
   d. Neighborhood health center

Answer:_____   Rationale: _____

_____

_____

2. Among the communication skills needed to provide nursing care to community clients is the ability to:
   a. Clarify client values and care expectations
   b. Follow medical prescriptions in many settings
   c. Manage generational interfamilial conflict
   d. Speak client's language or dialects

Answer:_____   Rationale: _____

_____

_____

3. Which of the following is an example of intrinsic risk factors for homelessness?
   a. Living below the poverty line
   b. Psychotic mental disorders
   c. Severe anxiety disorders
   d. Progressive chronic alcoholism

Answer:_____   Rationale: _____

_____

_____

4. When the community health nurse refers clients to appropriate resources and monitors and coordinates the extent and adequacy of services to meet family health care needs, the nurse is functioning in the role of:
   a. Collaborator
   b. Advocate
   c. Counselor
   d. Case manager

Answer:_____   Rationale: _____

_____

_____

5. The first step in community assessment is determining the community's:
   a. Set factors
   b. Goals
   c. Boundaries
   d. Throughputs

Answer:_____   Rationale: _____

_____

_____

Leadership, Delegation, and Quality Management

Chapter 4

 Health service organizations will require strong, innovative leaders, who can foster and implement change without compromising its mission of quality health care services.

PRELIMINARY READING
Chapter 4, pp. 64-85

COMPREHENSIVE UNDERSTANDING

LEADERSHIP AND MANAGEMENT
- Briefly explain the differences between leadership and management:
  a. Leadership: _____
  _____

  b. Management: _____
  _____

- Change and the ability to manage it in a constructive and proactive manner is central to the concept of leadership.

- A *management focus* is: _____.

LEADERSHIP IN CHANGE
- Identify the three types of change occurring in health care organizations.
  a. _____
  b. _____
  c. _____

TYPES OF LEADERSHIP
- Define the following two types of leadership and give an example of each.
  a. *Transactional:* _____
  _____

  b. *Transformational:* _____
  _____

LEADERSHIP BEHAVIOR AND STYLES

- Explain the two major dimensions of leadership behavior.
  - a. Initiating structure: _____
    _____
    _____
  - b. Consideration: _____
    _____
    _____

- List the ways to establish a considerate work behavior. _____
  _____
  _____

- Briefly describe the following *leadership styles* and when they are most appropriate.
  - a. *Autocratic:* _____
    _____
    _____
  - b. *Democratic:* _____
    _____
    _____
  - c. *Situational:* _____
    _____
    _____
  - d. *Laissez-faire:* _____
    _____
    _____

- Explain the four typical styles for situational leadership.
  - a. Directing: _____
    _____
  - b. Coaching: _____
    _____
  - c. Supporting: _____
    _____
  - d. Delegating: _____
    _____

- Define *empowerment:* _____
  _____

BUILDING A NURSING TEAM

- An empowering work environment is one that brings out the best in a professional, _____, _____, _____, _____, _____, and _____.

- Briefly identify the characteristics of the nurse executive. _____
  _____
  _____

NURSING CARE DELIVERY MODELS

- Care delivery must be effective in helping nurses achieve desirable outcomes for their clients.

- Briefly explain the following delivery systems.
  - a. *Total patient care:* _____
    _____
    _____
  - b. *Functional nursing:* _____
    _____
  - c. *Team nursing:* _____
    _____
    _____
  - d. *Primary nursing:* _____
    _____
    _____
  - e. *Case management:* _____
    _____
    _____

- Care maps are: _____
  _____.

MANAGEMENT STRUCTURE

- Briefly explain the following management structures.
  - a. *Centralized management:* _____
    _____
  - b. *Decentralized management:* _____
    _____
  - c. *Matrix:* _____
    _____

CREATING AN EMPOWERED WORK ENVIRONMENT

- Identify the responsibilities of a nurse manager. _____
  _____

- *Decentralized decision making* is defined as: ___
  _____

- The following are key elements in empowering staff and establishing decentralized decision making. Briefly explain each one.
  a. *Responsibility:* _____
  _____
  _____

  b. *Authority:* _____
  _____
  _____

  c. *Accountability:* _____
  _____
  _____

- The nurse manager nurtures and supports staff involvement through the following approaches. Briefly explain each.
  a. *Shared governance:* _____
  _____
  _____

  b. *Nurse/physician collaborative practice:* _____
  _____
  _____

  c. *Interdisciplinary collaboration:* _____
  _____
  _____

  d. *Staff communication:* _____
  _____
  _____

  e. *Staff education:* _____
  _____
  _____

- Identify the leadership skills a student nurse may develop. _____
  _____
  _____

- Clinical care coordination includes the following. Summarize each.
  a. Clinical decision making: _____
  _____

  b. Priority setting: _____
  _____

  c. Organizational skills and use of resources:
  _____
  _____

  d. Time management: _____
  _____

  e. Evaluation: _____
  _____

- Summarize the following principles of time management.
  a. Goal setting: _____
  _____

  b. Time analysis: _____
  _____

  c. Set priorities: _____
  _____

  d. Interruption control: _____
  _____

  e. Evaluation: _____
  _____

- Give an example of team communication. ___
  _____
  _____

- *Delegation* is defined as: _____
  _____.

- Identify the five rights of delegation.
  a. _____
  b. _____
  c. _____
  d. _____
  e. _____

- The standards that help define the necessary level of competency for the assistive personnel are: _____,
  _____, and _____.

- Identify the purposes of delegation.

  _____

  _____

- Summarize the requirements for proper delegation.

  a. _____

  b. _____

  c. _____

  d. _____

  e. _____

  f. _____

  g. _____

  h. _____

- List some ways that professional nurses build on their current knowledge base.

  _____

  _____

  _____

QUALITY MANAGEMENT

- List the principles of total quality improvement (TQM).

  a. _____

  b. _____

  c. _____

  d. _____

  e. _____

  f. _____

QUALITY IN NURSING PRACTICE

- *Quality improvement* is defined as: _____

  _____

  _____.

- The quality of nursing practice is defined by each of the following.

  a. Professional standards: _____

  _____

  _____

  b. Care guidelines: _____

  _____

  _____

  c. Outcomes: _____

  _____

  _____

- Differentiate between the two types of *outcomes.*

  a. Professional outcomes: _____

  b. Client outcomes: _____

- Differentiate between the two different types of quality improvement teams.

  a. Organization-wide: _____

  b. Unit-based: _____

- Identify JCAHO's ten steps to quality improvement.

  a. _____

  b. _____

  c. _____

  d. _____

  e. _____

  f. _____

  g. _____

  h. _____

  i. _____

  j. _____

- Identify who is responsible for the QI program: _____

  _____

- A unit's scope of service includes:

  _____

  _____.

- Some key aspects of service include:

  _____

  _____.

- A *quality indicator* is defined as: _____

  _____

- Explain the following three types of quality indicators.

  a. *Structure:* _____

  _____

  _____

  b. *Process:* _____

  _____

  _____

  c. *Outcome:* _____

  _____

  _____

Chapter 4: Leadership, Delegation, and Quality Management   19

- List some processes and related outcomes that may be in need of improvement.

  _____

  _____

  _____

- Threshold is defined as: _____.

- When QI is an ongoing process, staff continuously work to improve outcomes or performance by raising thresholds.

- Explain the purpose of data collection and analysis.

  _____

  _____

  _____

- Explain the model FOCUS-PDCA.

  _____

  _____

- After evaluating quality problems, the staff needs to do the following. Explain each.

  a. Resolve problems: _____

  _____

  b. Evaluate improvement: _____

  _____

  c. Communicate results: _____

  _____

  _____

REVIEW QUESTIONS

The student should select the appropriate answer and cite the rationale for choosing that particular answer.

1. One difference between a leader and a manager is that a manager:
   a. Is responsible for day-to-day operations and stability
   b. Has a vision or a goal for the group
   c. Influences others to follow his or her direction
   d. Focuses on innovation and change

   Answer:_____   Rationale: _____

   _____

   _____

2. A student nurse practicing primary leadership skills would demonstrate all of the following *except:*
   a. Being sensitive to the group's feelings
   b. Recognizing others for their contribution
   c. Assuming primary responsibility for planning, implementation, follow-up, and evaluation
   d. Developing listening skills and being aware of personal motivation

   Answer:_____   Rationale: _____

   _____

   _____

3. Mr. Jones is the team leader on a busy surgical floor. The team members are upset with the evening client assignments. Mr. Jones tells the team members to work things out for themselves and that whatever they decide will be satisfactory. Mr. Jones's leadership style could best be described as:
   a. Authoritarian
   b. Democratic
   c. Laissez-faire
   d. Situational

   Answer:_____   Rationale: _____

   _____

   _____

4. The effective nurse manager is able to use different styles and leadership skills depending on the specific situation and the maturity of the employees. This is an example of which leadership style?
   a. Authoritarian
   b. Democratic
   c. Laissez-faire
   d. Situational

   Answer:_____   Rationale: _____
   _____
   _____

5. During a cardiac arrest, which leadership style would be most effective?
   a. Authoritarian
   b. Democratic
   c. Laissez-faire
   d. Situational

   Answer:_____   Rationale: _____
   _____
   _____

Theoretical Foundations of Nursing Practice

Chapter 5

Application of nursing theory in practice depends on nurses having knowledge of the theories as well as an understanding of how the theories relate to one another.

PRELIMINARY READINGS

Chapter 5, pp. 86-99

COMPREHENSIVE UNDERSTANDING
THEORY

- Define *nursing theory*: _____

- Theory provides nurses with a perspective to view client situations and a method to analyze and interpret information.

COMPONENTS OF A THEORY

- Explain the following components of a theory.

  a. *Concepts:* _____
  _____

  b. *Definitions:* _____
  _____

  c. *Assumptions:* _____
  _____

  d. *Phenomena:* _____

TYPES OF THEORY

- Briefly explain the following classifications of theories.
  a. *Grand theories:* _____
  _____
  _____

  b. *Middle-range theories:* _____
  _____
  _____

  c. *Descriptive theories:* _____
  _____
  _____

  d. *Prescriptive theories:* _____
  _____
  _____

THEORETICAL MODELS

- A *theoretical model* refers to: _____
  _____
  _____

- Define the following components of nursing theoretical models.
  a. *Domain:* _____
  b. *Paradigm:* _____

- Briefly explain the four linkages of interest in the nursing paradigm.
  a. *Person:* _____
     _____
  b. *Health:* _____
     _____
  c. *Environment/situation:* _____
     _____
  d. *Nursing:* _____
     _____

HISTORICAL PERSPECTIVE

- Historically, nursing theories were studied in an isolated environment independent of nursing practice. The move now is toward nursing science or evidenced-based practice.

- Theoretical nursing models are used to _____, _____, and _____.

- Explain the historical review of the growing body of nursing knowledge.
  a. 1860: _____
     _____
  b. 1952: _____
     _____
  c. Mid-1950's: _____
     _____
  d. 1960's: _____
     _____
  e. 1970's: _____
     _____

RELATIONSHIP OF THEORY TO THE NURSING PROCESS AND CLIENT NEEDS

- Theory is the _____.
  Process is the method for _____.

- Summarize the nursing process as a tool for nursing practice.
  _____
  _____

INTERDISCIPLINARY THEORIES

- An *interdisciplinary theory* is: _____
  _____.

SYSTEMS THEORY

- A system is: _____
  _____.

- Define *input:* _____
  _____

- Define *output:* _____
  _____

- Define *feedback:* _____
  _____

BASIC HUMAN NEEDS

- List the five levels of the hierarchy of human needs.
  a. _____
  b. _____
  c. _____
  d. _____
  e. _____

HEALTH AND WELLNESS MODELS

- Health and wellness models are designed to:
  _____
  _____.

STRESS AND ADAPTATION

- The models that explain the stress response are: _____
  _____

DEVELOPMENTAL THEORIES

- The developmental theories explain the:
  _____
  _____.

- Give some examples of psychosocial theories. _____
_____
_____.

SELECTED NURSING THEORIES

- Briefly summarize the basic concepts relevant to the following nursing theories.

a. Nightingale: _____
_____
_____
_____
_____

b. Peplau: _____
_____
_____
_____
_____

c. Henderson: _____
_____
_____
_____
_____

d. Abdellah: _____
_____
_____
_____
_____

e. Levine: _____
_____
_____
_____
_____

f. Johnson: _____
_____
_____
_____
_____

g. Roger: _____
_____
_____
_____

h. Orem: _____
_____
_____
_____

i. King: _____
_____
_____
_____
_____

j. Neuman: _____
_____
_____
_____
_____

k. Roy: _____
_____
_____
_____

l. Watson: _____
_____
_____
_____
_____

m. Parse: _____
_____
_____
_____

n. Benner and Wrubel: _____
_____
_____
_____
_____

THE LINK BETWEEN THEORY AND KNOWLEDGE DEVELOPMENT IN NURSING

- Differentiate between theoretical knowledge and practical knowledge.

a. Theoretical knowledge: _____
_____
_____

b. Practical knowledge: _____
_____
_____

- Briefly explain each of the following:
a. Theory-generating research: _____
b. Theory-testing research: _____

REVIEW QUESTIONS

The student should select the appropriate answer and cite the rationale for choosing that particular answer.

1. Which of the following is a borrowed theory that has been applied to nursing?
   a. Orem's model of self-care
   b. Erickson's theory of psychosocial development
   c. Roger's theory of integrality
   d. Roy's adaptation model

Answer:_____ Rationale: _____
_____
_____

2. Which of the following conceptual models views the person and the environment as energy fields coextensive with the universe?
   a. King's model of personal, interpersonal, and social systems
   b. Orem's model of self-care
   c. Roy's adaptation model
   d. Roger's life process interactive person-environmental model

Answer:_____ Rationale: _____
_____
_____

3. Who is considered to have been the first nursing theorist?
   a. Florence Nightingale
   b. Virginia Henderson
   c. Adelaide Nutting
   d. Linda Richards

Answer:_____ Rationale: _____
_____
_____

4. How would you distinguish between theories and assumptions?
   a. Assumptions are tested, and theories are not
   b. Assumptions are assumed to be true, but theories are not
   c. Theories organize reality, but assumptions are not real
   d. Theories test hypotheses, but assumptions need no scientific proof.

Answer:_____ Rationale: _____
_____
_____

5. The development of nursing knowledge depends on:
   a. Science and philosophy
   b. Logic and reasoning
   c. Observation and verification
   d. Definitions and hypothesis

Answer:_____ Rationale: _____
_____
_____

Nursing Healing and Caring

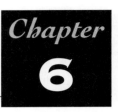

Chapter
6

The nurse that is able to engage clients in a caring and compassionate manner and recognize the therapeutic gain in caring will make enormous contributions to the health and well being of those clients.

PRELIMINARY READING
Chapter 6, pp. 101-111

COMPREHENSIVE UNDERSTANDING
THEORETICAL VIEWS ON CARING

- *Caring* is a universal phenomenon that influences the ways in which people _____, _____, and _____ in relation to one another.

- Caring in nursing has been studied from a variety of philosophical and ethical perspectives.

CARING IS PRIMARY

- Dr. Pat Benner does not try to predict or control phenomena but attempts to give nurses a rich, holistic understanding of nursing practice and caring through the interpretation of _____.

- Define *caring:* _____
_____

- Benner's theory of nursing practice focuses on: _____
_____.

- Briefly summarize how Benner describes the relationship between health, illness, and disease.
_____
_____
_____

THE ESSENCE OF NURSING AND HEALTH

- Leininger describes the concept of care as: _____
_____.

- Define acts of caring according to Leininger: _____

- Caring according to Leininger is a universal phenomenon, but the expressions, processes, and patterns of caring vary among cultures.

26   Chapter 6: Nursing Healing and Caring

TRANSPERSONAL CARING

- Summarize Watson's transpersonal caring theory. _____
_____
_____
_____

SWANSON'S THEORY OF CARING

- Swanson's theory of caring, consists of five categories. Explain each.
  a. Knowing: _____
  _____
  b. Being with: _____
  _____
  c. Doing for: _____
  _____
  d. Enabling: _____
  _____
  e. Maintaining belief: _____
  _____

SUMMARY OF THEORETICAL VIEWS

- Identify the common themes among the many nursing theorists.
_____
_____
_____

CLIENTS' PERCEPTIONS OF CARING

- Establishing a _____,
_____, and _____,
are recurrent caring behaviors that researchers have identified.

- When clients sense that health care providers are interested in them as people, clients will be more willing to follow recommendations and therapeutic plans.

- The nurse needs to focus on building a relationship that allows him or her to learn what is important to the client.

ETHICS OF CARE

- Caring is interpreted by many as being a moral imperative.

- In any client encounter, a nurse must know what behavior is ethically appropriate.

- Define *ethics of care*: _____
_____

CARING IN NURSING PRACTICE

- As nurses deal with health and illness in their practice, they grow in their ability to care.

- Expert nurses understand the differences and relationships among health, illness, and disease and become able to see clients in their own context, interpret their needs, and offer caring acts that improve client's health.

PROVIDING PRESENCE

- Summarize the concept of *presence*. _____
_____
_____

- Identify ways a nurse can establish presence with his or her clients. _____
_____
_____

COMFORTING

- Comforting provides both an emotional and physical calm.

- Give some examples of comforting approaches a nurse may use. _____
_____
_____

LISTENING

- Listening conveys the nurse's full attention and interest. Listening to the meaning of what a client says helps create a mutual relationship.

- A nurse must be able to give clients their full, focused attention as their stories are told.

- When an ill person chooses to tell their story, it involves reaching out to another human being.

Chapter 6: Nursing Healing and Caring   27

- Briefly summarize Frank's view of the clinical relationship the nurse and client share.
  _____
  _____

- Describe what listening involves. _____
  _____
  _____

KNOWING THE CLIENT

- To know a client means that the nurse
  _____ ,
  _____ ,
  and _____ .

- Knowing the client is at the core of the process by which nurses make clinical decisions. By establishing a caring relationship, the mutuality that develops helps the nurse to better know the client as a unique individual and to then choose the most appropriate and efficacious nursing therapies.

- Describe the following nurses and how they differ in knowing their clients.
  a. Expert nurse: _____
     _____
     _____
  b. Novice nurse: _____
     _____
     _____

SPIRITUAL CARING

- Spiritual health is achieved when: _____
  _____.

- Spirituality offers a sense of _____ ,
  _____ , and _____ .

- When a caring relationship is established, the client and nurse come to know one another so that both move toward a healing relationship by:
  a. _____
  b. _____
  c. _____

FAMILY CARE

- Success with nursing interventions often depends on the family's willingness to
  _____ ,
  _____ ,
  _____ ,
  and _____ .

- List the ten caring behaviors that are perceived as most hopeful by families of cancer clients.
  a. _____
  b. _____
  c. _____
  d. _____
  e. _____
  f. _____
  g. _____
  h. _____
  i. _____
  j. _____

THE CHALLANGE OF CARING

- The profession of nursing, unlike that of medicine, can care and assist people without medical diagnoses or new technologies and treatments.

- Caring motivates people to become nurses, and it becomes the source of satisfaction when we know we have made a difference in our client's lives.

- Summarize the challenges facing nursing in today's health care system.
  _____
  _____
  _____

REVIEW QUESTIONS

The student should select the appropriate answer and cite the rationale for choosing that particular answer.

1. Leininger's care theory states that the client's caring values and behaviors are derived largely from:
   a. Experience
   b. Gender
   c. Culture
   d. Religious beliefs

   Answer:_____ Rationale: _____
   _____
   _____

2. The central common theme of the caring theories is:
   a. Pathophysiology and self-care abilities
   b. Compensation for client disabilities
   c. The nurse-client relationship and psychosocial aspects of care
   d. Maintenance of client homeostasis

   Answer:_____ Rationale: _____
   _____
   _____

3. In order for the nurse to effectively listen to the client, he or she needs to:
   a. Sit with their legs crossed
   b. Lean back in the chair
   c. Respond quickly with appropriate answers to the client
   d. Maintain good eye contact

   Answer:_____ Rationale: _____
   _____
   _____

4. The nurse demonstrates caring by:
   a. Helping family members become active participants in the care of the client
   b. Doing all the necessary tasks for the client
   c. Following all of the physician's orders accurately
   d. Maintaining professionalism at all costs

   Answer:_____ Rationale: _____
   _____
   _____

5. According to Benner, the major characteristic that separates a "proficient" nurse from a novice nurse is:
   a. The ability to understand situations holistically
   b. An advanced educational preparation
   c. An intuitive understanding of situations
   d. Performance that is competitive

   Answer:_____ Rationale: _____
   _____
   _____

Diversity in Caring

Chapter
7

In light of the rapidly changing demographic profile of the United States, it is imperative that nurses develop an understanding about culture and its relevance to competent care.

PRELIMINARY READING
Chapter 7, pp. 112-137

COMPREHENSIVE UNDERSTANDING

IMPORTANT DEFINITIONS

- To understand transcultural nursing, the nurse must understand the following concepts. Briefly explain each.

  a. *Culture:* _____

  _____

  b. *Cultural values:* _____

  _____

  c. *Cultural behavior:* _____

  _____

  d. *Ethnicity:* _____

  _____

  e. *Ethnic minority:* _____

  _____

  f. *People of color:* _____

  _____

  g. *Biracial:* _____

  _____

  h. *Minority:* _____

  _____

  i. *Ethnocentrism:* _____

  _____

  j. *Stereotyping:* _____

  _____

TRANSCULTURAL NURSING

- Define transcultural nursing: _____

- To deliver culturally sensitive care, the nurse must remember that each individual is unique and a product of _____, _____, and _____ that have been learned and passed down from one generation to the next.

- Nurses must continually assess and evaluate each client's responses and never assume that all individuals within a specific cultural group will think and behave in a similar manner.

- State the goal of transcultural nursing.

  _____
  _____
  _____
  _____

- Define *cultural competence*: _____
  _____
  _____
  _____

CULTURALLY DIVERSE NURSING CARE

- *Culturally diverse nursing care* refers to:

  _____
  _____
  .

- Culturally diverse nursing care must take into account six cultural phenomena. Identify them.
  a. _____
  b. _____
  c. _____
  d. _____
  e. _____
  f. _____

COMMUNICATION

- Identify some common ways that nurses might *communicate* with clients of a different culture.

  _____
  _____
  _____

SPACE

- *Personal space* is: _____
  _____.

- Identify the common behaviors found in the following zones:
  a. Intimate zone: _____
  _____
  b. Personal zone: _____
  _____
  c. Social or public zone: _____
  _____

SOCIAL ORGANIZATION

- *Social organization* refers to: _____
  _____.

- Patterns of cultural behavior are important to the nurse because they provide explanations for behavior related to life events.

- In most cultures, next to the family, religion is the second most important social organization.

TIME

- Cultural groups construct systems of time that measure social events and agricultural activities.

- The sense of time is not innate but is developed early as a result of experiences linked to the individual's culture.

ENVIRONMENTAL CONTROL

- *Environmental control* refers to:
  _____.

- Briefly explain how the environment and people have a reciprocal relationship.

  _____
  _____

- Culture influences health-related behavior and has a profound effect on expectations and perceptions of sickness.

- Cultural health practices are categorized by western medicine as the following. Explain each.
  a. Efficacious: _____
  _____
  b. Neutral: _____
  _____
  c. Dysfunctional: _____
  _____
  d. Uncertain: _____
  _____

- Summarize the practice of folk medicine.
  _____
  _____

- The folk medicine system classifies illness as natural or unnatural. Explain.
  a. Natural illnesses: _____
  _____
  b. Unnatural illnesses: _____
  _____

- The ecological model is closely related to the folk medicine system. Identify the three areas on which it focuses.
  a. _____
  b. _____
  c. _____

- Identify some "alternative therapies."
  _____
  _____

- Summarize how religion can influence the cultural beliefs of the individual.
  _____
  _____

BIOLOGICAL VARIATIONS

- Define *biological variations*: _____
  _____

- The purpose of biocultural ecology is:
  _____
  _____.

APPLICATION OF GIGER AND DAVIDHIZAR'S TRANSCULTURAL ASSESSMENT MODEL

- Summarize the *Giger-Davidhizer* model, and explain how it identifies unique health care needs. _____
  _____
  _____

AFRICAN-AMERICANS

- Identify the three variables that affect the health of African-Americans.
  a. _____
  _____
  _____
  b. _____
  _____
  _____
  c. _____
  _____
  _____

- Summarize the following variables as they pertain to the African-American culture.
  a. Communication: _____
  b. Space: _____
  c. Social organization: _____
  d. Time: _____
  e. Environmental control: _____
  f. Cultural health variables: _____

- Explain the following biological variations in relation to the diseases that occur with higher incidence among the African-American population.
  a. Human immunodeficiency virus (HIV) infection: _____
  _____
  _____
  b. Hypertension: _____
  _____
  _____
  c. Cardiovascular disease: _____
  _____
  _____

d. Sickle cell anemia: _____

_____

e. Alcoholism: _____

_____

HISPANICS

- Identify the major issue that confronts Hispanic Americans._____

_____

- Summarize the following variables as they pertain to the Hispanic culture.
  a. Communication: _____

  _____

  _____

  b. Space: _____

  _____

  _____

  c. Social organization: _____

  _____

  _____

  d. Time: _____

  _____

  _____

  e. Environmental control: _____

  _____

  _____

- Summarize the specific cultural health practices of the Hispanic population.

  _____

  _____

- Explain the following biological variations in relation to the diseases that occur with a higher incidence among the Hispanic population.
  a. Diabetes mellitus: _____

  _____

  _____

  b. Hypertension: _____

  _____

  _____

c. Cardiovascular disease: _____

_____

d. Communicable diseases: _____

_____

e. Obesity: _____

_____

f. Human immunodeficiency virus (HIV) infection: _____

_____

_____

ASIANS-AMERICANS

- Summarize the following variables in relation to the Asian-American population.
  a. Communication: _____

  _____

  _____

  b. Space: _____

  _____

  c. Social organization: _____

  _____

  d. Stress of role reversal: _____

  _____

  _____

  e. Religion: _____

  _____

  _____

  f. Time: _____

  _____

  g. Environmental control: _____

  _____

  _____

- Describe the specific cultural health practices among Asian-Americans. _____

  _____

  _____

- Explain the following biological variations in relation to the diseases that occur with higher incidence among the Asian-American population.
  a. Cancer: _____

  _____
  _____

  b. Diabetes mellitus: _____

  _____
  _____

  c. Cardiovascular diseases: _____

  _____
  _____

NATIVE AMERICAN

- Summarize the following variables as they pertain to the Native American culture.
  a. Communication: _____

  _____
  _____

  b. Space: _____

  _____
  _____

  c. Social organization: _____

  _____
  _____

  d. Time: _____

  _____
  _____

  e. Environmental control: _____

  _____
  _____

- Summarize the cultural health practices of the Native American population. _____

  _____
  _____

- Explain the following biological variations in relation to the diseases that occur with higher incidence among the Native American population.
  a. Diabetes mellitus: _____

  _____
  _____

  b. Sexually transmitted diseases (STDs):

  _____
  _____
  _____

  c. Alcoholism: _____

  _____
  _____

  d. Suicide: _____

  _____
  _____

REVIEW QUESTIONS

The student should select the appropriate answer and cite the rationale for choosing that particular answer.

1. Which of the following is *not* included in evaluating the degree of heritage consistency in a client?
   a. Gender
   b. Culture
   c. Ethnicity
   d. Religion

Answer: _____   Rationale: _____

_____
_____

2. When providing care to clients with varied cultural backgrounds, it is imperative for the nurse to recognize that:
   a. Cultural considerations must be put aside if basic needs are in jeopardy
   b. Generalizations about the behavior of a particular group may be inaccurate
   c. Current health standards should determine the acceptability of cultural practices
   d. Similar reactions to stress will occur when individuals have the same cultural background

Answer: _____   Rationale: _____

_____
_____

3. To respect a client's personal space and territoriality, the nurse:
   a. Avoids the use of touch
   b. Explains nursing care and procedures
   c. Keeps the curtains pulled around the client's bed
   d. Stands 8 feet away from the bed, if possible

Answer:_____   Rationale: _____
_____
_____

4. To be effective in meeting various ethnic needs, the nurse should:
   a. Treat all clients alike
   b. Be aware of client's cultural differences
   c. Act as if he or she is comfortable with the client's behavior
   d. Avoid asking questions about the client's cultural background

Answer:_____   Rationale: _____
_____
_____

5. The most important factor in providing nursing care to clients in a specific ethnic group is:
   a. Communication
   b. Time orientation
   c. Biological variation
   d. Environmental control

Answer:_____   Rationale: _____
_____
_____

Caring in Families

Many changes have occurred in the concept and structure of the family, but it is clear that it remains the central institution in American society.

PRELIMINARY READING
Chapter 8, pp. 138-153

COMPREHENSIVE UNDERSTANDING
THE FAMILY
- Define the three important attributes that characterize contemporary families.
   a. Durability: _____
   b. Resiliency: _____
   c. Diversity: _____

CONCEPT OF FAMILY
- A *family* is a: _____
_____.

DEFINITION: WHAT IS A FAMILY?
- The family can be defined as _____, _____, or
   as a _____.

- To effectively provide care, nurses must understand that individual attitudes about family are deeply ingrained and deserve respect.

- To provide individualized care, the nurse must understand that families take many forms and have diverse cultural and ethnic orientations.

FAMILY FORMS
- Summarize the various family forms.
   a. Nuclear family: _____
   _____
   b. Extended family: _____
   _____
   c. Single-parent family: _____
   _____
   d. Blended family: _____
   _____
   e. Alternative: _____
   _____

CURRENT TRENDS AND NEW FAMILY FORMS

- Identify at least four current trends that challenge the family.
  a. _____
  b. _____
  c. _____
  d. _____

- Explain the following threats and concerns facing the family.
  a. Changing economic status: _____
  _____
  _____
  b. Homelessness: _____
  _____
  _____
  c. Family violence: _____
  _____
  _____
  d. Human immunodeficiency virus (HIV):
  _____
  _____
  _____

THEORETICAL APPROACHES: AN OVERVIEW

- Summarize the following three general perspectives when working with or studying families.
  a. Functional theory, or functionalism: ____
  _____
  _____
  b. Social conflict approach: _____
  _____
  _____
  c. Symbolic interactionism: _____
  _____
  _____

GENERAL SYSTEMS THEORY

FAMILY AS AN OPEN SOCIAL SYSTEM

- The family is viewed as an open social system that exists and interacts with the larger systems _____ of the community.

- The family system consists of interrelated parts _____ that form a variety of interaction patterns _____.

STRUCTURE

- Structure and function are closely related and continually interact with one another.

- Structure is based on organization, the _____.

- Structure may enhance or detract from the family's ability to respond to stressors. Briefly explain each of the following.
  a. Rigid structure: _____
  _____
  _____
  b. Open structure: _____
  _____
  _____

FUNCTION

- Family functioning focuses on the processes used by the family to achieve its goals. Identify these processes. _____
  _____
  _____
  _____

DEVELOPMENTAL STAGES THEORY

- Societal changes and an aging population have precipitated changes in the stages and transitions of the family life cycle.

THE FAMILY AND HEALTH

- The health of the family is influenced by its relative position in society.

- Identify the variables that affect the structure, function, and health of a family.
  _____
  _____
  _____
  _____

- The family strongly influences the health behaviors of its members. In turn the health status of each individual influences how the family unit functions and its ability to achieve goals.

- Family environment is crucial because health behavior reinforced in early life has a strong influence on later health practices.

ATTRIBUTES OF HEALTHY FAMILIES

- The crisis-proof or effective family is able to integrate the need for stability with the need for growth and change.

- Define *family hardiness*: _____
  _____

FAMILY NURSING

- The goal of family nursing is to: _____
  _____
  _____

- Identify the three levels and focuses proposed for family nursing practice. Briefly explain each.
  a. *Family as context:* _____
  _____
  _____
  b. *Family as client:* _____
  _____
  _____
  c. *Family as system:* _____
  _____
  _____

NURSING PROCESS FOR THE FAMILY

- Three beliefs underlie the family approach to the nursing process. Name them.
  a. _____
  b. _____
  c. _____

ASSESSING THE NEEDS OF THE FAMILY

- Identify areas to include in the family assessment.
  _____
  _____
  _____
  _____

FAMILY-FOCUSED CARE

- Collaboration with family members is an essential component of family-focused care, whether the family is the client or the context of care. Briefly explain each.
  a. Family as client: _____
  _____
  _____
  b. Family as context: _____
  _____
  _____

IMPLEMENTING FAMILY-CENTERED CARE

- Interventions aim to _____,
  _____, and to
  do _____.

HEALTH PROMOTION

- Health promotion behaviors that the nurse needs to encourage are often tied to the developmental stage of the family.

- Family strengths include _____,
  _____, _____,
  _____, and _____.

CHALLENGES FOR FAMILY NURSING

- Summarize the challenges for family nursing in relation to each of the following.
  a. Discharge planning: _____
  _____
  b. Cultural diversity: _____
  _____
  c. Communication techniques: _____
  _____

ACUTE CARE

- Summarize the challenges of family nursing in the acute care setting. _____
_____
_____
_____

RESTORATIVE CARE

- In restorative care settings, the challenge in family nursing is to _____.
Give some examples: _____
_____

- Whenever an individual becomes dependent on another family member for care and assistance, there is significant stress affecting both the caregiver and the recipient. Explain.
_____
_____

- Caregiving occurs within the context of the family.

- Explain the concept of *reciprocity*.
_____
_____

- Identify available family and community resources.
_____
_____
_____

REVIEW QUESTIONS

The student should select the appropriate answer and cite the rationale for choosing that particular answer.

1. Family functioning can best be described as:
   a. The processes that a family uses to meet its goal
   b. The way the family members communicate with each other
   c. Interrelated with family structure
   d. Adaptive behaviors that foster health

   Answer:_____   Rationale: _____
   _____
   _____

2. Family structure can best be described as:
   a. A basic pattern of predictable stages
   b. Flexible patterns that contribute to adequate functioning
   c. The pattern of relationships and ongoing membership
   d. A complex set of relationships

   Answer:_____   Rationale: _____
   _____
   _____

3. The majority of families today:
   a. Consist of a mother, father, and one or more children
   b. Include stepchildren
   c. Include a woman who works outside the home
   d. Are very similar to families of the past

   Answer:_____   Rationale: _____
   _____
   _____

Chapter 8: Caring in Families   39

4. When planning care for a client and using the concept of family as client, the nurse:
   a. Understands that the client's family will always be a help to the client's health goals.
   b. Considers the developmental stage of the client and not the family.
   c. Realizes that cultural background is an important variable when assessing the family.
   d. Includes only the client and his or her significant other.

   Answer:_____   Rationale: _____
   _____
   _____

5. Interventions used by the nurse when providing care to a rigidly structured family include:
   a. Exploring with them the benefits of moving toward more flexible modes of action
   b. Attempting to change the family structure
   c. Providing solutions for problems as they rise
   d. Administering nursing care in a manner that provides minimal opportunity for change

   Answer:_____   Rationale: _____
   _____
   _____

Developmental Theories

Chapter 9

Understanding developmental theories provides the basis for nurses to understand the client's responses to illness.

PRELIMINARY READING
Chapter 9, pp. 154-171

COMPREHENSIVE UNDERSTANDING

GROWTH VERSUS DEVELOPMENT
- Define growth: _____
- Define development: _____

FOUR AREAS OF THEORY DEVELOPMENT
- Identify the four main areas of theory development.
   a. _____
   b. _____
   c. _____
   d. _____

BIOPHYSICAL DEVELOPMENT THEORIES
- Define *biophysical development theories:* _____
  _____

GESELL'S THEORY OF DEVELOPMENT
- Briefly summarize Gesell's theory. _____
  _____
  _____

GENETIC THEORIES OF AGING
- The genetic theories of aging try to define how the DNA molecules transfer information to the formation of proteins, which determines the function and life-span of specific cells. Give an example. _____
  _____

NONGENETIC CELLULAR THEORIES

- Nongenetic cellular theories look at the cellular level and at how changes that take place in the molecules and structural elements of cells impair their effectiveness. Give an example. _____
_____
_____

- Explain the cross-linking theory. _____
_____
_____

- Explain the free radical theory. _____
_____
_____

PHYSIOLOGICAL THEORIES OF AGING

- Physiological theories of aging look at either the breakdown in the performance of a single organ or in the impairment of the physiological control mechanisms. Give an example.
_____
_____
_____

PSYCHOSOCIAL THEORY

- The psychosocial theories attempt to describe human development from the perspective of _____,
_____, and
_____.

SIGMUND FREUD

- Briefly explain *Freud's theory* regarding personality development.
_____
_____
_____

- Explain the five psychosexual developmental stages of Freud's theory.
  a. Stage 1: Oral: _____
  _____
  _____

  b. Stage 2: Anal: _____
  _____
  _____

  c. Stage 3: Phallic: _____
  _____

  d. Stage 4: Latency: _____
  _____

  e. Stage 5: Genital: _____
  _____

- Freud believed that three components of the personality govern adult life. Identify the functions of each.
  a. Id: _____
  b. Ego: _____
  c. Superego: _____

- The goal of the development as seen by Freud was the development of balance between the pleasures of the world and the domination of guilt and shame.

ERIK ERICKSON

- Erickson extended Freud's model by placing psychoanalytic theory within a social/cultural perspective.

- *Erickson* defined *eight stages of life*; each stage builds on a successful resolution of the previous development. Explain each.
  a. Trust vs. mistrust: _____
  _____
  _____

  b. Autonomy vs. shame and doubt: _____
  _____
  _____

  c. Initiative vs. guilt: _____
  _____
  _____

  d. Industry vs. inferiority: _____
  _____
  _____

  e. Identity vs. role confusion: _____
  _____
  _____

  f. Intimacy vs. isolation: _____
  _____
  _____

g. Generativity vs. stagnation: _____
_____
_____

h. Integrity vs. despair: _____
_____
_____

ROBERT HAVIGHURST'S DEVELOPMENT TASKS

- *Havinghurst* defined a series of essential tasks that arise from predictable and external pressures. These pressures include _____,
_____,
and _____.

- Identify a limitation to this theory.
_____
_____

ROGER GOULD'S THEMES OF ADULT DEVELOPMENT

- His research supports stage theory in adult development with a set of themes. Briefly explain the five themes identified.
  a. _____
  _____
  b. _____
  _____
  c. _____
  _____
  d. _____
  _____
  e. _____
  _____

STELLA CHESS AND ALEXANDER THOMAS'S TEMPERAMENT FACTOR

- Temperament is: _____.

- Explain the nine characteristics identified by Chess and Thomas.
  a. _____
  _____
  _____
  b. _____
  _____
  _____

c. _____
_____
_____
_____

d. _____
_____
_____

e. _____
_____

f. _____
_____
_____

g. _____
_____
_____

h. _____
_____
_____

i. _____
_____
_____

j. _____

- Three personality types were identified as _____, _____, and _____. One of the factors in the development of problems for these children was the ability of the parent and the environment to be flexible and understand the needs of the child given the personality structure.

COGNITIVE DEVELOPMENT THEORY

JEAN PIAGET THEORY OF COGNITIVE DEVELOPMENT

- *Jean Piaget* created a cognitive development theory that includes four periods and recognizes that children move through these specific periods at different rates but in the same sequence or order. Explain each of these periods.
  a. Sensori-motor intelligence: _____
  _____
  _____

b. Preoperational thought: _____

_____

_____

c. Concrete operations: _____

_____

_____

d. Formal operations: _____

_____

_____

MORAL DEVELOPMENTAL THEORY

• Moral development theories try to explain:

_____.

JEAN PIAGET'S MORAL DEVELOPMENTAL THEORY

• Explain the two stages of Piaget's moral development theory.

a. Heteronomous morality: _____

_____

b. Autonomous morality: _____

_____

LAWRENCE KOHLBERG'S MORAL DEVELOPMENTAL THEORY

• *Kohlberg* identified six stages of moral development under three levels. Briefly explain each.

a. Level I: Preconventional level: _____

_____

Stage 1: _____

_____

Stage 2: _____

_____

b. Level II: Conventional level: _____

_____

Stage 3: _____

_____

Stage 4: _____

_____

c. Level III: Postconventional level: _____

_____

Stage 5: _____

_____

Stage 6: _____

_____

• Identify the limitations to Kohlberg's research. _____

_____

_____

• Briefly explain Gilligan's argument with Kohlberg's theory.

_____

_____

REVIEW QUESTIONS

The student should select the appropriate answer and cite the rationale for choosing that particular answer.

1. According to Piaget, the school-age child is in the third stage of cognitive-development, which is characterized by:
   a. Conventional thought
   b. Concrete operations
   c. Identity versus role diffusion
   d. Postconventional thought

   Answer: _____   Rationale: _____

   _____

   _____

2. According to Erickson, the developmental task of adolescence is:
   a. Autonomy versus shame and doubt
   b. Self-identity versus role confusion
   c. Industry versus inferiority
   d. Role acceptance versus role confusion

   Answer: _____   Rationale: _____

   _____

   _____

3. According to Erickson's developmental theory, the primary developmental task of the middle years is to:
   a. Achieve generativity
   b. Achieve intimacy
   c. Establish a set of personal values
   d. Establish a sense of personal identity

Answer:_____   Rationale: _____
_____
_____

4. Which of the following behaviors is most characteristic of the concrete operations stage of cognitive development?
   a. Progression from reflex activity to imitative behavior
   b. Inability to put oneself in another's place
   c. Thought processes become increasingly logical and coherent
   d. Ability to think in abstract terms and draw logical conclusions

Answer:_____   Rationale: _____
_____
_____

5. According to Kohlberg, children develop moral reasoning as they mature. Which of the following is most characteristic of a preschooler's stage of moral development?
   a. Obeying the rules of correct behavior
   b. Showing respect for authority is important behavior
   c. Behavior that pleases others is considered good.
   d. Actions are determined as good or bad in terms of their consequences.

Answer:_____   Rationale: _____
_____
_____

Conception Through Adolescence

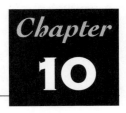

The nurse must have a clear understanding of normal or expected growth and development in all stages. This chapter discusses principles and concepts of growth and development and their application to health promotion from conception through adolescence.

PRELIMINARY READING

Chapter 10, pp. 172-223

COMPREHENSIVE UNDERSTANDING

GROWTH AND DEVELOPMENT

- Human growth and development are orderly, predictable processes that begin with conception and continue until death.

- All persons progress through definite phases of growth and development, but the pace and behavior of this progression are highly individualized.

- The ability to progress through each developmental phase influences the holistic health of the individual.

DEFINITIONS

- A person experiences quantitative and qualitative changes in growth and development. Summarize the following:
  a. *Physical growth:* _____
  _____
  b. *Development:* _____
  _____
  c. *Maturation:* _____
  _____
  d. *Differentiation:* _____
  _____

STAGES OF GROWTH AND DEVELOPMENT

Although chronological division is arbitrary, it is based on the timing and sequence of developmental tasks that the individual must accomplish to progress to the next stage.

MAJOR FACTORS INFLUENCING GROWTH AND DEVELOPMENT

- The human being is a complex, open system that is influenced by natural forces from within and from the environment. Give two examples of each.

  a. Forces of nature: _____

  _____

  _____

  _____

  b. External forces: _____

  _____

  _____

  _____

  _____

SELECTING A DEVELOPMENTAL FRAMEWORK FOR NURSING

- Providing nursing care that is appropriate developmentally is easier when planning on a theoretical framework.

- A developmental approach encourages organized care directed at the child's current level of functioning to motivate self-direction and health promotion.

CONCEPTION

INTRAUTERINE LIFE

- Define the following terms/events.

  a. *Nagele's rule:* _____

  b. *Fertilization:* _____

  _____

  c. *Zygote:* _____

  d. *Morula:* _____

  _____

  e. *Blastocyst:* _____

  f. *Embryo:* _____

  g. *Placenta:* _____

  _____

  h. *Implantation:* _____

  _____

- Explain the development process and health concerns for the following trimesters:

Trimesters	Developmental Process	Health Promotion
First trimester		
Second trimester		
Third trimester		

- Define the following terms.
  - a. First trimester

    Teratogens: _____

    _____

    Organogenesis: _____

    _____

    Fetus: _____

    _____

  - b. Second trimester

    Fundus: _____

    _____

    Quickening: _____

    _____

    Vernix caseosa: _____

    _____

    Lanugo: _____

    _____

    Prematurity: _____

    _____

    Tocolysis: _____

    _____

  - c. Third trimester

    VBAC: _____

    _____

    _____

    Temperament: _____

    _____

- Identify two prenatal events that are related to cognitive development.

    _____

    _____

TRANSITION FROM INTRAUTERINE TO EXTRAUTERINE LIFE

- _____, _____, and _____ influence adjustment to the external environment.

PHYSICAL CHANGES

- An immediate assessment of the neonate's condition is performed because the first concern is the _____.

- List the five physiological parameters evaluated through the Apgar assessment.
  - a. _____
  - b. _____

  - c. _____
  - d. _____
  - e. _____

PSYCHOSOCIAL CONCERNS

- What two factors are most important in promoting closeness of the parents and neonate?

    _____

    _____

- Define *bonding:*

    _____

    _____

HEALTH RISKS

- Briefly explain the three physical needs of the newborn that are most important.
  - a. Airway _____

    _____

  - b. Temperature _____

    _____

  - c. Prevention of infection _____

    _____

THE NEWBORN

- The *neonatal period* is defined as:

    _____

    _____.

PHYSICAL CHANGES

- Identify the normal characteristics of the newborn:
  - a. Height: _____
  - b. Weight: _____
  - c. Head circumference: _____
  - d. Vital signs: _____
  - e. Physical characteristics: _____

    _____

  - f. Neurological function: _____

    _____

  - g. Behavioral characteristics: _____

    _____

    _____

- Five distinct states that are highly influenced by environmental stimuli characterize infant behavioral responses. List these states.
  a. _____
  b. _____
  c. _____
  d. _____
  e. _____

COGNITIVE CHANGES

- Early cognitive development begins with innate behavior, reflexes, and sensory functions.
- Identify the sensory functions that contribute to cognitive development in the newborn.

  _____
  _____
  _____

PSYCHOSOCIAL CHANGES

- Explain the interactions that foster deep attachment between the infant and parents.

  _____
  _____
  _____

HEALTH RISKS

- Define *hyperbilirubinemia:* _____

  _____

HEALTH CONCERNS

- Screening for *inborn errors of metabolism* applies to: _____

  _____

- Circumcision is a common and controversial procedure. Identify the risks and benefits of this procedure.
  a. Risks: _____
  b. Benefits: _____

THE INFANT

- *Infancy* is the period from _____ to _____.

PHYSICAL CHANGES

- Summarize the normal characteristics of the infant.
  a. Physical growth: _____
  _____

  b. Vital signs: _____
  _____

  c. Gross motor skills: _____
  _____
  _____

  d. Fine motor skills: _____
  _____
  _____

COGNITIVE CHANGES

- Summarize the cognitive development of an infant. _____
  _____
  _____

PSYCHOSOCIAL DEVELOPMENT

- During the first year, infants begin to differentiate themselves from others as separate beings capable of acting on their own.

- Erickson describes the psychosocial developmental crisis for the infant as _____ versus _____.

- Define *play:* _____

- Identify activities appropriate at this stage of development. _____
  _____

HEALTH RISKS

- Identify the common types of injury and possible prevention strategies. _____
  _____
  _____

- Child maltreatment includes: _____
  _____

HEALTH CONCERNS

- The foundation for children's perceptions of their health status is laid early in life.

Chapter 10: Conception Through Adolescence   49

- Internal body sensations and experiences with the outside world affect self-perceptions.

- The quality of nutrition influences the infant's growth and development.

- Identify the feeding alternatives for an infant. _____ _____

- Identify some supplementation needs of an infant. _____ _____

- Briefly explain health concerns related to the following:
  a. Dentition: _____

  b. Immunizations: _____ _____

  c. Sleep: _____ _____

THE TODDLER

- *Toddlerhood* ranges from _____ to _____.

PHYSICAL CHANGES

- Summarize the normal characteristics of the toddler.
  a. Self-care activities: _____
  b. Motor skills: _____
  c. Vital signs: _____
  d. Head circumference: _____
  e. Weight: _____
  f. Height: _____
  g. *Physiological anorexia:* _____

COGNITIVE CHANGES

- Summarize Piaget's *preoperational thought stage.* _____ _____

- Describe language ability at this stage.

  _____ _____

PSYCHOSOCIAL CHANGES

- Identify Erickson's psychosocial development stage. _____ _____

- Explain the parental implications of the following developmental states:
  a. Independence: _____ _____

  b. Social interactions: _____ _____

  c. Play: _____ _____

HEALTH RISKS

- Describe some developmental abilities for this age period. _____ _____

- Identify injury prevention strategies. _____ _____ _____

HEALTH CONCERNS

- Children increasingly recognize internal body sensations but have difficulty pinpointing their location.

- Children who deviate radically from their usual patterns of eating, sleeping, or playing require assessment to determine whether or not these alterations result from illness.

- Children begin to internalize the labels that parents or health care professionals give to the somatic stages.

- Briefly explain the nutrition requirements for this age group. _____ _____

THE PRESCHOOLER

- The *preschool period* refers to _____.

PHYSICAL CHANGES

- Summarize the normal characteristics of the preschooler.
  - a. Vital signs: _____
  - b. Weight: _____
  - c. Height: _____
  - d. Coordination: _____

COGNITIVE CHANGES

- Preschoolers continue to master the preoperational stage of cognition.

- The first phase of this period, _____ (2 to 4 years), is characterized by _____.

- Define *artificialism:* _____
  _____

- Define *animism:* _____

- Summarize the intuitive phase of preconceptional thought (4 years). _____
  _____

- The greatest fear of this age-group is
  _____.

- Summarize this group's moral development.
  _____
  _____

- Describe the language ability for this age group: _____
  _____

PSYCHOSOCIAL CHANGES

- The preschooler's world expands beyond the family into the neighborhood where they meet other children and adults.

- Identify some dependent behaviors reverted to during stress or illness. _____
  _____

- Summarize the pattern of play for the preschooler. _____
  _____
  _____
  _____

HEALTH RISKS

- Guidelines for injury prevention in the toddler also apply to the preschooler. _____ and _____ are the top priorities for this age group.

HEALTH CONCERNS

- Parental beliefs about health, children's bodily sensations, and the ability to perform daily activities help children develop attitudes about their health.

- Explain the nutritional requirements of this age group. _____
  _____

SCHOOL-AGE CHILDREN AND ADOLESCENTS

- Summarize the developmental behavior typical of school-age children and adolescents.
  - a. Coping patterns: _____
    _____
    _____
  - b. Morals: _____
    _____
    _____
  - c. Diversity activity: _____
    _____
    _____
  - d. Nutrition: _____
    _____
    _____

THE SCHOOL AGE CHILD

- The school-age years range from _____ to _____.

- _____ signals the end of middle childhood.

- The school and home influence growth and development, and adjustments by the parents and child are required.

- Parents must learn to allow their child to make decisions, accept responsibility, and learn from life's experiences.

Chapter 10: Conception Through Adolescence   51

PHYSICAL CHANGES

- Summarize the normal characteristics of the school-age child.
  a. Weight: _____
  b. Height: _____
  c. Cardiovascular functioning: _____
  _____
  d. Neuromuscular functioning: _____
  _____
  e. Skeletal growth: _____
  _____

COGNITIVE CHANGES

- Cognitive changes provide the school-age child with the ability to think in a logical manner about the here and now. They are not yet capable of abstract thinking.

- Define the following cognitive skills that are developing in this group:
  a. *Concrete operations*: _____
  _____
  b. *Decenter*: _____
  _____
  c. *Reversibility*: _____
  _____
  d. *Seriation*: _____
  _____
  e. *Classification*: _____
  _____

- Describe the language development during middle childhood. _____
  _____
  _____

PSYCHOSOCIAL CHANGES

- The developmental task for school-age children is _____
  versus _____.

- Summarize psychosocial development in relation to the following:
  a. Moral development: _____
  _____
  _____
  b. Peer relationships: _____
  _____
  _____
  c. Sexual identity: _____
  _____
  _____

HEALTH RISKS

- _____ and _____ are the leading causes of death or injury.

- Infections account for the majority of all childhood illnesses; respiratory infections are the most prevalent.

- Identify the specific health concerns of children living in poverty. _____
  _____
  _____

HEALTH CONCERNS

- Perception of wellness is based on
  _____.

- Identify five critical functions of a school-based health promotion program.
  a. _____
  b. _____
  c. _____
  d. _____
  e. _____

- Accidents are the leading cause of death and injury in the school-age period. Children should be encouraged to take responsibility for their own safety.

- Identify at least five health promotion activities that are appropriate for the school-age child.
  - a. _____
  - b. _____
  - c. _____
  - d. _____
  - e. _____

- Identify the nutritional requirements for the school-age child. _____
_____

PREADOLESCENT

- *Preadolescence* refers to _____.

- Physically, preadolescence begins _____.

THE ADOLESCENT

- *Adolescence* is the period of development
_____.

- Define *puberty,* and explain the changes that occur at this time. _____
_____

- Identify the three subphases that exist within adolescence.
  - a. _____
  - b. _____
  - c. _____

PHYSICAL CHANGES

- List the four major physical changes associated with sexual maturation.
  - a. _____
  - b. _____
  - c. _____
  - d. _____

- Summarize the weight and skeletal changes that occur during adolescence. _____
_____
_____

- The hormones responsible for the development of secondary sex characteristics are _____ and _____.

- Explain the effects of physical changes on peer interactions. _____
_____
_____

- Identify the changes that occur during puberty in relation to the following:
  - a. Timing: _____
  - b. Sequence: _____
  - c. Hormonal changes: _____

COGNITIVE CHANGES

- Changes that occur within the mind and the widening social environment of the adolescent result in _____, the highest level of intellectual development.

- During this period of cognitive development, the adolescent develops the ability to solve problems through logical operations.

- For the first time the young person can move beyond the physical or concrete properties of a situation and use reasoning powers to understand the abstract.

- Elkind describes two characteristics of cognitive function. Briefly explain each one.
  - a. Imaginary audience: _____
  _____
  - b. Personal fable: _____
  _____
  - c. Adolescents have the capability to think as well as adults but do not have experiences on which to build: _____
  _____

- Describe the language skills of the adolescent. _____
_____

PSYCHOSOCIAL CHANGES

- The search for _____ is the major task of adolescent psychosocial development.

- Teenagers must establish close peer relationships or remain socially isolated.

- Explain identity versus role confusion (Erickson): _____
  _____

- Behaviors indicating negative resolution are _____, and _____.

- Explain the following components of total identity:
  a. Sexual identity: _____
     _____

  b. Group identity: _____
     _____

  c. Family identity: _____
     _____

  d. Vocational identity: _____
     _____

  e. Health identity: _____
     _____

  f. Moral identity: _____
     _____

- Define Erickson's *"psychosocial moratorium."*
  _____
  _____

HEALTH RISKS

- Identify the leading cause of death among adolescents and its sources. _____
  _____

- _____ is the second leading cause of death.

- Suicide is the third leading cause of death among adolescents. List the six warning signs of suicide for this group.
  a. _____
     _____

  b. _____
     _____

  c. _____
     _____

  d. _____
     _____

  e. _____
     _____

  f. _____
     _____

- Substance abuse is a major concern. Adolescents at risk are _____.

- In formation of healthy habits of daily living, emphasis is on exercise, sleep, nutrition, and stress reduction habits.

- Define the two eating disorders that follow:
  a. Anorexia nervosa: _____
     _____

  b. Bulimia nervosa: _____
     _____

- _____ and _____ expectations contribute to early heterosexual and homosexual relations.

- Briefly explain the two prominent consequences of adolescent sexual activity.
  a. Sexually transmitted disease (STD): ____
     _____
     _____

  b. Pregnancy: _____
     _____
     _____

- Identify health promotion interventions for the adolescent in regard to the following:
  a. Unintentional injuries: _____

  b. Substance abuse: _____
     _____

  c. Sexual activity: _____

  d. Firearms: _____
     _____

- Identify the concerns of the following adolescents:
  a. Rural adolescents: _____
     _____
     _____

  b. Minority adolescents: _____
     _____
     _____

REVIEW QUESTIONS

The student should select the appropriate answer and cite the rationale for choosing that particular answer.

1. Which statement about human growth and development is accurate?
   a. Growth and development processes are unpredictable.
   b. Growth and development begins with birth and ends after adolescence.
   c. All individuals progress through the same phases of growth and development.
   d. All individuals accomplish developmental tasks at the same pace.

Answer:_____   Rationale: _____
_____
_____

2. The mother of a 2-year-old expresses concern that her son's appetite has diminished and that he seems to prefer milk to other solid foods. Which response by the nurse reflects knowledge of principles of communication and nutrition?
   a. "Oh, I wouldn't be too worried; children tend to eat when they're hungry. I just wouldn't give him dessert unless he eats his meal."
   b. "That is not uncommon in toddlers. You might consider increasing his milk to 2 quarts per day to be sure he gets enough nutrients."
   c. "Have you considered feeding him when he doesn't seem interested in feeding himself?"
   d. "A toddler's rate of growth normally slows down. It's common to see a toddler's appetite diminish in response to decreased calorie needs."

Answer:_____   Rationale: _____
_____
_____

3. Which neonatal assessment finding would be considered abnormal?
   a. Cyanosis of the hands and feet during activity
   b. Palpable anterior and posterior fontanels
   c. Soft protuberant abdomen

Answer:_____   Rationale: _____
_____
_____

4. To stimulate cognitive and psychosocial development of the toddler, it is important for parents to:
   a. Set firm and consistent limits
   b. Foster sharing of toys with playmates and siblings
   c. Provide clarification about what is right and wrong
   d. Limit confusion by restricting exploration of the environment

Answer:_____   Rationale: _____
_____
_____

5. Which of the following is true of the developmental behaviors of school-age children?
   a. Formal and informal peer group membership is the key in forming self-esteem.
   b. Fears center on the loss of self-control.
   c. Positive feedback from parents and teachers is crucial to development.
   d. A full range of defense mechanisms is used including rationalization and intellectualization.

Answer:_____   Rationale: _____
_____
_____

6. Adolescents have mastered age-appropriate sexuality when they feel comfortable with their sexual:
   a. Behaviors
   b. Choices
   c. Relationships
   d. All of the above

Answer:_____   Rationale: _____
_____
_____

Young to Middle Adult

 Young and middle adulthood is a period of challenges, rewards, and crises.

PRELIMINARY READING
Chapter 11, pp. 224-242

COMPREHENSIVE UNDERSTANDING
- Developmental changes are based on earlier characteristics that help shape subsequent behavior and characteristics. Young adults pass through alternating periods of stability and change.

- Young adulthood is the period from _____ to _____.

- Individuals in young adulthood _____, _____, and _____.

- Middle age occurs from _____ to _____.

- The transition into middle age occurs _____.

- Briefly describe the characteristics of the *mature* adult. _____
_____
_____

- Briefly describe the intellectual and moral developmental differences between men and women during this time. _____
_____

THE YOUNG ADULT

PHYSICAL CHANGES
The young adult has completed physical growth by the age of _____.

- Identify the personal lifestyle assessment of a young adult. _____
_____
_____
_____
_____

COGNITIVE CHANGES

- Briefly explain the cognitive development of the period in relation to educational, life, and occupational experiences. _____
_____
_____

PSYCHOSOCIAL CHANGES

- The emotional health of the young adult is related to the individual's ability to address and resolve personal and social tasks. Explain the patterns of the following age groups:

  a. 23 to 28 years: _____
  _____
  _____

  b. 29 to 34 years: _____
  _____
  _____

  c. 35 to 43 years: _____
  _____
  _____

- The young adult must make decisions concerning a career, marriage, and parenthood. Briefly explain the general principles involved.

  a. Lifestyle: _____
  _____
  _____

  b. Career: _____
  _____
  _____

  c. Sexuality: _____
  _____

  d. Childbearing cycle: _____
  _____

  e. Lactation: _____
  _____
  _____

- Describe the following types of families:

  a. Singlehood: _____
  _____
  _____
  _____

  b. Marriage: _____
  _____
  _____
  _____

- Identify five tasks to be completed prior to marriage.

  a. _____
  b. _____
  c. _____
  d. _____
  e. _____

- Identify six tasks in the establishment of a household.

  a. _____
  b. _____
  c. _____
  d. _____
  e. _____
  f. _____

- Identify the hallmarks of emotional health for the young adult.
  _____
  _____

HEALTH RISKS

- Briefly explain the risk factors for young adults in regard to the following:

  a. Family history: _____
  _____
  _____
  _____

  b. Personal hygiene habits: _____
  _____
  _____

  c. Violent death and injury: _____
  _____
  _____

  d. Substance abuse: _____
  _____
  _____
  _____

e. Unplanned pregnancies: _____

_____

_____

_____

f. Sexually transmitted diseases: _____

_____

_____

_____

g. Environmental and occupational risks:

_____

_____

_____

_____

HEALTH CONCERNS

- Briefly explain the following:
  a. *Infertility:* _____

  _____

  _____

  b. Exercise: _____

  _____

  _____

  c. Routine health screening: _____

  _____

  d. Psychosocial health: _____

  _____

  _____

  _____

- The psychosocial concerns of the young adult are often related to stress. Briefly explain each of the following sources of stress.
  a. Job stress: _____

  _____

  _____

  _____

  b. Family stress: _____

  _____

  _____

  _____

- Explain the physiological changes that occur during pregnancy and childbirth.
  a. Prenatal care: _____

  _____

  _____

  b. First trimester: _____

  _____

  c. Second trimester: _____

  _____

  d. Third trimester: _____

  _____

  _____

  _____

- Define *Braxton Hicks contractions:* _____

  _____

- Define *puerperium:* _____

  _____

- Explain the cognitive changes that occur during pregnancy. _____

  _____

- Explain the sensory changes that occur during pregnancy. _____

  _____

- The childbearing family needs education about _____, _____,

  _____, _____,

  and _____.

- Explain the psychosocial changes that occur during pregnancy: _____

  _____

  _____

- Acute care for young adults is frequently related to: _____

  _____

- Causes of chronic illness and disability in the young adult are: _____
_____

THE MIDDLE ADULT

- Briefly explain the characteristics of the middle adult years. _____
_____
_____

PHYSICAL CHANGES

- Briefly explain the major physiological changes that occur between 30 and 65 years of age:
_____
_____
_____
_____
_____

- Define *menopause:* _____
_____

- Define *climacteric:* _____
_____

COGNITIVE CHANGES

- Changes in cognitive function of middle adults are rare except in cases of illness or trauma.

PSYCHOSOCIAL CHANGES

- Summarize the psychosocial development of the middle adult in the following areas:
  a. Career transition: _____
  _____
  _____
  b. Sexuality: _____
  _____
  _____
  c. Singlehood: _____
  _____
  _____
  d. Marital changes: _____
  _____
  _____

  e. Family transitions: _____
  _____
  _____
  f. Care of aging parents: _____
  _____
  _____

- Define *sandwich generation:* _____
_____
_____

HEALTH CONCERNS

- The following are physiological concerns for the middle adult. Briefly explain each one:
  a. Stress and stress reduction: _____
  _____
  _____
  b. Level of wellness: _____
  _____
  _____
  c. Forming positive health habits: _____
  _____
  _____

- Summarize two psychosocial concerns of the middle adult:
  a. Anxiety: _____
  _____
  _____
  b. Depression: _____
  _____
  _____

- Identify some common community health programs for the middle adult. _____
_____
_____

ACUTE CARE

- Identify the acute illness and injuries that occur in middle adulthood. _____
_____
_____
_____

RESTORATIVE AND CONTINUING CARE

- Identify some of chronic illnesses and/or issues that occur in middle adulthood.

  _____

  _____

REVIEW QUESTIONS

The student should select the appropriate answer and cite the rationale for choosing that particular answer.

1. The greatest cause of illness and death in the young adult population is:
   a. Sexually transmitted disease
   b. Violence
   c. Cardiovascular disease
   d. Substance abuse

   Answer:_____   Rationale: _____

   _____

   _____

2. Psychosocial changes of pregnancy commonly involve all of the following areas _except:_
   a. Body image
   b. Anxiety and depression
   c. Role changes
   d. Sexuality

   Answer:_____   Rationale: _____

   _____

   _____

3. Which physiological change would be a normal assessment finding in a middle adult?
   a. Increased breast size
   b. Abdominal tenderness and organomegaly
   c. Increased anteroposterior diameter of thorax
   d. Reduced auditory acuity

   Answer:_____   Rationale: _____

   _____

   _____

4. Which of the following characteristics would the nurse have to consider in planning care for a client in middle adulthood?
   a. Declining sexual interest
   b. Declining motor coordination
   c. Decreasing creativity
   d. Declining thinking ability

   Answer:_____   Rationale: _____

   _____

   _____

5. In planning patient education for Mrs. Smith, a 45-year-old woman who had an ovarian cyst removed, which of the following facts is true about the sexuality of the middle-aged adult?
   a. Menstruation ceases after menopause.
   b. Estrogen is produced after menopause.
   c. After reaching climacteric, a male is unable to father a child.
   d. With removal of the ovarian cyst, pregnancy cannot occur.

   Answer:_____   Rationale: _____

   _____

   _____

Chapter 11: Young to Middle Adult   61

Older Adult

Chapter 12

 Older adulthood traditionally begins after retirement, usually between 65 and 75 years of age.

PRELIMINARY READING

Chapter 12, pp. 243-272

COMPREHENSIVE UNDERSTANDING

- Older adulthood begins after retirement, usually between _____.

- Identify the common chronic conditions of this age group. _____.

- According to Lueckenotte, nursing assessment of an older adult takes into account the following points. Briefly explain each one.

  a. The interrelationship between physical and psychosocial aspects of aging: _____
  _____
  _____

  b. The effects of disease and disability on functional status: _____
  _____
  _____

  c. The decreased efficiency of homeostatic mechanisms: _____
  _____
  _____

  d. The lack of standards for health and illness norms: _____
  _____
  _____

TERMINOLOGY

- Define *geriatrics:* _____
  _____

- Define *gerontological nursing:* _____
  _____

- Define *gerontic nursing:* _____
  _____

MYTHS AND STEREOTYPES

- Identify at least five myths and/or stereotypes regarding the older adult. _____
  _____

- Define *ageism:* _____
  _____

NURSES' ATTITUDES TOWARD OLDER ADULTS

- Negative attitudes may result in a reduction in clients' sense of security, adequacy, and well-being.

- The attitude of the nurse toward older adults comes in part from _____,
  _____, _____,
  and _____.

THEORIES OF AGING

- Aging is not a simple progression, so there is no universally accepted theory that can predict and explain the complexities of older adults.

BIOLOGICAL THEORIES

- Give a brief description of the following theories:
  a. *Stochastic theories:* _____
     _____
     _____

  b. *Nonstochastic theories:* _____
     _____
     _____

PSYCHOSOCIAL THEORIES

- Describe the three classic psychosocial theories of aging:
  a. *Disengagement theory:* _____
     _____
     _____

  b. *Activity theory:* _____
     _____
     _____

  c. *Continuity theory:* _____
     _____
     _____

DEVELOPMENTAL TASKS FOR OLDER ADULTS

- List the seven developmental tasks of the older adult.
  a. _____
  b. _____
  c. _____
  d. _____
  e. _____
  f. _____
  g. _____

COMMUNITY-BASED AND INSTITUTIONAL HEALTH CARE SERVICES

Briefly describe the following health services that are used by the older population.
  a. Retirement communities: _____
     _____
     _____

  b. Home care: _____
     _____
     _____

  c. Day care: _____
     _____
     _____

  d. Respite care: _____
     _____
     _____

  e. Long-term care: _____
     _____
     _____

ASSESSING THE NEEDS OF OLDER ADULTS

PHYSIOLOGICAL CHANGES

- Identify the physiological changes that occur in the older adult with regard to the following:
  a. General survey: _____
     _____
     _____

b. Integumentary system: _____

_____

_____

c. Head and neck: _____

_____

_____

d. Thorax and lungs: _____

_____

_____

e. Heart and vascular system: _____

_____

_____

f. Breasts: _____

_____

_____

g. Gastrointestinal system and abdomen:

_____

_____

h. Reproductive system: _____

_____

_____

i. Urinary system: _____

_____

_____

j. Musculoskeletal system: _____

_____

_____

k. Neurological system: _____

_____

_____

COGNITIVE CHANGES

• The structural and physiological changes that occur in the brain during aging do not necessarily affect adaptive and functional abilities.

• Define *dementia*: _____

_____

• Identify the three stages of Alzheimer's disease.
  a. _____
  b. _____
  c. _____

• Identify some behavioral responses of a client with Alzheimer's disease: _____

_____

_____

• Define *multiinfarct dementia:* _____

_____

• Multiinfarct dementia may be related to vascular disorders in the brain. List two conditions from which it results:
  a. _____
  b. _____

• Define *delirium:* _____

_____

• Long-term abuse of alcohol and drugs can affect cognitive functioning. Identify these effects.

_____

_____

_____

PSYCHOSOCIAL CHANGES

• Identify at least five areas that should be addressed when counseling an older adult about retirement:
  a. _____
  b. _____
  c. _____
  d. _____
  e. _____

- Briefly describe the four patterns of social isolation experienced by older adults.

  Type I: _____

  _____

  Type II: _____

  _____

  Type III: _____

  _____

  Type IV: _____

  _____

- Briefly describe the sexual changes that occur in the older adult. _____

  _____

  _____

- List four factors to assess when assisting older adults with housing needs:

  a. _____

  b. _____

  c. _____

  d. _____

- A common misconception is that the death of an older adult is a blessing and the culmination of a full life.

- Many dying older adults still have goals and are not emotionally prepared to die.

HEALTH RISKS

- The three most common causes of death in the older adult are _____,

  _____, and _____.

ADDRESSING THE HEALTH CONCERNS OF OLDER ADULTS

HEALTH PROMOTION AND MAINTENANCE: PHYSIOLOGICAL CONCERNS

- Summarize the physiological health concerns related to each of the following:

  a. Heart disease: _____

  _____

  _____

  b. Cancer: _____

  _____

  _____

  c. Stroke: _____

  _____

  _____

  d. Smoking cessation: _____

  _____

  e. Nutrition: _____

  _____

  f. Dental problems: _____

  _____

  g. Exercise: _____

  _____

  h. Arthritis: _____

  _____

  i. Falls: _____

  _____

  j. Sensory impairments: _____

  _____

  k. Medication use: _____

  _____

  _____

- Briefly explain the age related changes affecting drug therapy in adults over the age of 65. _____

  _____

  _____

HEALTH PROMOTION AND MAINTENANCE: PSYCHOSOCIAL HEALTH CONCERNS

- Briefly describe the interventions used to maintain the psychosocial health of the older adult.

  a. Therapeutic communication: _____

  _____

  _____

  b. Touch: _____

  _____

  _____

  c. Reality orientation: _____

  _____

  _____

d. Validation therapy: _____

_____

_____

e. Reminiscence: _____

_____

_____

f. Body-image interventions: _____

_____

_____

OLDER ADULTS AND THE ACUTE CARE SETTING

- Older adults in the acute care setting are at increased risk for adverse events such as _____, _____, _____, _____, _____, and _____.

- Explain why the older adult is at risk for each of the following:

  a. Delirium: _____

  _____

  _____

  b. Dehydration: _____

  _____

  _____

  c. Malnutrition: _____

  _____

  _____

  d. Nosocomial infections: _____

  _____

  _____

  e. Urinary incontinence: _____

  _____

  _____

  f. Falls: _____

  _____

  _____

OLDER ADULTS AND RESTORATIVE CARE

- Summarize the two types of ongoing care for the older adult and identify the the focus of each. _____

  _____

  _____

  _____

REVIEW QUESTIONS

The student should select the appropriate answer and cite the rationale for choosing that particular answer.

1. Which statement about older adults is accurate?
   a. Older adults are institutionalized.
   b. Most older adults live on a fixed income.
   c. Most older adults cannot learn to care for themselves.
   d. Most older adults have no sexual desire.

Answer: _____ Rationale: _____

_____

_____

2. Which statement describing delirium is correct?
   a. Persons with delirium may experience illusions and hallucinations.
   b. The onset of delirium is slow and insidious.
   c. Symptoms of delirium are stable and unchanging.
   d. Symptoms of delirium are irreversible.

Answer: _____ Rationale: _____

_____

_____

3. Nutritional needs of the older adult:
   a. Are exactly the same as those of young and middle adults
   b. Include increased amounts of vitamin C, vitamin A, and calcium
   c. Include increased kilocalories to support metabolism and activity
   d. Include increased proteins and carbohydrates

Answer: _____ Rationale: _____

_____

_____

4.   Ms. Dale states that she does not need the TV turned on because she cannot see very well. Visual changes in older adults include all of the following *except:*
a. Decreased visual acuity
b. Decreased accommodation to darkness
c. Double vision
d. Sensitivity to glare

Answer:_____   Rationale: _____
_____
_____

5. Mr. DeLone states that he is worried about his parents' plans to retire. All of the following would be appropriate responses regarding retirement of the elderly *except:*
a. Positive adjustment is often related to how much a person planned for the retirement.
b. Retirement for most persons represents a sudden shock that is irreversibly damaging to self-image and self-esteem.
c. Reactions to retirement are influenced by the importance that has been attached to the work role.
d. Retirement may affect an individual's physical and psychological functioning.

Answer:_____   Rationale: _____
_____
_____

Critical Thinking and Nursing Judgment

Chapter 13

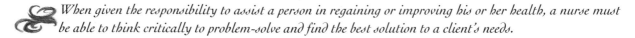
When given the responsibility to assist a person in regaining or improving his or her health, a nurse must be able to think critically to problem-solve and find the best solution to a client's needs.

PRELIMINARY READING
Chapter 13, pp. 273-289

COMPREHENSIVE UNDERSTANDING

CRITICAL THINKING IN NURSING PRACTICE

- The nurse must be able to think critically in order to problem solve and find the best solution for a client's needs.

- Describe the process of critical thinking in nursing. _____
  _____

- To think critically, the nurse must be able to:
  a. _____
  b. _____
  c. _____
  d. _____
  e. _____

CRITICAL THINKING DEFINED

- Define *critical thinking*: _____

- Identify the APA core critical thinking skills that apply to nursing:
  a. _____
  b. _____
  c. _____
  d. _____
  e. _____
  f. _____

- Learning to think critically helps a nurse to care for clients as their advocate and to make better informed choices about their care.

REFLECTION

- Define *reflection:* _____

- Briefly summarize nine tips to facilitate critical thinking:
    a. _____
    b. _____
    c. _____
    d. _____
    e. _____
    f. _____
    g. _____
    h. _____
    i. _____

- Provide some examples of how a nurse can use reflection. _____

- Identify a common approach to reflection that a student nurse may use. _____

LANGUAGE

- To become a critical thinker, a nurse must be able to use language precisely and clearly. It is important to not only communicate clearly with clients and families but to be able to clearly communicate findings to other health professionals.

INTUITION

- Define *intuition:* _____

- Site some examples of how a nurse gains intuitive knowledge. _____

LEVELS OF CRITICAL THINKING IN NURSING

- There are three levels of critical thinking in nursing that have been identified. Briefly describe each.
    a. Basic: _____

    b. Complex: _____

    c. Commitment: _____

CRITICAL THINKING COMPETENCIES

- There are three types of critical thinking competencies: _____, _____, and _____.

SCIENTIFIC METHOD

- Define *scientific method:* _____

- List the steps of the scientific method:
    a. _____
    b. _____
    c. _____
    d. _____
    e. _____

PROBLEM SOLVING

- Define *problem solving:* _____

- Solving a problem in one situation allows the nurse to apply the knowledge to future client situations.

DECISION MAKING

- Define *decision making:* _____

- Explain the process that an individual needs to go through to make a decision. _____

DIAGNOSTIC REASONING AND INFERENCES

- Explain the process of diagnostic reasoning. _____

CLINICAL DECISION MAKING

- The clinical decision making process requires _____.

- List the criteria for decision making (Strader, 1992):
    a. _____
    b. _____
    c. _____

- After considering each of the criteria, the nurse sets priorities as they relate to the client's situation.

- Once the nurse prioritizes the client's problems, the nurse chooses the nursing interventions most likely to relieve each problem.

- Site some examples of how nurse's make decisions about their client's. _____
  _____

NURSING PROCESS AS A COMPETENCY

- The nursing process is a systematic and comprehensive approach for nursing care. List the five steps of the nursing process:
    a. _____
    b. _____
    c. _____
    d. _____
    e. _____

THINKING AND LEARNING

- Our intellectual and emotional growth involves _____
  _____

- As new knowledge becomes available, professional nurses must challenge traditional ways of doing things and discover _____, _____, and _____.

CRITICAL THINKING MODEL

- Summarize the critical thinking model and list its five components: _____
  _____
  _____

SPECIFIC KNOWLEDGE BASE

- Identify what constitutes a nurse's knowledge base. _____
  _____

EXPERIENCE

- Identify the ways that critical thinking is developed through experience. _____
  _____

ATTITUDES FOR CRITICAL THINKING

- The following attributes are important for critical thinking. Briefly explain each of them.
    a. Confidence: _____
    _____
    _____

    b. Thinking independently: _____
    _____
    _____

    c. Fairness: _____
    _____

    d. Responsibility and accountability: _____
    _____

    e. Risk taking: _____
    _____

    f. Discipline: _____
    _____

    g. Perseverance: _____
    _____
    _____

    h. Creativity: _____
    _____

    i. Curiosity: _____
    _____

    j. Integrity: _____
    _____
    _____

    k. Humility: _____
    _____
    _____

- The fifth component of critical thinking includes _____ and _____.

- Intellectual standards refer to: _____.

- Professional standards refer to _____.

CRITICAL THINKING SYNTHESIS

- *Critical thinking* is defined as: _____ _____.

- The nursing process is the traditional critical thinking competency which allows nurses to make clinical judgements and take actions based on reason.

- Briefly explain how the nursing process and the critical thinking model work together.
  _____
  _____

NURSING PROCESS OVERVIEW

- The three characteristics of a process are purpose, organization, and creativity. Briefly describe how the nursing process addresses each one of these characteristics.
  a. Purpose: _____
  _____
  _____
  b. Organization: _____
  _____
  _____
  c. Creativity: _____
  _____
  _____

REVIEW QUESTIONS

The student should select the appropriate answer and cite the rationale for choosing that particular answer.

1. Clinical decision-making requires the nurse to:
   a. Improve a client's health
   b. Establish and weigh criteria in deciding the best choice of therapy for a client
   c. Follow the physician's orders for client care
   d. Standardize care for the client

   Answer:_____   Rationale: _____
   _____
   _____

2. Which of the following is not one of the five steps of the nursing process?
   a. Planning
   b. Evaluation
   c. Hypothesis testing
   d. Assessment

   Answer:_____   Rationale: _____
   _____
   _____

3. Gathering, verifying, and communicating data about the client to establish a database is an example of which component of the nursing process?
   a. Assessment
   b. Planning
   c. Evaluation
   d. Nursing diagnosis
   e. Implementation

   Answer:_____   Rationale: _____
   _____
   _____

4. Completing nursing actions necessary for accomplishing a care plan is an example of which component of the nursing process?
   a. Assessment
   b. Planning
   c. Evaluation
   d. Nursing diagnosis
   e. Implementation

Answer: _____ Rationale: _____
_____
_____

Nursing Assessment

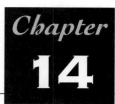

Chapter

14

Assessment begins with the nurse applying knowledge and experience to collect data about a client. Accurate assessment is crucial to ensure that needs are properly identified and that the right course of action is implemented by the nurse.

PRELIMINARY READING
Chapter 14, pp. 290-309

COMPREHENSIVE UNDERSTANDING

NURSING PROCESS OVERVIEW

• The nursing process is used to _____, _____, and _____.

• The nursing process is one variation of scientific reasoning that allows nurses to _____, _____, and _____ nursing practice.

A CRITICAL APPROACH TO ASSESSMENT

• Nursing *assessment* is the systematic process of _____, _____, and _____ data about a client.

• This phase of the nursing process includes two steps. Name them.
  a. _____
  b. _____

• Identify the purpose of the assessment. _____
_____

• As the nurse initiates the assessment component for a specific client, the nurse is also synthesizing critical knowledge, experience, standards, and attitudes simultaneously.

• A comprehensive database includes: _____

- List Gordon's eleven functional health patterns.
  a. _____
  b. _____
  c. _____
  d. _____
  e. _____
  f. _____
  g. _____
  h. _____
  i. _____
  j. _____
  k. _____

- Briefly explain the problem-focused approach to assessment. _____
  _____
  _____

- Whichever approach is used, the nurse must cluster cues of information and identify emerging patterns and potential problems.

ORGANIZATION OF DATA GATHERING

- Accurate assessment makes it possible to develop appropriate nursing diagnoses and to devise appropriate goals and strategies.

- It is important for the nurse's assessment to first consider the _____.

- Identify some nonverbal behavior that a nurse may observe during an assessment.
  _____
  _____
  _____

DATA COLLECTION

- Assessment does not include inferences or interpretative statements that are unsupported with data.

- Descriptive data originate in:
  a. _____
  b. _____
  c. _____
  d. _____

- The collection of inaccurate, incomplete, or inappropriate data leads to incorrect identification of the client's health care needs and subsequent inaccurate, incomplete, or inappropriate nursing diagnoses. Data are incomplete if the nurse _____,
  _____, or _____.

TYPES OF DATA

- Define each of the following:
  a. *Subjective* data: _____
  _____
  _____

  b. *Objective* data: _____
  _____
  _____

SOURCES OF DATA

- Each source provides information about the client's level of wellness, anticipated prognosis, risk factors, health practices and goals, and patterns of health and illness.

CLIENT

- Identify the types of information a client can provide.
  a. _____
  b. _____
  c. _____
  d. _____
  e. _____

FAMILY AND SIGNIFICANT OTHERS

- Families can be an important secondary source of information about the client's health status. Give an example. _____
  _____
  _____

- Identify the ways that health care team members identify data.
  a. _____
  b. _____
  c. _____

MEDICAL RECORDS

- By reviewing medical records, the nurse can _____, _____, and _____.

OTHER RECORDS

- Identify records that may contain pertinent health care information. _____ _____

LITERATURE REVIEW

- Reviewing nursing, medical, and pharmacological literature about an illness helps the nurse complete the database.

NURSE'S EXPERIENCE

- A nurses's ability to make an assessment will improve as he or she uses _____, applies _____, and focuses _____.

METHODS OF DATA COLLECTION

INTERVIEW

- The first step in establishing the database is to interview the client. Identify the major purposes of an interview.
  a. _____
  b. _____
  c. _____

- Identify the six objectives of the nursing interview.
  a. _____
  b. _____
  c. _____
  d. _____
  e. _____
  f. _____

- Define *nurse-client relationship*: _____ _____

- The nurse uses various types of interview techniques. Define the following types:
  a. *Open-ended questions:* _____
  _____
  b. *Back-channeling:* _____
  _____
  c. *Problem-seeking:* _____
  _____
  d. *Closed ended questions:* _____
  _____

- There are three phases of the interview. Briefly explain each one.
  a. Orientation phase: _____
  _____
  b. Working phase: _____
  _____
  c. Termination phase: _____
  _____

- Identify ten communication strategies used to facilitate communication between the nurse and client.
  a. _____
  b. _____
  c. _____
  d. _____
  e. _____
  f. _____
  g. _____
  h. _____
  i. _____
  j. _____

NURSING HEALTH HISTORY

- The nursing health history is data collected about:
  a. _____
  b. _____
  c. _____
  d. _____
  e. _____

- Identify the four purposes (objectives) for obtaining a nursing health history.
  a. _____
  b. _____
  c. _____
  d. _____

- Briefly explain each of the following components of a health history.
  a. Biographical information: _____
  _____
  _____

  b. Reason for seeking health care: _____
  _____
  _____

  c. Client expectations: _____
  _____
  _____

  d. Present illness: _____
  e. Past health history: _____
  f. Family history: _____
  g. Environmental history: _____
  g. Psychosocial history: _____
  h. Spiritual health: _____
  i. Review of Systems (ROS): _____

PHYSICAL EXAMINATION

- The physical examination and the collection of diagnostic and laboratory data involve the _____ _____.

- Define *standard:* _____

- Define *norm:* _____

ORDER OF EXAMINATION

- The exam is carried out in a systematic manner. Explain: _____ _____

- Define the following physical examination techniques:
  a. *Inspection:* _____
  _____

  b. *Palpation:* _____
  _____

  c. *Percussion:* _____
  _____

  d. *Auscultation:* _____
  _____

- Identify at least two contributions that laboratory data make to the nursing assessment.
  a. _____
  b. _____

FORMULATING NURSING JUDGMENTS

- Through a process of inferential reasoning and judgment, the nurse decides what information has meaning in relation to the client's health status.

DATA INTERPRETATION

- Define *inferential reasoning:* _____ _____

DATA CLUSTERING

- After collecting and validating subjective and objective data and interpreting the data, the nurse organizes the information into meaningful clusters. This depends on recognizing _____.

- During data clustering, the nurse organizes data and focuses attention on client functions needing support and assistance for recovery.

DATA DOCUMENTATION

- Identify the two essential reasons for thoroughness in data documentation.
  a. _____
  b. _____

REVIEW QUESTIONS

The student should select the appropriate answer and cite the rationale for choosing that particular answer.

1. In most circumstances, the best source of information for nursing assessment of the adult client is the:
   a. Nursing literature
   b. Physician
   c. Client
   d. Medical record

   Answer:_____   Rationale: _____
   _____
   _____

2. The interview technique that is most effective in strengthening the nurse-client relationship by demonstrating the nurse's willingness to hear the client's thoughts is:
   a. Open-ended question
   b. Direct question
   c. Problem-solving
   d. Problem-seeking

   Answer:_____   Rationale: _____
   _____
   _____

3. While obtaining a health history, the nurse asks Mr. Jones if he has noted any change in his activity tolerance. This is an example of which interview technique?
   a. Direct question
   b. Problem-seeking
   c. Problem-solving
   d. Open-ended question

   Answer:_____   Rationale: _____
   _____
   _____

4. Mr. Davis tells the nurse that he has been experiencing more frequent episodes of indigestion. The nurse asks if the indigestion is associated with meals or a reclining position and about what relieves the indigestion. This is an example of which interview technique?
   a. Problem-seeking
   b. Problem-solving
   c. Direct question
   d. Open-ended question

   Answer:_____   Rationale: _____
   _____
   _____

5. The information obtained in a review of systems (ROS) is:
   a. Objective
   b. Subjective
   c. Based on physical examination findings
   d. Based on the nurse's perspective

   Answer:_____   Rationale: _____
   _____
   _____

Nursing Diagnosis

The nursing diagnosis is a clinical judgment about individual, family, or community responses to actual or potential health problems or life processes.

PRELIMINARY READING

Chapter 15 pp. 310-325

COMPREHENSIVE UNDERSTANDING

- Define *nursing diagnosis:* _____

EVOLUTION OF NURSING DIAGNOSIS

- Nursing has attempted to define itself professionally and functionally since the writings of Florence Nightingale. Briefly summarize the evolution of nursing diagnosis. _____

- Explain the purpose of *NANDA:* _____

CRITICAL THINKING AND THE NURSING DIAGNOSTIC PROCESS

DIAGNOSTIC PROCESS

- The *diagnostic process* includes: _____

- The nursing diagnosis deals with the client's response to the illness or condition rather than the medical diagnosis, it distinguishes the nurse's role from the physician's role, and it helps the nurse to focus on the role of nursing.

ANALYSIS AND INTERPRETATION OF DATA

- Data analysis involves recognizing _____, comparing _____, and drawing _____.

- *Defining characteristics* are: _____

- *Clinical criteria* are: _____

- Defining characteristics that are beyond healthy norms form the basis for problem-identification.

IDENTIFICATION OF CLIENT NEEDS

- An *actual health problem* is defined as: _____
  _____

- An *at-risk health problem* is defined as: _____
  _____

FORMULATION OF THE NURSING DIAGNOSIS

- NANDA has identified five types of nursing diagnoses. Briefly explain each one.
  a. Risk nursing diagnosis: _____
     _____
  b. Actual nursing diagnosis: _____
     _____
  c. Possible nursing diagnosis: _____
     _____
  d. Syndrome diagnosis: _____
     _____
  e. Wellness nursing diagnosis: _____
     _____

NURSING DIAGNOSIS STATEMENT

- Nursing diagnoses are stated in a two-part format. The _____ followed by a _____.

- Nursing interventions are directed toward altering or resolving etiologic or related factors. The problem is _____; the related factors are _____.

- The etiology, or cause, of the nursing diagnosis must be within the domain of _____ and a condition that responds to _____.

- The modification of nursing diagnoses is ongoing. As the level of nursing care and the level of wellness change, these changes are reflected in the nursing diagnosis statement.

SUPPORT OF THE DIAGNOSTIC STATEMENT

- Nursing assessment data must support the diagnostic label and related factors must support the etiology.

SOURCES OF DIAGNOSIS ERROR

ERRORS IN DATA COLLECTION

- Identify the four practices that are essential during assessment to avoid data collection errors.
  a. _____
  b. _____
  c. _____
  d. _____

ERRORS IN INTERPRETATION AND ANALYSIS OF DATA

- Identify three ways the nurse can determine if data are accurate and complete.
  a. _____
  b. _____
  c. _____

ERRORS IN DATA CLUSTERING

- Identify three ways that incorrect data clustering occurs.
  a. _____
  b. _____
  c. _____

ERRORS IN THE DIAGNOSTIC STATEMENT

- Identify some common guidelines developed to reduce errors in the diagnostic statement.
  a. _____
  b. _____
  c. _____
  d. _____

NURSING DIAGNOSIS AND MEDICAL DIAGNOSIS

- Compare the characteristics of medical and nursing diagnoses in each of the following areas:

NURSING DIAGNOSIS: APPLICATION TO CARE PLANNING

- The formulated nursing diagnoses provide direction for the planning process and the selection of nursing interventions to achieve the desired outcomes.

	Medical Diagnosis	Nursing Diagnosis
Nature of Diagnosis	_____ _____ _____	_____ _____ _____
Goal	_____ _____ _____	_____ _____ _____
Objective	_____ _____ _____	_____ _____ _____

ADVANTAGES OF NURSING DIAGNOSES

- Explain the advantages of nursing diagnoses to each of the following:
  a. Communication tool: _____
     _____
     _____
  b. Documentation: _____
     _____
     _____
  c. Discharge teaching: _____
     _____
     _____
  d. Quality assurance and improvement: ____
     _____
     _____
  e. Professionally: _____
     _____
     _____

LIMITATIONS OF NURSING DIAGNOSES

- List two limitations of nursing diagnoses.
  a. _____
  b. _____

REVIEW QUESTIONS

The student should select the appropriate answer and cite the rationale for choosing that particular answer.

1. A nursing diagnosis:
   a. Is a statement of a client response to a health problem that requires nursing intervention
   b. Identifies nursing problems
   c. Is derived from the physician's history and physical examination
   d. Is not changed during the course of a client's hospitalization

Answer: _____   Rationale: _____
_____
_____

2. The first part of the nursing diagnosis statement:
   a. Identifies an actual or potential health problem
   b. Identifies the cause of the client problem
   c. May be stated as a medical diagnosis
   d. Identifies appropriate nursing interventions

Answer: _____   Rationale: _____
_____
_____

3. The second part of the nursing diagnosis statement:
   a. Is connected to the first part of the statement with the phrase "due to"
   b. Identifies the probable cause of the client problem
   c. Identifies the expected outcomes of nursing care
   d. Is usually stated as a medical diagnosis

Answer: _____   Rationale: _____
_____
_____

4. Which of the following is the correctly stated nursing diagnosis?
   a. Needs to be fed related to broken right arm
   b. Abnormal breath sounds caused by weak cough reflex
   c. Impaired physical mobility related to rheumatoid arthritis
   d. Impaired skin integrity related to fecal incontinence

Answer: _____   Rationale: _____
_____
_____

5. Mr. Margauz, a 52-year-old business executive, is admitted to the coronary care unit. During his admission interview he denies chest pain or shortness of breath. His pulse and blood pressure are normal. He appears tense and does not want the nurse to leave his bedside. When questioned, he states that he is very nervous. At this moment, which nursing diagnosis is most appropriate?

a. Alteration in comfort, chest pain

b. Alteration in bowel elimination related to restricted mobility

c. High risk for altered cardiac output related to heart attack

d. Anxiety related to intensive care unit admission

Answer:_____   Rationale: _____

_____

_____

Planning for Nursing Care

> *Planning is the category of nursing in which client-centered goals and expected outcomes are established. Nursing interventions are then designed to achieve those goals.*

PRELIMINARY READING
Chapter 16, pp. 326-346

COMPREHENSIVE UNDERSTANDING

ESTABLISHING PRIORITIES

- After formulating specific nursing diagnoses, the nurse uses critical thinking skills to establish priorities for the client's diagnoses by ranking them in order of importance.

- Priority selection is the method the nurse and client use to mutually rank the diagnoses in order of importance based on the client's _____, _____, and _____.

- Maslow's hierarchy of needs arranges basic needs in five levels of priority. Give an example of each.
  a. Physiological: _____
  b. Safety and security: _____
  c. Love and belonging: _____
  d. Self-esteem: _____
  e. Self-actualization: _____

- Priorities depend on the urgency of the problem, the nature of the treatment indicated, and the interactions among the nursing diagnoses. Explain each one.
  a. High: _____
  b. Intermediate: _____
  c. Low: _____

CRITICAL THINKING IN ESTABLISHING GOALS
AND EXPECTED OUTCOMES

- Establishing goals and expected outcomes requires that the nurse critically evaluate the _____, the _____, and the _____.

- Goals and expected outcomes are specific statements of client _____ or _____ that the nurse anticipates from the nursing care.

- Identify the two purposes for writing goals and expected outcomes.
  a. _____
  b. _____

- Each goal and expected outcome statement must have a time frame for evaluation.

GOALS OF CARE

- Define the following:
  a. *Goals:* _____
  _____
  b. *Mutual goal setting:* _____
  _____
  c. *Client-centered goal:* _____
  _____
  d. *Short-term goal:* _____
  _____
  e. *Long-term goal:* _____
  _____

EXPECTED OUTCOMES

- Define *expected outcomes:* _____
  _____

- Outcomes are desired responses of the client's condition in the _____, _____, _____, _____, or _____ dimensions.

- The expected outcomes should be written in measurable behavioral terms sequentially, with time frames.

- Identify the functions of an expected outcome.
  a. _____
  b. _____
  c. _____
  d. _____

- The rationale for several expected outcomes is _____
  _____.

GUIDELINES FOR WRITING GOALS AND EXPECTED OUTCOMES

- There are seven guidelines to follow when writing goals and expected outcomes. Define and give an example of each.
  a. *Client-centered factors:* _____
  _____
  b. *Singular factors:* _____
  _____
  c. *Observable factors:* _____
  _____
  d. *Measurable factors:* _____
  _____
  e. *Time-limited factors:* _____
  _____
  f. *Mutual factors:* _____
  _____
  g. *Realistic factors:* _____
  _____

CRITICAL THINKING IN DESIGNING NURSING INTERVENTIONS

- Nursing interventions are those actions designed to assist the client in moving from the present level of health to that described in the expected outcome.

TYPES OF INTERVENTIONS

- There are three categories of interventions, and category selection is based on the client's needs. Define and give an example of each.
  a. *Nurse-initiated:* _____
  _____
  b. *Physician-initiated:* _____
  _____
  c. *Collaborative:* _____
  _____

SELECTION OF INTERVENTIONS

- Identify the six factors the nurse uses to select nursing interventions for a specific client.

  a. _____

  b. _____

  c. _____

  d. _____

  e. _____

  f. _____

- Define *collaboration:* _____

  _____

- The advantages of the taxonomy of nursing interventions are:

  a. _____

  b. _____

  c. _____

  d. _____

PLANNING NURSING CARE

- Define the following methods for planning nursing care:

  a. *Nursing care plan:* _____

  _____

  b. *Critical pathways:* _____

  _____

PURPOSE OF CARE PLANS

- Briefly explain the purpose of a nursing care plan in relation to the following:

  a. Communication: _____

  b. Identification and coordination of resources:

  _____

  c. Continuity of care: _____

  d. Change-of-shift reports: _____

  e. Long-term needs of client: _____

  f. Expected outcome criteria: _____

- The complete care plan is the blueprint for nursing action. It provides direction for implementation of the plan and a framework for evaluation of the client's response to nursing actions.

CARE PLANS IN VARIOUS SETTINGS

- The structure of the care plan varies depending on the setting. Its overall purpose is to provide a written guideline for care so that the health care needs of the client and subsequent therapies are communicated among the members of the health care team. Briefly explain each of the following:

  a. Institutional care plans: _____

  _____

  _____

  b. Computerized care plans: _____

  _____

  _____

  c. Student care plans: _____

  _____

  _____

  d. Care plans for community-based settings:

  _____

  _____

  _____

  e. Critical pathways _____

  _____

  _____

WRITING THE NURSING CARE PLAN

- The nursing diagnosis with the highest priority is the beginning point for the nursing care plan and is followed by other nursing diagnoses in order of assigned priority.

- Using the five-column plan, identify the information in each column.

  Column 1: _____

  Column 2: _____

  Column 3: _____

  Column 4: _____

  _____

  Column 5: _____

  _____

Chapter 16: Planning for Nursing Care   85

WRITING CRITICAL PATHWAYS

- Critical pathways are a case management tool that delineates client outcomes within specific time frames. They are multidisciplinary, outcome-based care plans.

- Critical pathways are written so that all members of the health care team can document delivery of care or changes in status.

CONSULTING OTHER HEALTH CARE PROFESSIONALS

- Consultation is a process in which _____ _____.

- Consultation is based on the problem-solving approach, and the consultant is the stimulus for change.

WHEN TO CONSULT

- The need to consult occurs when the nurse has identified a problem that cannot be solved using personal knowledge, skills, and resources.

HOW TO CONSULT

- List the six responsibilities of the nurse when seeking consultation.
  a. _____
  b. _____
  c. _____
  d. _____
  e. _____
  f. _____

REVIEW QUESTIONS

The student should select the appropriate answer and cite the rationale for choosing that particular answer.

1. Well-formulated, client-centered goals should:
   a. Meet immediate client needs
   b. Include preventive health care
   c. Include rehabilitation needs
   d. All of the above

   Answer:_____   Rationale: _____
   _____
   _____

2. The following statement appears on the nursing care plan for an immunosuppressed client: The client will remain free from infection throughout hospitalization. This statement is an example of a (an):
   a. Nursing diagnosis
   b. Short-term goal
   c. Long-term goal
   d. Expected outcome

   Answer:_____   Rationale: _____
   _____
   _____

3. The following statements appear on a nursing care plan for a client after a mastectomy: Incision site approximated; absence of drainage or prolonged erythema at incision site; and client remains afebrile. These statements are examples of:
   a. Nursing interventions
   b. Short-term goals
   c. Long-term goals
   d. Expected outcomes

   Answer:_____   Rationale: _____
   _____
   _____

4. The planning step of the nursing process includes which of the following activities?
   a. Assessing and diagnosing
   b. Evaluating goal achievement
   c. Performing nursing actions and documenting them
   d. Setting goals and selecting interventions

Answer:_____   Rationale: _____
_____
_____

5. The nursing care plan is:
   a. A written guideline for implementation and evaluation
   b. A documentation of client care
   c. A projection of potential alterations in client behaviors
   d. A tool to set goals and project outcomes

Answer:_____   Rationale: _____
_____
_____

Implementing Nursing Care

Implementation is a category of nursing behavior in which the actions necessary for achieving the goals and expected outcomes of nursing care are initiated and completed.

PRELIMINARY READING
Chapter 17, pp. 347-361

COMPREHENSIVE UNDERSTANDING

- *Implementation* describes _____.

- A *nursing intervention* is _____.

TYPES OF NURSING INTERVENTIONS

INDEPENDENT NURSING INTERVENTIONS

- Describe an independent nursing intervention: _____

PROTOCOLS AND STANDING ORDERS

- Nursing interventions can be based on protocols and standings orders. Briefly explain each and provide and example of where they are commonly used.
  a. *Protocols:* _____
  _____
  b. *Standing orders:* _____
  _____

CRITICAL THINKING IN IMPLEMENTING NURSING INTERVENTIONS

- Identify the factors that make decision making more difficult when choosing among nurse-initiated interventions.
  a. _____
  b. _____

- Identify the sequence of activities in the information-processing model.
  a. _____
  b. _____
  c. _____
  d. _____

IMPLEMENTATION PROCESS

REASSESSING THE CLIENT

- When new data are obtained and a new need is identified, the nurse modifies nursing care. This provides a mechanism for the nurse to determine if the proposed nursing action is appropriate.

REVIEWING AND REVISING THE EXISTING NURSING CARE PLAN

- If the client's status has changed and the nursing diagnosis and related nursing interventions are no longer appropriate, the nursing care plan needs to be modified.

- Modification of the existing care plan includes several steps. Identify them.
  a. _____
  b. _____
  c. _____
  d. _____

ORGANIZING RESOURCES AND CARE DELIVERY

- Before implementing care, the nurse evaluates the plan to determine the need for assistance and the type of assistance required. List the areas of preparation that allows the nurse to implement the nursing care plan appropriately.
  a. _____
  b. _____
  c. _____
  d. _____
  e. _____
  f. _____

IMPLEMENTING NURSING INTERVENTIONS

- Describe the five different methods for implementing nursing interventions.
  a. _____
  b. _____
  c. _____
  d. _____
  e. _____

- Nursing practice is composed of three skills. Define and give an example of each.
  a. *Cognitive:* _____
  _____
  _____
  b. *Interpersonal:* _____
  _____
  _____
  c. *Psychomotor:* _____
  _____
  _____

IMPLEMENTATION METHODS

ASSISTING WITH ACTIVITIES OF DAILY LIVING

- Define *activities of daily living (ADL):* _____
  _____

- Conditions that result in the need for assistance with ADLs can be acute, chronic, temporary, permanent, or rehabilitative.

COUNSELING

- *Counseling* is defined as: _____
  _____

- Identify some areas in which clients or families may need counseling.
  a. _____
  b. _____
  c. _____

TEACHING

- Define the following:
  a. *Teaching:* _____
  _____
  b. *Teaching-learning process:* _____
  _____

PROVIDING DIRECT NURSING CARE

- To achieve the therapeutic goals for the client, the nurse initiates interventions to:
  a. _____
  b. _____
  c. _____
  d. _____

Chapter 17: Implementing Nursing Care   89

COMPENSATION FOR ADVERSE REACTIONS

- An *adverse reaction* is: _____
  _____

PREVENTIVE MEASURES

- *Preventive nursing actions* are: _____.

CORRECT TECHNIQUES IN ADMINISTERING CARE AND PREPARING A CLIENT FOR PROCEDURES

- When techniques are integrated within a procedure the ultimate outcome is safe and effective. To carry out a procedure, the nurse must be knowledgeable about _____, _____, _____, and _____.

LIFESAVING MEASURES

- The purpose of a lifesaving measure is _____.

ACHIEVING GOALS OF CARE

- The client's health care goals can be achieved by:
  a. _____
  b. _____
  c. _____
  d. _____

DELEGATING, SUPERVISING, AND EVALUATING THE WORK OF OTHER STAFF MEMBERS

- The nurse assigning tasks is responsible for ensuring that each task is assigned appropriately and completed according to the standard of care.

COMMUNICATING NURSING INTERVENTIONS

- Nursing interventions are written (via the nursing care plan and medical record) or communicated orally (one nurse to another or to another health care professional).

REVIEW QUESTIONS

The student should select the appropriate answer and cite the rationale for choosing that particular answer.

1. Which of the following is *not* true of standing orders?
   a. Standing orders are approved and signed by the physician in charge of care before implementation.
   b. With standing orders, the nurse relies on the physician's judgment to determine if the intervention is appropriate.
   c. Standing orders are commonly found in critical care and community health settings.
   d. With standing orders, nurses have the legal protection to intervene appropriately in the client's best interest.

   Answer: _____   Rationale: _____
   _____
   _____

2. The nursing care plan calls for the client, a 300-lb woman, to be turned every 2 hours. The client is unable to assist with turning. The nurse knows that she may hurt her back if she attempts to turn the client by herself. The nurse should:
   a. Rewrite the care plan to eliminate the need for turning
   b. Ignore the intervention related to turning in the care plan
   c. Turn the client by herself
   d. Ask another nurse to help her turn the client

   Answer: _____   Rationale: _____
   _____
   _____

3. Being alert to the possibility of the client becoming nauseated after general anesthesia is an example of which type of nursing skill?
   a. Cognitive
   b. Interpersonal
   c. Technical
   d. Psychosocial

Answer:_____ Rationale: _____
_____
_____

4. Mrs. Kay comes to the family clinic for birth control. The nurse obtains a health history and performs a pelvic examination and Pap smear. The nurse is functioning according to:
   a. Protocol
   b. Standing order
   c. Nursing care plan
   d. Intervention strategy

Answer:_____ Rationale: _____
_____
_____

5. Mary Jones is a newly diagnosed diabetic patient. The nurse shows Mary how to administer an injection. This intervention activity is:
   a. Counseling
   b. Communicating
   c. Teaching
   d. Managing

Answer:_____ Rationale: _____
_____
_____

Evaluation

The evaluation phase of the nursing process measures the client's response to nursing actions and his or her progress toward achieving goals.

PRELIMINARY READING
Chapter 18, pp. 362-374

COMPREHENSIVE UNDERSTANDING
- Identify the focus of the *professional standards review organizations (PSROs)*. _____
_____

CRITICAL THINKING SKILLS AND EVALUATION
- Evaluation of care requires the nurse to reflect on the client's responses to nursing interventions and to determine their effectiveness in promoting the client's well being.

- If outcomes are met, the overall goals for the client are also met.

- Evaluation is the step in the nursing process whereby the nurse continually redirects nursing care to meet client needs.

- Explain the two types of evaluations.
  a. Positive: _____
  b. Negative: _____

- A client whose health status changes continuously requires frequent evaluation.

GOALS
- A goal specifies the behavior or response that _____
_____.

EXPECTED OUTCOMES
- Explain the purpose of the Nursing Outcomes Classification (NOC) project:
  a. _____
  b. _____
  c. _____

- Expected outcomes are the expected results of a goal-oriented process. They are statements of progressive, step-by-step _____ _____ or _____ that the client needs to accomplish to achieve the goals of care provided.

- If the client achieves the expected outcome, the nurse either continues the care plan or discontinues interventions because the goal of care is met.

EVALUATION OF GOAL ACHIEVEMENT

- The purpose of nursing care is to:
  a. _____
  b. _____
  c. _____

- Describe the steps in the objective evaluation of client goal achievement.
  a. _____
  b. _____
  c. _____
  d. _____
  e. _____

- Identify the three degrees of goal attainment.
  a. _____
  b. _____
  c. _____

EVALUATIVE MEASURES AND SOURCES

- Evaluative measures are _____

- The new data collected from evaluation measures are critically analyzed and compared with expected outcomes to determine whether or not changes occurred.

- The primary source of data for evaluation is the _____.

- Documentation and reporting in the evaluation process are of critical importance. Give some examples.
  a. _____
  b. _____

c. _____
d. _____

CARE PLAN REVISION AND CRITICAL THINKING

- Accurate evaluation leads to the appropriate revision of ineffective care plans and discontinuation of therapy that has been successful.

DISCONTINUING A CARE PLAN

- After determining that expected outcomes and goals have been achieved, the nurse confirms this evaluation with the client and discontinues that care plan.

MODIFYING A CARE PLAN

- When goals are not met, the nurse identifies the factors that interfered with goal achievement.

- Lack of goal achievement may also result from an error in nursing judgment or failure to follow each step of the nursing process.

- When there is failure to achieve a goal, the entire _____ sequence is repeated to discover changes that need to be made to _____ or _____ the client's health.

- A complete reassessment of all client factors relating to the nursing diagnosis and etiology is the first step in reevaluating the nursing process. Briefly explain the following:
  a. Reassessment: _____
  _____
  b. Nursing diagnosis: _____
  _____
  c. Goals and expected outcomes: ____
  _____
  d. Interventions: _____
  _____
  e. Evaluation: _____
  _____

QUALITY IMPROVEMENT

- The evaluation of health care is a process used to determine the quality of care and service provided to clients.

- JCAHO defines *quality improvement (QI)* as:

  _____

  _____

- Explain the following steps in relation to improving the quality of nursing care and taking appropriate action to resolve any problems.
  a. Evaluation of care: _____
  b. Evaluation of improvement: _____

REVIEW QUESTIONS

The student should select the appropriate answer and cite the rationale for choosing that particular answer.

1. Measuring the client's response to nursing interventions and his or her progress toward achieving goals occurs during which phase of the nursing process?
   a. Planning
   b. Nursing diagnosis
   c. Evaluation
   d. Assessment

   Answer:_____   Rationale: _____
   _____
   _____

2. Evaluation is:
   a. Begun immediately before the client's discharge
   b. Only necessary if the physician orders it
   c. An integrated, ongoing nursing care activity
   d. Performed primarily by nurses in the quality assurance department

   Answer:_____   Rationale: _____
   _____
   _____

3. The criteria used to determine the effectiveness of a nursing action are based on the:
   a. Nursing diagnosis
   b. Expected outcomes
   c. Client's satisfaction
   d. Nursing interventions

   Answer:_____   Rationale: _____
   _____
   _____

4. The primary source of data for evaluation is the:
   a. Physician
   b. Client
   c. Nurse
   d. Medical record

   Answer:_____   Rationale: _____
   _____
   _____

5. When a client-centered goal has not been met in the projected time frame, the most appropriate action by the nurse would be to:
   a. Repeat the entire sequence of the nursing process to discover needed changes
   b. Conclude that the goal was inappropriate or unrealistic and eliminate it from the plan
   c. Continue with the same plan until the goal is met
   d. Rewrite the plan using different interventions

   Answer:_____   Rationale: _____
   _____
   _____

Professional Nursing Roles

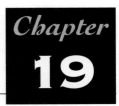

Chapter
19

The profession of nursing evolves as society, health care needs, and policies change. Nursing responds and adapts to changes, meeting new challenges as they arise.

PRELIMINARY READING
Chapter 19, pp. 375-400

COMPREHENSIVE UNDERSTANDING

HISTORICAL PERSPECTIVE

- Nursing was distinguished in its early history as a form of community service and was originally related to a strong instinct to preserve and protect the family.

- Throughout history, nursing and medicine have been interdependent.

- Briefly explain how each of the following have influenced nursing:
  a. Ancient Egyptians: _____
  _____
  b. Hebrews: _____
  _____
  c. Greeks: _____
  _____
  d. Christianity: _____
  _____
  e. Middle ages: _____
  _____
  f. Crusades: _____
  _____
  g. Sisters/Daughters of Charity: _____
  _____
  h. Florence Nightingale: _____
  _____
  i. Civil War: _____
  _____
  j. Twentieth century: _____
  _____

NATIONAL COMMISSION ON NURSING AND NURSING EDUCATION

• Identify the issues the National Commission explored. _____
_____
_____
_____

• The 1926 ANA Code of Ethics proposed _____
_____
_____

NURSING THEORIES

• Conceptual and theoretical nursing models are used to _____,
_____, and
_____.

NURSING AS A PROFESSION

PROFESSIONALISM

• List the five primary characteristics of a profession.
a. _____
b. _____
c. _____
d. _____
e. _____

• Briefly explain the profession of nursing in relation to the following:
a. Education: _____
_____
b. Theory: _____
_____
c. Service: _____
_____
d. Autonomy: _____
_____
e. Code of Ethics: _____
_____

EDUCATIONAL PREPARATION

PROFESSIONAL REGISTERED NURSE EDUCATION

• As the profession of nursing grew, various educational routes for becoming an RN were developed. Briefly explain the following:
a. Associate degree education: _____
_____
b. Diploma education: _____
_____
c. Baccalaureate education: _____
_____
_____

ACCREDITATION

• To be accredited, nursing programs must meet certain criteria established by the National League for Nursing (NLN). Briefly explain the purpose of accreditation. _____
_____
_____

LICENSURE

• In the United States, RN candidates must pass the National Council Licensure Examination for Registered Nurses (NCLEX-RN). This provides a standardized minimum knowledge base for the client population nurses serve.

CERTIFICATION

• The nurse may choose to work toward certification in a specific area of nursing practice. Minimal requirements are set based on the specific certification.

• Explain the two advanced educational preparations that a nurse may seek.
a. Master's: _____
_____
b. Doctorate: _____
_____

CONTINUING AND IN-SERVICE EDUCATION

• The goals of continuing education are to:

_____

_____

• An *in-service education* program is: _____

_____

LICENSED PRACTICAL NURSE EDUCATION

• An *LPN* or *LVN* is trained in _____ and _____ and practices under the supervision of a registered nurse in a hospital or community health practice setting.

NURSING PRACTICE

AMERICAN NURSES ASSOCIATION (ANA) DEFINITION OF NURSING PRACTICE

• Briefly describe the focus of the ANA definition of nursing practice for the following dates:

a. 1955: _____

_____

b. 1965: _____

_____

c. 1979: _____

_____

d. 1980: _____

_____

CANADIAN NURSES ASSOCIATION (CNA) DEFINITION OF NURSING PRACTICE

• Briefly explain the CNA definition of nursing. _____

_____

STANDARDS OF NURSING PRACTICE

• Standards of practice are important for the following reasons.

a. _____
b. _____
c. _____
d. _____
e. _____

STANDARDS OF CARE

• Competent levels of nursing care are demonstrated through the _____.

• Standards of care are important in legal disputes over whether a nurse practiced appropriately in a particular case.

NURSE PRACTICE ACTS

• Nurse practice acts regulate the licensure and practice of nursing. Each state or province defines for itself the scope of nursing practice but most have similar practice acts.

PRACTICE SETTINGS

• Nursing practice settings are expanding because of the changes in the health care delivery system. Briefly explain the following practice settings for nurses.

a. Hospitals: _____

_____

_____

b. Skilled nursing facilities: _____

_____

_____

c. Long-term care facilities: _____

_____

_____

d. Restorative care facilities: _____

_____

_____

COMMUNITY-BASED PRACTICE SETTINGS

• Nursing in community-based settings is focused on health promotion and maintenance, education and management, and coordination and continuity of restorative care within the client's community. Explain the following community based settings:

a. Community health centers: _____

_____

b. Schools: _____

_____

_____

c. Occupational health settings: _____
_____
_____

d. Home health care agencies: _____
_____
_____

ROLES AND FUNCTIONS OF THE NURSE

- The contemporary nurse functions in the following roles. Briefly explain each one.

  a. Care giver: _____
  _____
  _____

  b. Clinical decision maker: _____
  _____
  _____

  c. Protector and client advocate: _____
  _____
  _____

  d. Case manager: _____
  _____
  _____

  e. Rehabilitator: _____
  _____
  _____

  f. Comforter: _____
  _____
  _____

  g. Communicator: _____
  _____
  _____

  h. Teacher/educator: _____
  _____
  _____

CAREER ROLES

- Explain the following career roles and functions.

  a. Clinician: _____
  _____

  b. Nurse educator: _____
  _____

  c. Advanced practice nurse (APN): _____
  _____

  d. Clinical nurse specialist (CNS): _____
  _____

  e. Nurse practitioner: _____
  _____

- Describe the five types of nurse practitioners:

  a. _____
  b. _____
  c. _____
  d. _____
  e. _____

- Explain the following nurse roles:

  a. Certified nurse-midwife (CNM): _____

  b. Certified registered nurse anesthetist (CRNA): _____

  c. Nurse administrator: _____

  d. Nurse researcher: _____

  e. Military nurse: _____
  _____

HEALTH CARE TEAM

- The health care team is made up of four general types of professionals. Briefly explain each role.

  a. Physician: _____
  _____

  b. Physician assistant: _____
  _____

  c. Allied and other health professionals: ___
  _____

  d. Pharmacist: _____
  _____

  e. Social worker: _____
  _____

  f. Pastoral care: _____
  _____

  g. Assistive personnel/nursing assistant: ___
  _____

  h. Clerical/secretarial staff: _____
  _____

PROFESSIONAL NURSING ORGANIZATIONS

- Briefly identify the issues with which the following organizations deal:

  a. ANA and CAN: _____

  _____

  b. ICN: _____

  _____

  c. NLN: _____

  _____

  d. NSNA: _____

  _____

  e. AORN: _____

  _____

  f. AWHONN: _____

  _____

  g. NAPNAP: _____

  _____

  h. AACN: _____

  _____

SOCIETAL INFLUENCES ON NURSING

- Explain how the following issues have affected nursing practice:

  a. Demographic changes: _____

  _____

  _____

  b. Cultural diversity: _____

  _____

  _____

  c. Consumer's movement: _____

  _____

  _____

  d. Health promotion and wellness: _____

  _____

  _____

  e. Women's movement: _____

  _____

  _____

  f. Human rights movement: _____

  _____

  _____

TRENDS IN NURSING

- Nursing grows and evolves as changes occur in society, in health care emphases and methods, in life styles, and among nurses themselves. Explain the following trends and their influence:

  a. Education: _____

  _____

  _____

  b. Employment settings: _____

  _____

  _____

  c. Political: _____

  _____

  _____

NURSING'S INFLUENCE ON HEALTH CARE POLICY AND PRACTICE

- Nursing's Agenda for Health Care Reform supports the creation of a health care system that ensures _____,

  _____, _____,

  and _____.

- *Healthy People 2010* is a document for _____

  _____.

REVIEW QUESTIONS

The student should select the appropriate answer and cite the rationale for choosing that particular answer.

1. The factor that best advanced the practice of nursing in the first century was:
   a. Teachings of Christianity
   b. Growth of cities
   c. Better education of nurses
   d. Improved conditions for women

   Answer: _____   Rationale: _____

   _____

   _____

2. Nursing education programs may seek voluntary accreditation by the appropriate council of the:
   a. American Nurses Association
   b. International Council of Nurses
   c. Congress for Nursing Practice
   d. National League for Nursing

   Answer:_____ Rationale: _____
   _____
   _____

3. The graduate nurse must pass a licensure examination administered by the:
   a. Accredited school of nursing
   b. American Nurses Association
   c. State boards of nursing
   d. National League for Nursing

   Answer:_____ Rationale: _____
   _____
   _____

4. When Mr. Jones had his leg amputated, the nurse assisted him as he learned to cope with the artificial limb and new routine. The nurse's primary role at this time was:
   a. Rehabilitator
   b. Manager
   c. Friend
   d. Advisor

   Answer:_____ Rationale: _____
   _____
   _____

5. A group that lobbies at the state and federal levels for advancement of the nurse's role, economic interest, and health care is the:
   a. American Nurses Association
   b. State boards of nursing
   c. National Student Nurses' Association
   d. American Hospital Association

   Answer:_____ Rationale: _____
   _____
   _____

Ethics and Values

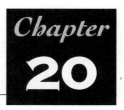
Resolution of ethical issues often incorporates not only the nurse's personal values but also the interpretation of the client's personal values, based on the unique perspective of nurses.

PRELIMINARY READING
Chapter 20, pp. 401-422

COMPREHENSIVE UNDERSTANDING
• Define a *code of ethics*. _____

• Explain the field of bioethics. _____
_____

ETHICS
• Define *ethics:* _____
_____

• Define the following basic terms within the context of ethics.
a. *Autonomy:* _____
_____

b. *Beneficence:* _____
_____

c. *Nonmaleficence:* _____
_____

d. *Justice:* _____
_____

e. *Fidelity:* _____
_____

PROFESSIONAL NURSING
• A code of ethics is a set of _____, which serve to
_____.

• *Accountability* refers to _____.

- Professional accountability serves the following purposes.
  - a. _____
  - b. _____
  - c. _____
  - d. _____

- *Responsibility* refers to _____ .

- Describe the concept of *confidentiality*. _____
  _____

- *Veracity* means: _____
  _____

VALUES

- A *value* is defined as: _____
  _____ .

- Briefly explain the following modes of values formation.
  - a. Modeling: _____
    _____
  - b. Moralizing: _____
    _____
  - c. Laissez-faire: _____
    _____
  - d. Responsible choice: _____
    _____
  - e. Reward and punishment: _____
    _____

- The process of *value clarification* is: _____
  _____

- Identify and explain the three steps of values clarification.
  - a. _____
  - b. _____
  - c. _____

- Define the following terms:
  - a. *Cultural values:* _____
    _____
  - b. *Ethnocentrism:* _____
    _____

- Briefly explain the following professional values and behaviors essential to nursing.
  - a. Altruism: _____
    _____
  - b. Equality: _____
    _____
  - c. Esthetics: _____
    _____
  - d. Freedom: _____
    _____
  - e. Human dignity: _____
    _____
  - f. Justice: _____
    _____
  - g. Truth: _____
    _____
    _____

BIOETHICS

- The notion of autonomy was developed to explain and define a society's growing desire to protect clients from scientific endeavors. The notion of client autonomy reflects a change in society's definition of power and knowledge.

PHILOSOPHICAL CONSTRUCTIONS

- Briefly explain the following philosophical constructs in relation to ethical systems.
  - a. Deontology: _____
    _____
    _____
  - b. Utilitarianism/consequentialism: _____
    _____
  - c. Feminist ethics: _____
    _____
  - d. Ethics of care: _____
    _____
    _____

CONSENSUS IN BIOETHICS

- Consensus bioethics proposes _____
  _____

NURSING POINT OF VIEW

- Briefly summarize the nurse's point of view in relation to addressing an ethical dilemma.
  _____
  _____
  _____

HOW TO PROCESS AN ETHICAL DILEMMA

- Processing an ethical dilemma differs from the nursing process as _____
  _____ .

- To distinguish an ethical problem from questions of procedure, legality, or medical diagnosis the nurse must decide whether the problem has one or more of the following characteristics.
  a. _____
  b. _____
  c. _____

- The nurse uses the following guidelines for ethical processing and decision-making. Briefly describe each one.
  a. Is this an ethical dilemma? _____
  _____
  _____
  b. Gather the relevant information. _____
  _____
  _____
  c. Examine and determine one's own values.
  _____
  _____
  _____
  d. Articulate the problem. _____
  _____
  _____

e. Propose alternative courses of action. ____
_____
_____

f. Negotiate the outcome. _____
_____
_____

g. Evaluate the action. _____
_____
_____

INSTITUTIONAL ETHICS COMMITTEES

- To help facilitate ethical dialogue and provide the educational and policy resources necessary to create a climate sensitive to ethical challenges, health care institutions have developed ethics committees.

- Identify the functions of institutional ethics committees. _____
  _____
  _____

ISSUES IN BIOETHICS

- Briefly describe the following issues that are common in health care settings.
  a. Informed consent: _____
  _____
  _____
  b. Advance directives: _____
  _____
  _____
  c. Quality of life: _____
  _____
  _____
  d. Allocation of scarce resources: _____
  _____
  _____

REVIEW QUESTIONS

The student should select the appropriate answer and cite the rationale for choosing that particular answer.

1. A health care issue often becomes an ethical dilemma because:
   a. A client's legal rights coexist with a health professional's obligations.
   b. Decisions must be made quickly, often under stressful conditions.
   c. Decisions must be made based on value systems.
   d. The choices involved do not appear to be clearly right or wrong.

   Answer:_____ Rationale: _____
   _____
   _____

2. A document that lists the medical treatment a person chooses to refuse if unable to make decisions is the:
   a. Durable power of attorney
   b. Informed consent
   c. Living Will
   d. Advance directives

   Answer:_____ Rationale: _____
   _____
   _____

3. Which statement about an institutional ethics committee is correct?
   a. The ethics committee is an additional resource for clients and health care professionals.
   b. The ethics committee relieves health care professionals from dealing with ethical issues.
   c. The ethics committee would be the first option in addressing an ethical dilemma.
   d. The ethics committee replaces decision-making by the client and health care providers.

   Answer:_____ Rationale: _____
   _____
   _____

4. The nurse is working with parents of a seriously ill newborn. Surgery has been proposed for the infant, but the chances of success are unclear. In helping the parents resolve this ethical conflict, the nurse knows that the first step is:
   a. Exploring reasonable courses of action
   b. Collecting all available information about the situation
   c. Clarifying values related to the cause of the dilemma.
   d. Identifying people who can solve the difficulty

   Answer:_____ Rationale: _____
   _____
   _____

5. Mrs. G, an 88-year-old woman, believes that life should not be prolonged when hope is gone. She has decided that she does not want extraordinary measures taken when her life is at its end. Because she feels this way, she has talked with her daughter about her desires, completed a living will, and left directions with her physician. This is an example of:
   a. affirming a value
   b. choosing a value
   c. prizing a value
   d. reflecting a value

   Answer:_____ Rationale: _____
   _____
   _____

Legal Implications in Nursing Practice

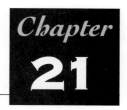

Chapter

21

Nurses must understand the law not only to protect themselves from liability but also to protect their client's rights.

PRELIMINARY READING
Chapter 21, pp. 423-443

COMPREHENSIVE UNDERSTANDING

LICENSURE

- All states use the NCLEX for registered nurse and licensed practical nurse examinations.

- Licensure permits persons to offer special skills to the public and provides legal guidelines for protection of the public.

- A license can be suspended or revoked by the Board of Nursing if a nurse's conduct violates a provision in the licensing statute.

LEGAL LIMITS OF NURSING

- Professional nurses must understand the legal limits influencing their daily practice.

SOURCES OF LAW

- The legal guidelines that nurses must follow are derived from the following. Briefly explain each one:

  a. Statutory law: _____
  _____

  b. Nurse Practice Acts: _____
  _____

  c. Regulatory law: _____
  _____

  d. Common law: _____
  _____

- Define the following:
  a. *Criminal law:* _____
  _____
  _____
  _____

  b. *Crimes:* _____
  _____
  _____
  _____

  c. *Felony:* _____
  _____
  _____
  _____

  d. *Misdemeanor:* _____
  _____
  _____
  _____

  e. *Civil laws:* _____
  _____
  _____
  _____

TORTS

- Define the following:
  a. *Tort:* _____

  b. *Malpractice:* _____
  _____

  c. *Assault:* _____
  _____

  d. *Battery:* _____
  _____

  e. *Invasion of privacy:* _____
  _____

  f. *Defamation of character:* _____
  _____

  g. *Malice:* _____
  _____

  h. *Slander:* _____
  _____

  i. *Libel:* _____
  _____

  j. *Negligence:* _____
  _____

- List the criteria by which nurses can be found liable for malpractice.
  a. _____
  b. _____
  c. _____
  d. _____

- Identify some common negligent acts involving nurses. _____
  _____
  _____
  _____

STUDENT NURSES

- If a client is harmed as a direct result of a nursing student's actions or lack of action, the liability for the incorrect action is generally shared by the student, instructor, hospital or health care facility, and university or educational institution.

- When students are employed as nursing assistants or nurse's aides when not attending classes, they should not perform tasks that do not appear in a job description for a nurses' aide or assistant.

LEGAL LIABILITY IN NURSING

MINIMIZING LIABILITY THROUGH EFFECTIVE DOCUMENTATION AND CLIENT RELATIONSHIPS

- Nurses can reduce their chances of being named in lawsuits by following _____
  _____.

CONTRACTS

- A *contract* is: _____
  _____

- Briefly explain the following:
  a. Employment contracts: _____
  _____
  _____

  b. Insurance: _____
  _____
  _____

c. Health insurance: _____

_____

_____

d. Right to continue group health coverage:

_____

_____

_____

e. Portability of health insurance (HIPAA):

_____

_____

_____

f. Newborns and Mothers Health Protection
Act: _____

_____

_____

g. Mental health plan: _____

_____

_____

_____

GOOD SAMARITAN LAWS

- Good Samaritan laws protect _____

_____.

STANDARDS OF CARE

- *Standards of care* are the guidelines for nursing
practice and are defined by the _____

_____.

- The nurse practice acts establish: _____

_____

- In a malpractice lawsuit, these standards are
used to determine: _____

_____

- All nurses should know the standards of care
they are expected to meet within their specific specialty and work setting. Ignorance of
the law or of standards of care is not a
defense to malpractice.

- Briefly summarize the case of Darling v.
Charleston Community Memorial Hospital
and the Illinois Supreme Court's decision.

_____

_____

_____

CONSENT

- A signed consent form is required for all routine treatment, hazardous procedures, some
treatment programs such as chemotherapy,
and research involving clients.

- Identify the individuals who may consent to
medical treatment.
a. Adults: _____

_____

b. Minors: _____

_____

- The following factors must be verified for a
consent to be valid:
a. _____

_____

b. _____

_____

c. _____

_____

d. _____

_____

- The nurse assumes the responsibility for witnessing the client's signature on the consent
form but does not legally assume the duty of
obtaining consent.

- The nurse's signature witnessing the consent
means _____.

- Only a person who can understand the
explanations provided and who can truly
understand the decision they are making can
provide informed consent.

- A client who refuses surgery or any other
medical treatment must be informed of any
harmful consequences.

LEGAL RELATIONSHIPS IN NURSING PRACTICE

PHYSICIANS' ORDERS

- The physican is responsible for directing the
medical treatment.

- Nurses are obligated to follow the physician's orders unless _____
  _____.

- A nurse should not perform a physician's order if it is foreseeable that harm will come to the client.

VERBAL ORDERS

- If a verbal order is necessary, it should be written out and signed by the physician within 24 hours.

"DO NOT RESUSCITATE" ORDERS

- A "no code" order needs to be written, not given verbally. The physician needs to regularly review DNR orders in case the client's condition warrants a change.

- If resuscitative procedures are performed "more slowly" than recommended by the American Heart Association, they may by interpreted as below the standard of care and therefore be the basis for a lawsuit.

- Cardiopulmonary resuscitation is an emergency treatment that is provided without client consent. The statues assume that all clients will be resuscitated unless there is a DNR order in the chart in writing.

SHORT STAFFING

- The JCAHO requires institutions to establish guidelines for determining the number of nurses required to give care to a specific number of clients (staffing ratios).

- Nursing supervisors should be informed when a nurse is assigned to care for more clients than is reasonable, and a written protest should be filed to document such an assignment.

- When staffing is inadequate, nurses should not walk out because charges of abandonment can be made.

FLOATING

- Nurses who float should inform the supervisor of any lack of experience they may have caring for the type of clients on the nursing unit.

- A supervisor can be held liable if a staff nurse is given an assignment she cannot safely handle.

LEGAL ISSUES IN NURSING PRACTICE

- Legal issues reflect changing trends in the life styles of people in our society.

SURROGATE PREGNANCY CONTRACTS AND ADOPTION

- Identify the statutes in relation to the following:
  a. Surrogate parenting: _____
  _____
  b. Baby selling: _____
  _____
  c. Adoption: _____
  _____

ABORTION ISSUES

- Summarize the legal rights of women relative to abortion.
  a. Roe *v.* Wade: _____
  _____
  b. Webster *v.* Reproductive Health Services:
  _____
  _____
  c. Planned Parenthood of Southeastern Pennsylvania *v.* Casey: _____
  _____

AMERICANS WITH DISABILITIES ACT (ADA)

- Briefly explain the Americans with Disabilities act and the implications for practice.

  _____

  _____

HUMAN IMMUNODEFICIENCY VIRUS (HIV)

- Nurses must use Universal Precautions when caring for all clients.

- Co-workers who refuse to work with HIV-infected people can leave companies open to indirect charges of discrimination if the employer does not monitor the work environment.

- The ADA regulations _____.

- Briefly discuss the issues related to mandatory HIV testing for health care workers.

  _____

  _____.

DEATH AND DYING

- Identify the essential standards for the determination of death.

  a. _____

  b. _____

- Consent for an autopsy must be given by the decedent before death or may be given by a close family member at the time of death.

- Describe the reasons why a death may require investigation by a coroner. What role does the nurse play in this investigation?

  _____

  _____

RIGHT TO REFUSE TREATMENT

- The doctrine of informed consent ensures the client the right to refuse medical treatment.

- Explain court doctrine in relation to the following:

  a. Competent client's refusal: _____

  _____

  _____

  b. Incompetent client's refusal: _____

  _____

  _____

PHYSICIAN-ASSISTED SUICIDE

- Briefly summarize the Oregon Death with Dignity Act._____

  _____

- State the American Nurses Association (ANA) position on physician-assisted suicide. _____

  _____

ADVANCE DIRECTIVES

- The Patient's Self-Determination Act (1992) requires _____

  _____.

- _Living wills_ are defined as: _____

  _____.

- Health care surrogate statutes are sometimes referred to as _____

  _____

ORGAN DONATIONS

- Summarize the policies and procedures of the institution or the laws of a state regarding the nurse's role in organ donations.

  _____

  _____

  _____

  _____

- Summarize the Uniform Anatomical Gift Act. _____

  _____

  _____

  _____

LEGAL ISSUES IN NURSING SPECIALTIES

- Within every specialty of nursing there are legal issues that affect nursing practice. The more common legal issues are listed here. Explain each.

    a. Community health nursing: _____
    _____
    _____

    b. Emergency department: _____
    _____
    _____

    c. Nursing of children: _____
    _____
    _____

    d. Medical-surgical nursing and geriatrics:
    _____
    _____
    _____

    e. Critical care nursing: _____
    _____
    _____

    f. Operating room nursing: _____
    _____
    _____

    g. Psychiatric nursing: _____
    _____
    _____

    h. Home health nursing: _____
    _____
    _____

THE NURSE AS AN ADVOCATE

- Nurses serve as client advocates by
    _____
    _____.

THE NURSE AS RISK MANAGER

- Through minimizing the risk in providing care for clients, the nurse reduces the possibility that clients will be financially and emotionally devastated as a result of being injured by inappropriate care.

- *Risk management* is _____.

- The steps involved in risk management include:

    a. _____
    b. _____
    c. _____
    d. _____

- A tool used by risk managers is the
    _____.

- Risk management includes documentation. It should be _____
    _____

PROFESSIONAL INVOLVEMENT

- Nurses must be involved in their professional organizations and on committees that define the standards of care for nursing practice.

- Nurses become more powerful and more effective as a profession when they are organized and cohesive.

REVIEW QUESTIONS

The student should select the appropriate answer and cite the rationale for choosing that particular answer.

1. The scope of nursing practice is legally defined by:
    a. State nurse practice acts
    b. Professional nursing organizations
    c. Hospital policy and procedure manuals
    d. Physicians in the employing institutions

Answer:_____   Rationale: _____
_____
_____

2. A student nurse who is employed as a nursing assistant may perform any functions that:
a. Have been learned in school
b. Are expected of a nurse at that level
c. Are identified in the position's job description
d. Require technical rather than professional skill

Answer:_____   Rationale: _____
_____
_____

3. A confused client who fell out of bed because side rails were not used is an example of which type of liability?
a. Felony
b. Assault
c. Battery
d. Negligence

Answer:_____   Rationale: _____
_____
_____

4. The nurse puts a restraint jacket on a client without the client's permission and without a physician's order. The nurse may be guilty of:
a. Assault
b. Battery
c. Invasion of privacy
d. Neglect

Answer:_____   Rationale: _____
_____
_____

5. In a situation in which there is insufficient staff to implement competent care, a nurse should:
a. Organize a strike
b. Inform the clients of the situation
c. Refuse the assignment
d. Accept the assignment but make a protest in writing to the administration

Answer:_____   Rationale: _____
_____
_____

Communication

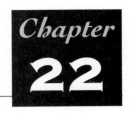

Chapter 22

Communication is part of the art of nursing-the intentional creative use of oneself, based on skill and expertise, to transmit emotion and meaning to another.

PRELIMINARY READING
Chapter 22, pp. 444-469

COMPREHENSIVE UNDERSTANDING

COMMUNICATION AND NURSING PRACTICE

- *Communication* is a process. This process allows _____.

- Competency in communication helps the nurse maintain effective relationships with the entire sphere of professional practice, and helps meet legal, ethical, and clinical standards of care.

COMMUNICATION AND INTERPERSONAL RELATIONSHIPS

- Communication is the means to establishing helping-healing relationships.

- Nurses with expertise in communication can express caring by: _____
  _____
  _____

- The nurse's ability to relate to others is _____
  _____.

- Briefly summarize how the nurse will look at communication in the 21st century. _____
  _____
  _____

DEVELOPING COMMUNICATION SKILLS

- Define the following qualities of critical thinking in relation to the communication process.

  a. *Inquisitive:* _____
  _____
  _____

  b. *Systematic:* _____
  _____
  _____
  _____

  c. *Analytical:* _____
  _____
  _____
  _____

  d. *Truth seeker:* _____
  _____
  _____
  _____

  e. *Open-minded:* _____
  _____
  _____
  _____

  f. *Self-confident:* _____
  _____
  _____

  g. *Mature:* _____
  _____
  _____
  _____

- Critical thinking can help the nurse overcome perceptual biases, _____
  _____.

- Nurses use communication skills to gather, analyze, and transmit information and to accomplish the work of each phase.

LEVELS OF COMMUNICATION

- Summarize the following communication interactions.

  a. *Intrapersonal:* _____
  _____
  _____

  b. *Interpersonal:* _____
  _____
  _____

  c. *Transpersonal:* _____
  _____

  d. *Small-group:* _____
  _____

  e. *Public:* _____
  _____

BASIC ELEMENTS OF THE COMMUNICATION PROCESS

- Briefly summarize the following elements of communication.

  a. *Referent:* _____
  _____
  _____

  b. *Sender:* _____
  _____
  _____

  c. *Receiver:* _____
  _____

  d. *Message:* _____
  _____

  e. *Channels:* _____
  _____

  f. *Feedback:* _____
  _____
  _____

  g. *Interpersonal variables:* _____
  _____
  _____

  h. *Environment:* _____
  _____
  _____

FORMS OF COMMUNICATION

- People send messages in verbal and nonverbal modes, which are bound together during interpersonal interaction.

VERBAL COMMUNICATION

- Verbal communication involves spoken or written words. Verbal language is a code that conveys specific meaning as words are combined.

- Briefly explain the important aspects of verbal communication listed below.
    a. Vocabulary: _____
    _____
    _____

    b. Denotative and connotative meaning: _____
    _____
    _____

    c. Pacing: _____
    _____

    d. Intonation: _____
    _____

    e. Clarity: _____
    _____

    f. Brevity: _____
    _____
    _____

NONVERBAL COMMUNICATION

- *Nonverbal communication* is: _____
    _____

- Nonverbal communication is much more powerful than verbal communication.

- Becoming an astute observer of nonverbal behavior takes practice, concentration, and sensitivity to others. Briefly explain the following nonverbal behaviors.
    a. Personal appearance: _____
    _____
    _____

    b. Posture and gait: _____
    _____
    _____

    c. Facial expression: _____
    _____
    _____

    d. Eye contact: _____
    _____

    e. Gestures: _____
    _____
    _____

    f. Sounds: _____
    _____

    g. Territoriality and personal space: _____
    _____
    _____

- Identify the zones of personal space. _____
    _____
    _____
    _____
    _____

- Identify the zones of touch. _____
    _____
    _____
    _____

SYMBOLIC COMMUNICATION

- Summarize symbolic communication.
    _____
    _____

METACOMMUNICATION

- Define *metacommunication*: _____
    _____

PROFESSIONAL NURSING RELATIONSHIPS

- Professional relationships are created through _____,
    _____, and
    _____.

NURSE-CLIENT HELPING RELATIONSHIPS

- The relationship is therapeutic, promoting a psychological climate that facilitates positive change and growth.

- Acceptance conveys a _____.

- Briefly explain the phases of a helping relationship.
  a. Preinteraction phase: _____
  _____
  _____

  b. Orientation phase: _____
  _____
  _____

  c. Working phase: _____
  _____
  _____

  d. Termination phase: _____
  _____
  _____

- Nurses often encourage clients to share personal stories. This is called _____.

NURSE-FAMILY RELATIONSHIPS

- Summarize the principles related to nurse-family relationships: _____
  _____
  _____

NURSE-HEALTH TEAM RELATIONSHIPS

- Communication in nurse-health team relationships is geared by: _____
  _____
  _____

NURSE-COMMUNITY RELATIONSHIPS

- Communication within the community occurs through channels such as
  _____.

ELEMENTS OF PROFESSIONAL COMMUNICATION

- Briefly explain the following elements of professional communication:
  a. Courtesy: _____
  _____
  _____

  b. Use of names: _____
  _____
  _____

c. Privacy and confidentiality: _____
_____

d. Trustworthiness: _____
_____

e. Autonomy and responsibility: _____
_____

f. Assertiveness: _____
_____

COMMUNICATION WITHIN THE NURSING PROCESS

✍ ASSESSMENT

- Assessment of a client's ability to communicate includes gathering data about the many contextual factors that influence communication.

- List the contextual factors that influence communication.
  a. _____
  b. _____
  c. _____
  d. _____
  e. _____

- Identify the psychophysiological factors that influence communication. _____
  _____

- Physical barriers cause _____,
  _____, or _____.

- Explain how developmental factors influence communication. _____
  _____

- Summarize how sociocultural factors influence communication: _____
  _____
  _____

- Gender influences communication. Explain how communication differs in regard to gender.
  a. Male: _____
  b. Female: _____

✍ NURSING DIAGNOSIS

- List three nursing diagnoses appropriate for a client with alterations in communication.
  a. _____
  b. _____
  c. _____

✍ PLANNING

- List three goals for effective interpersonal communication.
  a. _____
  b. _____
  c. _____

✍ IMPLEMENTATION

- Therapeutic communication techniques are specific responses that encourage the expression of feelings and ideas and convey the nurse's acceptance and respect. Briefly explain the following techniques.
  a. Active listening: _____
  _____
  _____
  b. Presence: _____
  _____
  _____
  c. Sharing observations: _____
  _____
  _____
  d. Sharing empathy: _____
  _____
  _____
  e. Sharing hope: _____
  _____
  _____
  f. Sharing humor: _____
  _____
  _____

g. Sharing feelings: _____
_____

h. Using touch: _____
_____
_____

i. Using silence: _____
_____
_____

j. Asking relevant questions: _____
_____

k. Providing information: _____
_____
_____

l. Paraphrasing _____
_____

m. Clarifying: _____
_____
_____

n. Focusing: _____
_____
_____

o. Summarizing: _____
_____

p. Self-disclosing: _____
_____
_____

q. Confronting: _____
_____
_____

- Certain communication techniques can hinder or damage professional relationships, these techniques are referred to as non-therapeutic. Briefly explain the following non-therapeutic techniques:
  a. Asking personal questions: _____
  _____
  _____
  b. Giving personal opinions: _____
  _____
  _____
  c. Changing the subject: _____
  _____
  _____

d. Automatic responses: _____

_____

e. False reassurance: _____

_____

f. Sympathy: _____

_____

g. Asking for explanations: _____

_____

h. Approval or disapproval: _____

_____

i. Defensive responses: _____

_____

j. Passive or aggressive responses _____

_____

k. Arguing _____

_____

_____

- Briefly identify the communication techniques to use with the client with special needs.
  a. Clients who cannot speak clearly: _____

  _____

  b. Clients who are cognitively impaired: _____

  _____

  c. Clients who are unresponsive: _____

  _____

  d. Clients who do not speak English: _____

  _____

  _____

EVALUATION

- List four expected outcomes for the client with impaired communication.
  a. _____
  b. _____
  c. _____
  d. _____

REVIEW QUESTIONS

The student should select the appropriate answer and cite the rationale for choosing that particular answer.

1. In demonstrating the method for deep breathing exercises, the nurse places his or her hands on the client's abdomen to explain diaphragmatic movement. This technique involves the use of which communication element?
   a. Feedback
   b. Tactile channel
   c. Referent
   d. Message

Answer:_____   Rationale: _____

_____

_____

2. Which statement about nonverbal communication is correct?
   a. It is easy for a nurse to judge the meaning of a client's facial expression.
   b. The nurse's verbal messages should be reinforced by nonverbal cues.
   c. The physical appearance of the nurse rarely influences nurse-client interaction.
   d. Words convey meanings that are usually more significant than nonverbal communication.

Answer:_____   Rationale: _____

_____

_____

3. The term referring to the sender's attitude toward the self, the message, and the listener is:
   a. Nonverbal communication
   b. Metacommunication
   c. Connotative meaning
   d. Denotative meaning

Answer:_____   Rationale: _____

_____

_____

4. The referent in the communication process is:
   a. That which motivates the communication
   b. The means of conveying messages
   c. Information shared by the sender
   d. The person who initiates the communication

Answer:_____   Rationale: _____
_____
_____

5. The nurse is conducting an admission interview with the client. To maintain the client's territoriality and maximize communication, the nurse should sit:
   a. 0 to 18 inches from the client
   b. 18 inches to 4 feet from the client
   c. 4 to 12 feet from the client
   d. 12 feet or more from the client

Answer:_____   Rationale: _____
_____
_____

Client Education

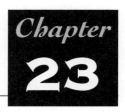

Chapter
23

Clients and family members have the right to health education so that they are able to make intelligent, informed decisions about their health and lifestyle. The nurse provides education by identifying clients' learning needs and by using the most appropriate teaching strategies.

PRELIMINARY READING

Chapter 23, pp. 470-499

COMPREHENSIVE UNDERSTANDING

STANDARDS FOR CLIENT EDUCATION

- Briefly summarize the standards for client and family education (JCAHO, 1998).

  Standard 1: _____

  _____

  Standard 2: _____

  _____

  Standard 3: _____

  _____

  Standard 4: _____

  _____

- Evidence of successful client education must be noted in the client's medical record.

PURPOSES OF CLIENT EDUCATION

- Comprehensive client education includes three important purposes, each involving a separate phase of health care.

MAINTENANCE AND PROMOTION OF HEALTH AND ILLNESS PREVENTION

- The nurse is a visible, competent resource for clients intent on improving their physical and psychological well-being. In the school, home, clinic, or workplace, the nurse provides information and skills that will allow clients to practice healthier behaviors.

- Promoting healthy behaviors through education increases self-esteem by allowing clients to assume more responsibility for their health.

- Greater knowledge can result in better health maintenance habits.

RESTORATION OF HEALTH

- Injured or ill clients need information and skills that will help them regain or maintain their levels of health.

- The family is a vital part of a client's return to health, and family members may need as much information as the client.

- The nurse should not assume that the family should be involved and must first assess the client-family relationship.

COPING WITH IMPAIRED FUNCTIONING

- In the case of a serious disability, the client's family role may change, making understanding and acceptance by family members necessary.

- The family's ability to provide support can result from education, which begins as soon as the client's needs are identified and the family displays a willingness to help.

TEACHING AND LEARNING

- Define the following:
  a. *Teaching:* _____
  _____
  b. *Learning:* _____
  _____

- Teaching is most effective when it responds to a learner's needs.

- Interpersonal communication is essential for successful teaching.

ROLE OF THE NURSE IN TEACHING AND LEARNING

- The nurse has an ethical responsibility to teach his or her clients.

- The nurse clarifies information provided by physicians and may become the primary source of information for adjusting to health problems.

TEACHING AS COMMUNICATION

- The teaching process closely parallels the communication process.

- A *learning objective* is: _____
  _____

- Define the following terms in relation to the teaching-learning process:
  a. *Referent:* _____
  _____
  b. *Sender:* _____
  _____
  c. *Message:* _____
  d. *Channels:* _____
  e. *Receiver:* _____
  f. *Feedback:* _____

DOMAINS OF LEARNING

- Learning occurs in _____
  (understandings), _____
  (attitudes), and _____
  (motor skills) domains.

- The characteristics of learning within each domain affect the teaching and evaluation methods used.

COGNITIVE LEARNING

- Bloom (1956) classifies *cognitive behaviors* in an ordered hierarchy. Summarize each one.
  a. Knowledge: _____
  _____
  b. Comprehension: _____
  _____
  c. Application: _____
  _____
  d. Analysis: _____
  _____
  e. Synthesis: _____
  _____
  f. Evaluation: _____
  _____

AFFECTIVE LEARNING

- *Affective learning* deals with the expression of feelings and the acceptance of attitudes, opinions, and values.

- Summarize the following hierarchy behaviors.
  a. Receiving: _____
  _____
  _____

  b. Responding: _____
  _____
  _____

  c. Valuing: _____
  _____
  _____

  d. Organizing: _____
  _____
  _____

  e. Characterizing: _____
  _____
  _____

PSYCHOMOTOR LEARNING

- *Psychomotor learning* involves acquiring skills that require the integration of mental and muscular activity.

- Summarize the following hierarchy behaviors.
  a. Perception: _____
  _____
  _____

  b. Set: _____
  _____
  _____

  c. Guided response: _____
  _____
  _____

  d. Mechanism: _____
  _____
  _____

  e. Complex overt response: _____
  _____
  _____

f. Adaptation: _____
_____
_____

g. Origination: _____
_____
_____

BASIC LEARNING PRINCIPLES

- Learning depends on the motivation to learn, the ability to learn, and the learning environment.

- The ability to learn depends on _____, _____, _____, and _____.

MOTIVATION TO LEARN

- An *attentional set* is: _____.

- Briefly explain how the following distractions influence the ability to learn.
  a. Physical discomfort: _____
  b. Anxiety: _____
  c. Environment: _____

- *Motivation* is: _____

- Briefly explain how the following can affect motivation.
  a. Social mastery: _____
  _____
  b. Task mastery: _____
  _____
  c. Physical mastery: _____
  _____

- *Compliance* is: _____

- The process of grieving gives clients time to adapt psychologically to the emotional and physical implications of illness.

- Readiness to learn is significantly related to the stage of grieving.

- When the client enters the stage of acceptance, which is compatible with learning, the nurse introduces a teaching plan.

Chapter 23: Client Education   121

- Teaching continues as long as the client remains in a stage conducive to learning.

- The client is not seen as a passive recipient or consumer of health care and education but as an active partner in the provision of care.

ABILITY TO LEARN

- Summarize how each of the following influence the ability to learn.
  a. Developmental capability: _____
  _____
  _____

  b. Learning in children: _____
  _____
  _____

  c. Adult learning: _____
  _____
  _____

  d. Physical capability: _____
  _____
  _____

LEARNING ENVIRONMENT

- Factors in the physical environment where teaching takes place can make learning a pleasant or a difficult. List five factors to consider when selecting the learning setting.
  a. _____
  b. _____
  c. _____
  d. _____
  e. _____

INTEGRATING THE NURSING AND TEACHING PROCESSES

- The teaching process requires assessment to _____. A diagnostic statement specifies _____.

- The nurse sets specific learning objectives and implements the teaching plan using teaching and learning principles to ensure _____.

- The teaching process requires an evaluation of learning based on _____.

- The nursing and teaching processes are not the same. The nursing process requires _____
_____.

- The teaching process focuses on _____
_____.

ASSESSMENT

- The client requires the nurse to assess the following factors. Summarize each one.

Learning needs
  a. _____
  b. _____
  c. _____
  d. _____

Motivation to learn
  a. _____
  b. _____
  c. _____
  d. _____
  e. _____
  f. _____
  g. _____
  h. _____
  i. _____

Ability to learn
  a. _____
  b. _____
  c. _____
  d. _____

Teaching environment
  a. _____
  b. _____
  c. _____

Resources for learning
  a. _____
  b. _____
  c. _____
  d. _____
  e. _____

NURSING DIAGNOSIS

• Classifying diagnoses by the three learning domains helps the nurse focus specifically on subject matter and teaching methods.

PLANNING

• After determining the nursing diagnoses that identify a client's learning needs, the nurse develops a teaching plan, determines goals and expected outcomes, and involves the client in selecting learning experiences. Expected outcomes guide the _____ _____.

• A learning objective identifies the _____ of a planned learning experience and helps _____ for learning.

• A learning objective includes the same criteria as goals or outcomes in a nursing care plan. These are:
  a. _____
  b. _____
  c. _____
  d. _____

• The principles of teaching are techniques that incorporate the principles of learning. Explain the following principles.
  a. Setting priorities: _____
  _____
  _____
  b. Timing: _____
  _____
  _____
  c. Organizing teaching material: _____
  _____
  _____
  d. Maintaining learning attention and participation: _____
  _____
  _____
  e. Building on existing knowledge: _____
  _____
  _____

f. Selection of teaching methods: _____
_____
_____

g. Availability of teaching resources: _____
_____
_____

h. Writing teaching plans: _____
_____
_____

IMPLEMENTATION

• Briefly explain the following teaching approaches.
  a. Telling: _____
  _____
  b. Selling: _____
  _____
  c. Participating: _____
  _____
  d. Entrusting: _____
  _____
  e. Reinforcing: _____
  _____

• Summarize the following instructional methods.
  a. One-to-one discussion: _____
  _____
  b. Group instruction: _____
  _____
  c. Preparatory instruction: _____
  _____
  d. Demonstrations: _____
  _____
  e. Analogies: _____
  _____
  f. Role playing: _____
  _____
  g. Discovery: _____
  _____

• Identify some teaching tools to be used with the following:
  a. Functional: _____

b. Illiteracy: _____

_____

c. Cultural diversity: _____

_____

d. Children's needs: _____

_____

e. Older adults: _____

_____

EVALUATION

- Evaluation reinforces correct behavior by the learner, helps learners realize how they should change incorrect behavior, and helps the teacher determine the adequacy of teaching.

- Identify some evaluation measures. _____

_____

_____

- List the three areas to be included when documenting client teaching.
    a. _____
    b. _____
    c. _____

REVIEW QUESTIONS

The student should select the appropriate answer and cite the rationale for choosing that particular answer.

1. An internal impulse that causes a person to take action is:
    a. Anxiety
    b. Motivation
    c. Compliance
    d. Adaptation

Answer: _____ Rationale: _____

_____

_____

2. Demonstration of the principles of body mechanics used when transferring clients from bed to chair would be classified under which domain of learning?
    a. Cognitive
    b. Social
    c. Psychomotor
    d. Affective

Answer: _____ Rationale: _____

_____

_____

3. Which of the following clients is most ready to begin a patient-teaching session?
    a. Ms. Hernandez, who is unwilling to accept that her back injury may result in permanent paralysis
    b. Mr. Frank, a newly diagnosed diabetic, who is complaining that he was awake all night because of his noisy roommate
    c. Mrs. Brown, a client with irritable bowel syndrome, who has just returned from a morning of testing in the GI lab
    d. Mr. Jones, a client who had a heart attack 4 days ago and now seems somewhat anxious about how this will affect his future

Answer: _____ Rationale: _____

_____

_____

4. The nurse works with pediatric clients who have diabetes. Which is the youngest age group to which the nurse can effectively teach psychomotor skills such as insulin administration?
    a. Toddler
    b. Adolescent
    c. School-age
    d. Preschool

Answer: _____ Rationale: _____

_____

_____

5. Which of the following is an appropriately stated learning objective for Mr. Ryan, a newly diagnosed diabetic?
   a. Mr. Ryan will be taught self administration of insulin by 5/2.
   b. Mr. Ryan will perform blood glucose monitoring with the EZ-Check Monitor by the time of discharge.
   c. Mr. Ryan will know the signs and symptoms of low blood sugar by 5/5.
   d. Mr. Ryan will understand diabetes.

Answer: _____   Rationale: _____
_____
_____

Documentation

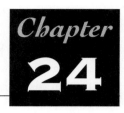

Chapter

24

The quality of care, the standards of regulatory agencies, the reimbursement structure in the health care system, and the legal guidelines for nursing practice make documentation and reporting an extremely important responsibility of a nurse.

PRELIMINARY READING

Chapter 24, pp. 500-523

COMPREHENSIVE UNDERSTANDING

MULTIDISCIPLINARY COMMUNICATION WITHIN THE HEALTH CARE TEAM

- Caregivers use a variety of ways to exchange information about clients. Briefly explain the following.
  a. *Reports:* _____
  b. *Client record:* _____
  c. *Consultations:* _____

DOCUMENTATION

- *Documentation* is defined as: _____

- Good documentation reflects not only quality of care but also evidence of each health care team member's accountability in giving care.

PURPOSES OF RECORDS

- Briefly explain the following purposes of a record.
  a. Communication: _____
  b. Financial billing: _____
  c. Education: _____
  d. Assessment: _____
  e. Research: _____
  f. Auditing: _____

- Identify four areas of common communication problems in malpractice that are caused by inadequate documentation.
  - a. _____
  - b. _____
  - c. _____
  - d. _____

GUIDELINES FOR QUALITY DOCUMENTATION AND REPORTING

- Five important guidelines must be followed to ensure quality documentation and reporting. Explain each one.
  - a. Factual: _____
  - b. Accurate: _____
  - c. Complete: _____
  - d. Current: _____
  - e. Organized: _____

STANDARDS

- Current standards require that all clients who are admitted to a health care institution have an assessment of physical, psychosocial, environmental, self-care, client education, and discharge-planning needs.

- The JCAHO requires documentation within the context of the nursing process, as well as evidence of client and family teaching and discharge planning.

NARRATIVE DOCUMENTATION

- Narrative documentation is a storylike format that documents information specific to client conditions and nursing care. The disadvantages of this style are:
  - a. _____
  - b. _____
  - c. _____

- *Problem-oriented medical records (POMR)* place emphasis on the client's problems. The method corresponds to the nursing process and facilitates communication of client needs. Explain the following major sections of the POMR.
  - a. Database: _____
  - b. Problem list: _____
  - c. Care plan: _____
  - d. Progress notes: _____

- *Focus charting* or *DAR* includes: _____

- Briefly explain the other forms of documentation.
  - a. Source records: _____
  - b. Charting by exception: _____
  - c. Case management and critical pathways: _____

COMMON RECORD-KEEPING FORMS

- Briefly explain the following formats used for record-keeping.
  - a. Nursing history forms: _____
  - b. Graphic sheets and flow sheets: _____
  - c. Nursing Kardex: _____
  - d. Acuity recording systems: _____
  - e. Standardized care plans: _____
  - f. Discharge summary forms: _____

HOME HEALTH CARE DOCUMENTATION

- Documentation in the home health care system has different implications than it does in other areas of nursing. The primary difference is _____.

- Documentation is both quality control and justification for reimbursement from Medicare, Medicaid, or private insurance companies.

- The nurse is the pivotal person in the documentation of home health care delivery.

LONG-TERM HEALTH CARE DOCUMENTATION

- Long-term care documentation supports a multidisciplinary approach in the _____ and _____ process.

COMPUTERIZED DOCUMENTATION

- Explain the many benefits of computerized documentation. _____ _____

REPORTING

- Nurses communicate information about clients so that all members of the health care team can make informed decisions about the client and their care.

CHANGE-OF-SHIFT REPORTS

- Identify the eight major areas to include in a change-of-shift report.
  a. _____
  b. _____
  c. _____
  d. _____
  e. _____
  f. _____
  g. _____
  h. _____

TELEPHONE REPORTS

- It is important that information in a telephone report be clear, accurate, and concise.

TELEPHONE ORDERS

- List the guidelines the nurse should follow when receiving telephone orders from physicians.
  a. _____
  b. _____
  c. _____
  d. _____
  e. _____
  f. _____

TRANSFER REPORTS

- List the seven major information areas in a transfer report.
  a. _____
  b. _____
  c. _____
  d. _____
  e. _____
  f. _____
  g. _____

INCIDENT REPORTS

- Define the purpose of an *incident report*: _____ _____

REVIEW QUESTIONS

The student should select the appropriate answer and cite the rationale for choosing that particular answer.

1. The primary purpose of a client's medical record is to:
   a. Satisfy requirements of accreditation agencies
   b. Communicate accurate, timely information about clients
   c. Provide validation for hospital charges
   d. Provide the nurse with a defense against malpractice

Answer: _____   Rationale: _____
_____
_____

128   Chapter 24: Documentation

2. Which of the following is correctly charted according to the six guidelines for quality recording?
   a. "Respirations rapid; lung sounds clear."
   b. "Was depressed today."
   c. "Crying. States she doesn't want visitors to see her like this."
   d. "Had a good day. Up and about in room."

Answer:_____ Rationale: _____
_____
_____

3. During a change-of-shift report:
   a. Two or more nurses always visit all clients to review their plan of care.
   b. Nurses should exchange judgments they have made about client attitudes.
   c. The nurse should identify nursing diagnoses and clarify client priorities.
   d. Client information is communicated from a nurse on a sending unit to a nurse on a receiving unit.

Answer:_____ Rationale: _____
_____
_____

4. An incident report is:
   a. A legal claim against a nurse for negligent nursing care
   b. A summary report of all falls occurring on a nursing unit
   c. A report of an event inconsistent with the routine care of a client
   d. A report of a nurse's behavior submitted to the hospital administration

Answer:_____ Rationale: _____
_____
_____

5. If an error is made while recording, the nurse should:
   a. Erase it or scratch it out
   b. Obtain a new nurse's note and rewrite the entries
   c. Leave a blank space in the note
   d. Draw a single line through the error and initial it

Answer:_____ Rationale: _____
_____
_____

Research as a Basis for Practice

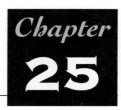

Chapter 25

The scientific knowledge base for professional practice is developed through scholarly inquiry of research literature and the actual conduct of research.

PRELIMINARY READING
Chapter 25, pp. 524-539

COMPREHENSIVE UNDERSTANDING
- *Nursing research* involves _____.

- Identify the priorities for nursing research, as stated by the National Center for Nursing Research and the International Council of Nurses are. _____
  _____
  _____
  _____

HISTORICAL PERSPECTIVE
- Briefly explain the significance of each of the following:
  a. Florence Nightingale: _____
  _____

  b. Goldmark report: _____
  _____

  c. 1940: _____
  _____

  d. 1950: _____
  _____

  e. 1960: _____
  _____

  f. 1970: _____
  _____

  g. 1981: _____
  _____

  h. 1993: _____
  _____

- Define *outcomes research*: _____

SCIENTIFIC RESEARCH IN NURSING

KNOWLEDGE ACQUISITION

- Knowledge is acquired in many ways. Scientific research is the most reliable and objective of all methods of gaining knowledge.

- The following are ways an individual acquires knowledge. Briefly explain each one.
  a. Tradition: _____
  _____
  b. Information seeking: _____
  _____
  c. Experience: _____
  _____
  d. Problem solving: _____
  _____
  e. Critical thinking: _____
  _____

SCIENTIFIC METHOD

- Define the *scientific method*: _____
  _____

- List the six characteristics of a scientific investigation.
  a. _____
  b. _____
  c. _____
  d. _____
  e. _____
  f. _____

NURSING AND THE SCIENTIFIC APPROACH

- The purpose of the scientific approach is to:
  _____
  _____

- Research provides a way for nursing questions and problems to be studied in greater depth within the context of nursing.

DEFINITIONS OF SCIENTIFIC AND NURSING RESEARCH

- Define the following:
  a. *Phenomena:* _____
  _____
  b. *Hypothesis:* _____
  _____
  c. *Biomedical research:* _____
  _____

RESEARCH METHODS

- The two broad approaches to research are _____ and _____.

QUANTITATIVE RESEARCH

- *Quantitative nursing research* is: _____

- Briefly explain the following quantitative approaches to answer research questions:
  a. Experimental study: _____
  _____
  b. Quasi-experimental: _____
  _____
  c. Surveys: _____
  _____
  d. Evaluation: _____
  _____
  e. Quantitative analysis: _____
  _____

QUALITATIVE RESEARCH

- *Qualitative research* is: _____

- Define the following design strategies that are used with qualitative research.
  a. *Ethnography:* _____
  _____
  b. *Phenomenology:* _____
  _____
  c. *Grounded theory:* _____
  _____

Chapter 25: Research as a Basis for Practice   131

NURSING RESEARCH AND THE NURSING PROCESS

- The research process consists of phases or steps that can be compared and contrasted with those of the nursing process. Briefly compare the two.
  - a. Nursing process: _____
  _____
  _____
  - b. Research process: _____
  _____
  _____

CONDUCTING NURSING RESEARCH

- Briefly explain the 1997 ANA position statement of nursing research. _____
  _____

- Briefly explain the expectations of the following levels of nursing preparation with clinical nursing research.
  - a. Associate degree: _____
  _____
  _____
  - b. Baccalaureate degree: _____
  _____
  _____
  - c. Master's degree: _____
  _____
  _____
  - d. Doctorally prepared: _____
  _____
  _____

ETHICAL ISSUES IN RESEARCH

RIGHTS OF HUMAN SUBJECTS

- *Informed consent* means that research subjects:
  - a. _____
  - b. _____
  - c. _____
  - d. _____

- *Confidentiality* is: _____

- *Anonymity* is: _____
  _____

- Briefly explain the responsibilities of the Institutional Review Board (IRB). _____
  _____

RIGHTS OF OTHER RESEARCH PARTICIPANTS

- All participants, including health care professionals caring for clients, have the right to be fully informed about the study, its procedures, and any physical or emotional injury that clients could experience as a result of participation.

- Any nurse or student nurse has the right to refuse to carry out any research procedures if he or she is concerned about their ethical aspects.

NURSING RESEARCH IN NURSING PRACTICE

RESEARCH REPORT VERSUS CLINICAL ARTICLE

- The typical research report has the following parts. Briefly explain each section:
  - a. Abstract: _____
  _____
  - b. Introduction: _____
  _____
  - c. Methods section: _____
  _____
  - d. Results section: _____
  _____
  - e. Discussion section: _____
  _____
  - f. Reference list: _____
  _____

- Explain the difference between a *primary* and *secondary* source: _____
  _____

- Identify some common sources of research studies. _____
  _____
  _____

ORGANIZING INFORMATION FROM A RESEARCH REPORT

- Define *citations*: _____
  _____

IDENTIFYING CLINICAL NURSING PROBLEMS

- List three characteristics of a clinical nursing problem with the potential to be researched.
  - a. _____
  - b. _____
  - c. _____

RESEARCH UTILIZATION

- To use findings in clinical practice, the nurse must be aware of the problems already studied.

- List four criteria used to determine if research findings should be applied to nursing practice.
  - a. _____
  - b. _____
  - c. _____
  - d. _____

- Define *research utilization*: _____
  _____

- Identify barriers to using research in clinical settings. _____
  _____

REVIEW QUESTIONS

The student should select the appropriate answer and cite the rationale for choosing that particular answer.

1. The researcher's refusal to disclose the names of subjects is:
   - a. Confidentiality
   - b. Anonymity
   - c. Informed consent
   - d. Protection of clients

   Answer: _____ Rationale: _____
   _____
   _____

2. The purpose of an institutional review board is to:
   - a. Ensure that federal funds are equitably appropriated
   - b. Conduct research benefiting the public
   - c. Determine the risk status of clients in research projects
   - d. Ensure that ethical principles are observed in human-subject research

   Answer: _____ Rationale: _____
   _____
   _____

3. Research studies can most easily be identified by:
   - a. Looking for the word "research" in the title of the report
   - b. Looking for the study only in research journals
   - c. Examining the contents of the report
   - d. Reading the abstract and conclusion of the report

   Answer: _____ Rationale: _____
   _____
   _____

4. Which statement concerning research reports is accurate?
   a. Nursing textbooks are primary sources of information.
   b. Primary sources are those written by one of the researchers in the study.
   c. The fact that a report is a primary source guarantees its accuracy.
   d. Secondary sources are the best source of information about the research study.

   Answer:_____   Rationale: _____
   _____
   _____

5. A research report includes all of the following *except:*
   a. A summary of literature used to identify the research problem
   b. The researcher's interpretation of the study results
   c. A summary of other research studies with the same results
   d. A description of methods used to conduct the study

   Answer:_____   Rationale: _____
   _____
   _____

Self-Concept

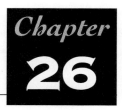

Chapter

26

   Self-concept is a subjective image of the self and a complex mixture of unconscious and conscious feelings, attitudes, and perceptions.

PRELIMINARY READING
Chapter 26, pp. 540-565

COMPREHENSIVE UNDERSTANDING

NURSING KNOWLEDGE BASE

OVERVIEW OF SELF-CONCEPT

- The four components of *self-concept* are _____, _____, _____, and _____.

- Self-concept is a dynamic combination that is based on the following.
  a. _____
  b. _____
  c. _____
  d. _____
  e. _____
  f. _____
  g. _____
  h. _____
  i. _____

- A healthy self-concept has a high degree of stability and generates positive or negative feelings toward the self.

- Define the following concepts.
  a. *Body image*: _____
  b. *Self-esteem*: _____.

- Briefly explain the four significant components of self-concept.
  a. *Identity:* _____
  _____
  _____
  _____

  b. *Body image:* _____
  _____
  _____
  _____

  c. *Self-esteem:* _____
  _____
  _____
  _____

  d. *Role performance:* _____
  _____
  _____
  _____

- List the processes through which a child learns appropriate behaviors.
  a. _____
  b. _____
  c. _____
  d. _____
  e. _____

STRESSORS AFFECTING SELF-CONCEPT

- Stressors challenge a person's adaptive capacities.

- A self-concept stressor is any _____.

- Being able to adapt to stressors is likely to lead to a positive sense of self, whereas failure to adapt often leads to a negative sense of self.

- Any change in health can be a stressor that affects self-concept.

- A physical change in the body leads to an altered body image. Identity and self-esteem can also be affected.

- A crisis occurs when a person cannot overcome obstacles with the usual methods of problem solving and adapting.

- *Identity* is defined as: _____

- Stressors throughout life affect identity. Give an example of a stressor for each developmental stage.
  a. Adolescence: _____
  _____
  b. Adulthood: _____
  _____
  c. Retirement: _____
  _____

- Changes in the appearance, structure, or function of a body part will require change in body image. Identify at least five stressors that affect body image.
  a. _____
  b. _____
  c. _____
  d. _____
  e. _____

- Having high self-esteem means that an individual sees himself or herself as being a good person worthy of respect and love. Identify at least three stressors that affect self-esteem.
  a. _____
  b. _____
  c. _____

- Roles involve expected behavior patterns associated with one individual's function in various social groups. Identify at least three stressors that affect roles.
  a. _____
  b. _____
  c. _____

- Define each of the following.
  a. *Role conflict:* _____
  _____
  b. *Role ambiguity:* _____
  _____
  c. *Role strain:* _____
  _____
  d. *Role overload:* _____
  _____

DEVELOPMENT OF SELF-CONCEPT

- Each stage of development has specific activities that assist the client in developing a positive self-concept. Identify some activities for each stage.

  a. Infancy: _____

  _____

  _____

  b. Toddler: _____

  _____

  _____

  c. Preschooler: _____

  _____

  _____

  d. School-age child: _____

  _____

  _____

  e. Adolescent: _____

  f. Young adult: _____

  _____

  _____

  g. Middle adult: _____

  _____

  _____

  h. Older adult: _____

  _____

  _____

FAMILY EFFECT ON SELF-CONCEPT DEVELOPMENT

- The family plays a key role in creating and maintaining its members' self-concepts.

- Children learn from their parents and siblings a basic sense of whom they are and how they are expected to live.

THE NURSE'S EFFECT ON THE CLIENT'S SELF-CONCEPT

- A nurse's acceptance of a client with an altered self-concept helps stimulate positive rehabilitation.

- List five areas the nurse must clarify and assess about themselves in order to promote a positive self-concept in clients.

  a. _____

  b. _____

  c. _____

  d. _____

  e. _____

SELF-CONCEPT AND THE NURSING PROCESS

ASSESSMENT

- In assessing self-concept, the nurse should focus on each component of self-concept (_____, _____, _____, and _____); behaviors suggestive of an altered self-concept; actual and potential self-concept stressors; and _____ patterns.

- Much of the data regarding self-concept are most effectively gathered through observation of a client's non-verbal behavior and by paying attention to the content of the client's conversation rather than through direct questioning.

- The nursing assessment should include consideration of previous coping behaviors: the _____, _____, and _____ of the stressors; and the client's _____ and _____ resources.

- As the nurse identifies previous coping patterns it is useful to consider if these patterns have contributed to healthy functioning or created more problems.

- Exploring resources and strengths, such as helpful significant others or prior use of community resources, can be important in formulating a realistic and effective plan.

- Asking the client how he or she believes interventions will make a difference in their problem can provide useful information regarding the client's expectations and provide an opportunity to discuss the client's goals. Give an example. _____
_____

🐍 NURSING DIAGNOSIS

- Accurate development of a nursing diagnosis requires discussing the problem with the client and the family.

- Before involving the family, the nurse needs to consider the _____ and
_____.

🐍 PLANNING

- The nurse, client, and family need to plan care directed at helping the client regain or maintain a healthy self-concept.

- Interventions focus on helping the client and on coping methods.

- The nurse looks for strengths in both the individual and the family and provides resources and education to turn limitations into strengths.

🐍 IMPLEMENTATION

Promoting a Healthy Self-Concept

Health Promotion
- List some healthy lifestyle measures that contribute to a healthy self-concept. _____
_____
_____

Acute Care
- In acute care, the nurse is likely to encounter clients who are experiencing _____ to their self-concept. Identify the stressors: _____, _____, and _____.

- Identify ways a nurse can assist a client in the adjustment to a change in physical appearance. _____
_____
_____
_____

Restorative Care
- Identify goals to help a client attain a more positive self-concept.
  a. _____
  b. _____
  c. _____
  d. _____
  e. _____

- Identify seven nursing interventions for the client to engage in self-exploration.
  a. _____
  b. _____
  c. _____
  d. _____
  e. _____
  f. _____
  g. _____

🐍 EVALUATION

- Client care evaluates the actual care delivered by the health team based on expected outcomes. Briefly explain the expected outcomes for a self-concept disturbance.
_____
_____
_____

- Client expectations evaluate care from the client's perspective. Give an example.
_____
_____
_____

REVIEW QUESTIONS

The student needs to select the appropriate answer and cite the rationale for choosing that particular answer.

1. Which developmental stage is particularly crucial for identity development?
   a. Infancy
   b. Preschool age
   c. Adolescence
   d. Young adult

   Answer:_____ Rationale: _____
   _____
   _____

2. Which of the following statements about body image is correct?
   a. Physical changes are quickly incorporated into a person's body image.
   b. Body image refers only to the external appearance of a person's body.
   c. Body image is a combination of a person's actual and perceived (ideal) body.
   d. Perceptions by other persons have no influence on a person's body image.

   Answer:_____ Rationale: _____
   _____
   _____

3. Robert, who is 2-years-old, is praised for using his potty instead of wetting his pants. This is an example of learning a behavior by:
   a. Identification
   b. Imitation
   c. Substitution
   d. Reinforcement-extinction

   Answer:_____ Rationale: _____
   _____
   _____

4. Mrs. Watson has just undergone a radical mastectomy. The nurse is aware that Mrs. Watson will probably have considerable anxiety over:
   a. Role performance
   b. Self-identity
   c. Body image
   d. Self-esteem

   Answer:_____ Rationale: _____
   _____
   _____

5. Which of the following statements demonstrates that the nurse's self-concept is positively affecting the client?
   a. "You've got to take a more active part in caring for your ostomy."
   b. "I know your ostomy is difficult to look at, but you will get used to it in time."
   c. (While grimacing) "Ostomy care isn't so bad."
   d. "Let me show you how to place the bag on your stoma."

   Answer:_____ Rationale: _____
   _____
   _____

Chapter 26: Self-Concept 139

SYNTHESIS MODEL FOR NURSING CARE PLAN ALTERATIONS IN SELF-CONCEPT

Imagine that you are the student nurse, Jan, in the Care Plan on page 556 of your text. Complete the *Assessment phase* of the synthesis model by writing in the appropriate boxes of the model below. Think about the following:

- In developing Mr. Johnson's plan of care, what **knowledge** did Jan apply?

- In what way might Jan's previous **experience** apply in this case?

- What intellectual or professional **standards** were applied to Mr. Johnson?

- What critical thinking **attitudes** did you use in assessing Mr. Johnson?

- As you review your **assessment** what key areas did you cover?

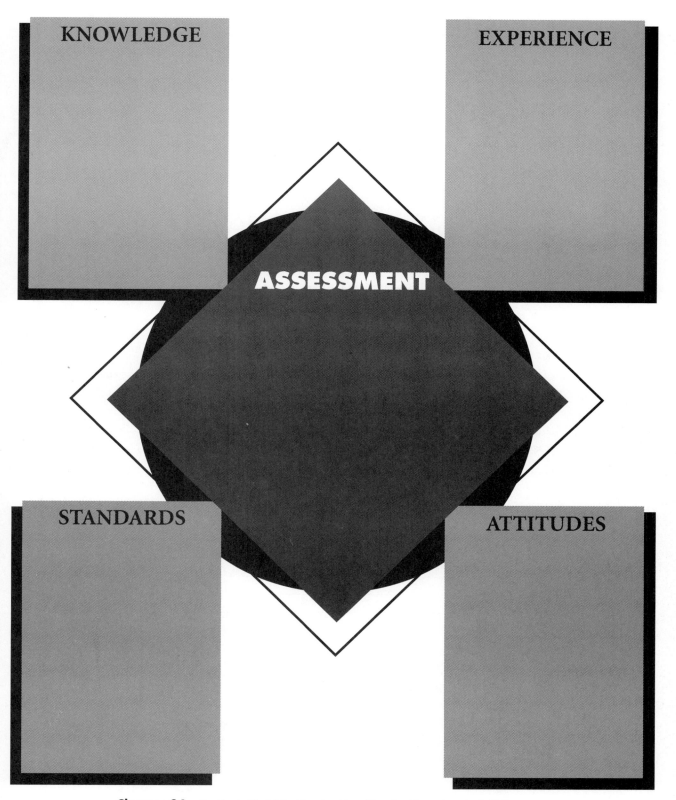

KNOWLEDGE

EXPERIENCE

ASSESSMENT

STANDARDS

ATTITUDES

Chapter 26 *Synthesis Model for Nursing Care Plan for* Alterations in Self-Concept.

See answers on p. 555.

Chapter 26: Self-Concept   141

Sexuality

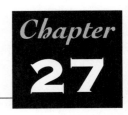
Chapter 27

 Sexuality encompasses our whole being. It includes biological, sociological, psychological, spiritual, and cultural dimensions of each person's being.

PRELIMINARY READING
Chapter 27, pp. 566-588

COMPREHENSIVE UNDERSTANDING
SCIENTIFIC KNOWLEDGE

SEXUAL DEVELOPMENT
- Each stage of development brings changes in sexual functioning and the role of sexuality in relationships. Explain each stage.
  a. Infancy: _____
  _____

  b. Toddler/preschool: _____
  _____

  c. School-aged: _____
  _____

  d. Puberty/adolescence: _____
  _____

  e. Adulthood: _____
  _____

  f. Older adult: _____
  _____

SEXUAL RESPONSE CYCLE
- The three phases of the sexual response are _____, _____, and _____.

- These phases are the result of vasocongestion and myotonia. Explain each of these physiological responses.
  a. Female: _____
  _____

  b. Male: _____
  _____

SEXUAL ORIENTATION

- *Sexual orientation* is defined as: _____
_____

- Human sexual orientation is a continuum between _____ and _____ orientations.

CONTRACEPTION

- There are numerous contraceptive options available. Briefly list the options available under the following categories.
  a. Nonprescriptive methods: _____
  _____
  b. Methods requiring a health care provider:
  _____
  _____

ABORTION

- Identify the issues that make the availability of abortions uncertain. _____
  _____
  _____

SEXUALLY TRANSMITTED DISEASES

- The highest prevalence is among _____ and _____.

- List the prevalent STDs.
  a. _____
  b. _____
  c. _____
  d. _____
  e. _____

- Identify the primary routes of HIV transmission. _____
  _____
  _____

- Those primarily vulnerable to HIV infections are _____, _____, _____, and _____.

NURSING KNOWLEDGE BASE

SOCIOCULTURAL DIMENSIONS OF SEXUALITY

- Global cultural diversity creates considerable variability in sexual norms and represents a wide spectrum of beliefs and values.

- Common areas of diversity include the following.
  a. _____
  b. _____
  c. _____
  d. _____
  e. _____
  f. _____

- Briefly summarize the impact of pregnancy and menstruation on sexuality. _____
  _____
  _____

- Identify the issues regarding the difficulty of the nurse from discussing sexuality with clients.
  a. _____
  b. _____
  c. _____
  d. _____

DECISIONAL ISSUES

- Briefly discuss the following decisional issues.
  a. Contraception: _____
  _____
  _____
  b. Abortion: _____
  _____
  _____
  c. STD prevention: _____
  _____
  _____

ALTERATIONS IN SEXUAL HEALTH

- Explain the following issues.
  a. Infertility: _____
  _____
  _____
  b. Sexual abuse: _____
  _____
  _____
  c. Personal and emotional conflicts: _____
  _____
  _____
  d. Sexual dysfunction: _____
  _____
  _____

SEXUALITY AND THE NURSING PROCESS

- A person's sexuality has physical, psychological, social, and cultural elements.

ASSESSMENT

- Briefly explain the following factors that affect sexuality.
  a. Physical: _____
  _____
  _____
  _____
  b. Self-concept: _____
  _____
  _____
  _____
  c. Relationship: _____
  _____
  _____
  _____
  d. Self-esteem: _____
  _____
  _____
  _____

- List five questions a nurse may use to elicit a brief sexual history from an adult.
  a. _____
  b. _____
  c. _____
  d. _____
  e. _____

- Explain how the nurse is able to anticipate when a client is at risk for sexual dysfunction.
  _____
  _____

- Briefly explain the physical assessment in evaluating the cause of sexual concerns or problems.
  a. Female: _____
  b. Male: _____

NURSING DIAGNOSIS

- Identify clues that may signal risk for or an actual nursing diagnosis related to sexuality.
  a. _____
  b. _____
  c. _____
  d. _____
  e. _____

PLANNING

- The PLISSIT model developed by Annon (1976) guides the planning phases. Explain each of the following:
  a. P _____
  b. LI _____
  c. SS_____
  d. IT _____

IMPLEMENTATION

Health Promotion

- Topics of education vary, depending on the defining characteristics and related factors. Describe some situations. _____
  _____
  _____
  _____
  _____
  _____

Acute Care

- Nursing interventions that address alterations in sexuality are aimed at _____, _____, and/or _____.

- The client should be encouraged to investigate and acknowledge social and ethical values and analyze the role of sexuality in his or her self-concept.

- Identify situational and developmental crises that prompt education._____
  _____
  _____
  _____
  _____
  _____

Restorative care
- In the home environment it is important to assist individuals in creating an environment comfortable for sexual activity.

- In the long-term care setting, facilities should make proper arrangements for privacy during resident's sexual experiences.

✍ EVALUATION
- Client care evaluates the actual care delivered by the health care team based on the expected outcomes.

- Client or spouse verbalizations determine if goals and outcomes have been achieved.

- Sexuality is felt more than observed, and sexual expression requires an intimacy not amenable to observation.

- All people involved may need to be reminded of the individual nature of sexual expression and the multiple factors that affect perceptions and responses.

- Client expectations evaluate care from the client's perspective. Briefly explain the client's perspective.
  _____
  _____
  _____
  _____
  _____

REVIEW QUESTIONS

The student should select the appropriate answer and cite the rationale for choosing that particular answer.

1. At what developmental stage is it particularly important for children reared in single-parent families to be exposed to same-sex adults?
   a. Infancy
   b. Toddlerhood and preschool years
   c. School-age
   d. Adolescence

   Answer:_____   Rationale: _____
   _____
   _____

2. In the school-age child, learning and reinforcement of gender-appropriate behaviors are most commonly derived from:
   a. Parents
   b. Teachers
   c. Siblings
   d. Peers

   Answer:_____   Rationale: _____
   _____
   _____

3. Which statement about sexual response in the older adult is correct?
   a. The resolution phase is slower.
   b. The orgasm phase is prolonged.
   c. The plateau phase is prolonged.
   d. The refractory phase is more rapid.

   Answer:_____   Rationale: _____
   _____
   _____

4. The least effective means of preventing pregnancy is:
   a. Coitus interruptus
   b. Calendar (rhythm) method
   c. Body temperature method
   d. Mucus method

   Answer:_____ Rationale: _____
   _____
   _____

5. The only 100% effective method to avoid contracting a disease through sex is:
   a. Using condoms
   b. Avoiding sex with partners at risk
   c. Knowing the sexual partner's health history
   d. Abstinence

   Answer:_____ Rationale: _____
   _____
   _____

SYNTHESIS MODEL FOR NURSING CARE PLAN FOR SEXUAL DYSFUNCTION

Imagine that you are Jack, the nurse in the Care Plan on page 582 of your text. Complete the *Assessment phase* of the synthesis model by writing your answers in the appropriate boxes of the model shown. Think about the following:

- In developing Mr. Clement's plan of care, what **knowledge** did Jack apply?

- In what way might Jack's previous **experience** assist in this case?

- What intellectual or professional **standards** were applied to Mr. Clement?

- What critical thinking **attitudes** did you utilize in assessing Mr. Clement?

- As you review your **assessment** what key areas did you cover?

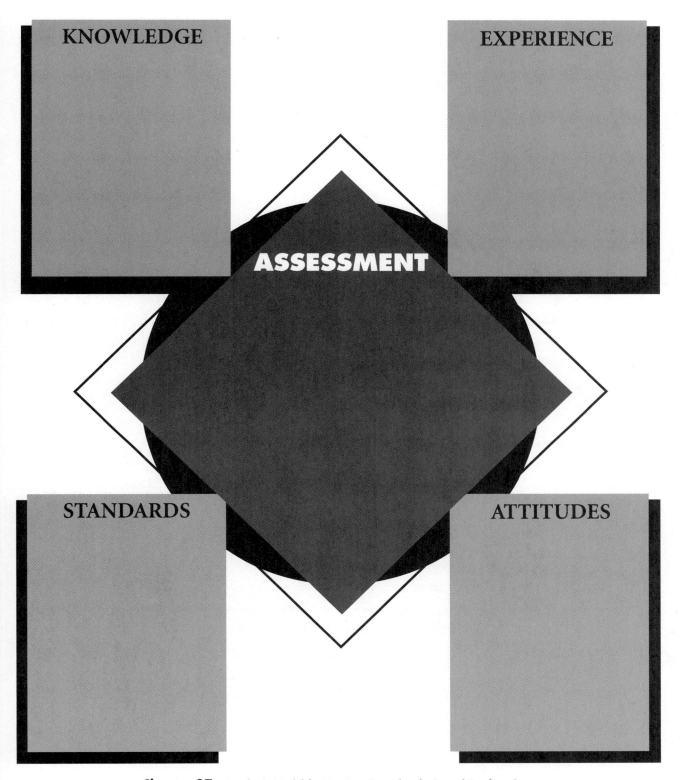

KNOWLEDGE

EXPERIENCE

ASSESSMENT

STANDARDS

ATTITUDES

Chapter 27   *Synthesis Model for Nursing Care Plan for Sexual Dysfunction.*

See answers on page 556.

Chapter 27: Sexuality   147

Spiritual Health

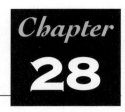

A person's health depends on a balance of physical, psychological, sociological, cultural, developmental, and spiritual factors.

PRELIMINARY READING
Chapter 28, pp. 589-611

COMPREHENSIVE UNDERSTANDING
- *Spirituality* is: _____

SCIENTIFIC KNOWLEDGE BASE
- Summarize the relationship of spirituality and healing. _____
_____

CONCEPTS IN SPIRITUAL HEALTH

- The concepts of _____, _____, _____, and
_____ give direction in understanding the views each individual has of life and its
value.

- Individuals' definitions of spirituality are influenced by their own _____,
_____, _____, and _____.

- Identify the two important characteristics of spirituality.
  a. _____
  b. _____

- Explain how the following view spirituality.
  a. Atheists:_____
  b. Agnostics: _____

- Explain the concept of faith. _____
_____
_____

- The belief that comes with faith involves _____, or an awareness of which one
cannot see or know in ordinary ways.

- Define *religion*: _____
  _____

- Religion serves different purposes in people's lives.

- Explain the differences between the terms *spirituality* and *religion*. _____
  _____
  _____

- Summarize the concept of hope. _____
  _____
  _____

- Define *spiritual health*: _____
  _____

- Identify how each of the following age-groups grow spiritually.
  a. Children: _____
  _____
  _____
  b. Adults: _____
  _____
  _____
  c. Older adults: _____
  _____
  _____

SPIRITUAL PROBLEMS

- *Spiritual distress* is: _____
  _____

- Briefly explain each of the following causes of spiritual distress.
  a. Acute illness: _____
  _____
  _____
  b. Chronic illness: _____
  _____
  _____
  c. Terminal illness: _____
  _____
  _____
  d. Near-death experience: _____
  _____
  _____

RELIGIOUS PROBLEMS

- Explain how the following can affect the client's sense of well-being.
  a. A change in denominational membership or religious conversion: _____
  _____
  _____
  b. Loss or questioning of faith: _____
  _____
  _____

CRITICAL THINKING SYNTHESIS

- Summarize how the use of intuition is different in the beginning nurse and the expert nurse. _____
  _____
  _____

NURSING PROCESS

- An element of quality health care is to exhibit caring for the client so that a relationship of trust forms. Trust is strengthened when the caregiver _____ and _____.

- Briefly explain shared community and compassion. _____
  _____
  _____
  _____

- It is important for nurses to sort out value-judgments about other people's belief systems.

- The nurse must be willing to share and discover another person's meaning and purpose in life, sickness, and health.

ASSESSMENT

- The assessment should focus on aspects of spirituality most likely to be influenced by life experiences, events, and questions in the case of illness and hospitalization.

Chapter 28: Spiritual Health   149

- The JAREL spirituality well-being scale provides nurses and other health care professionals with a tool for assessing client's spiritual well-being. Briefly summarize the three dimensions.
  a. Faith/belief dimension: _____
  _____
  _____

  b. Life/self responsibility: _____
  _____
  _____

  c. Life-satisfaction/self-actualization: _____
  _____
  _____

- Explain how the following can affect a client's spiritual health.
  a. Fellowship and community: _____
  _____
  _____

  b. Ritual and practice: _____
  _____
  _____

  c. Vocation: _____
  _____
  _____

NURSING DIAGNOSIS

- When reviewing a spiritual assessment and integrating the information into an appropriate nursing diagnosis, the nurse should consider the client's current health status from a holistic perspective, with spirituality as the unifying principle.

- State the defining characteristics for the following two diagnoses.
  a. Spiritual well-being: _____
  _____
  _____

  b. Spiritual distress: _____
  _____
  _____

PLANNING

- In order to develop an individualized plan of care, the nurse integrates knowledge gathered from the assessment and relating to resources and therapies available for spiritual care.

- Identify the three goals for spiritual caregiving.
  a. _____
  b. _____
  c. _____

IMPLEMENTATION

Health Promotion
- Spiritual care should be a central theme in promoting an individual's overall well-being.

- Briefly explain the following interventions and how they are helpful in maintaining or promoting a client's spiritual health:
  a. Establishing presence: _____
  _____

  b. Supporting a healing relationship: _____
  _____
  _____

Acute Care
- Within acute care settings, clients experience multiple stressors that threaten to overwhelm their coping resources.

- Explain how the following interventions are helpful in the client's therapeutic plan.
  a. Support systems: _____
  _____
  _____

  b. Diet therapies: _____
  _____
  _____

  c. Supporting rituals: _____
  _____
  _____

Restorative and Continuing Care

- Spiritual care becomes very important to clients who are recovering from a long-term illness or disability or who suffer chronic or terminal disease.

- Explain how the following interventions are helpful in maintaining or promoting a client's spiritual health.

  a. Prayer: _____

  _____

  _____

  b. Meditation: _____

  _____

  _____

  c. Supporting grief work: _____

  _____

  _____

🕮 EVALUATION

Client Care

- Client care evaluates the actual care delivered by the health team based on the expected outcomes. Give some examples. _____

  _____

  _____

  _____

  _____

Client Expectations

- A client's expectation evaluates care from the client perspective. Give some examples.

  _____

  _____

  _____

  _____

REVIEW QUESTIONS

The student should select the appropriate answer and cite the rationale for choosing that particular answer.

1. When planning care to include spiritual needs for a client of the Moslem faith, the religious practices the nurse should understand include all of the following *except*:

   a. A priest be present to conduct rituals
   b. Strength gained through group prayer
   c. Family members as a source of comfort
   d. Faith healing providing psychological support

   Answer:_____   Rationale: _____

   _____

   _____

2. When consulting with the dietary department regarding meals for a client of the Hindu religion, which of the following dietary items would not be included on the meal trays?

   a. Meats
   b. Dairy products
   c. Vegetable entrees
   d. Fruits

   Answer:_____   Rationale: _____

   _____

   _____

3. If an Islamic client dies, the nurse should be aware of what religious practice?

   a. Only relatives and friends may touch the body.
   b. Members of a ritual burial society cleanse the body.
   c. Last rites are mandatory.
   d. The body is always cremated.

   Answer:_____   Rationale: _____

   _____

   _____

4. If a nurse were to use a nursing diagnosis to relate concerns about spiritual health, which of the following would be used?
   a. Spiritual distress
   b. Inability to adjust
   c. Lack of faith
   d. Religious dilemma

Answer:_____   Rationale: _____
_____
_____

5. Mr. Phillips was recently diagnosed with a malignant tumor. The staff had observed him crying on several occasions, and now he cries as he reads from his Bible. Interventions to help Mr. Phillips cope with his illness would include:
   a. Asking the hospital chaplain to visit him daily
   b. Engaging Mr. Phillips in diversional activities to reduce feelings of hopelessness
   c. Supporting his use of inner resources by providing time for meditation
   d. Praying with Mr. Phillips as often as possible

Answer:_____   Rationale: _____
_____
_____

SYNTHESIS MODEL FOR NURSING CARE PLAN FOR SPIRITUAL WELL-BEING

Imagine that you are Leah, the nurse in the Care Plan on page 604 of your text. Complete the *Planning phase* of the synthesis model by writing your answers in the appropriate boxes of the model shown. Think about the following:

• In developing James' plan of care, what **knowledge** did Leah apply?

• In what way might Leah's previous **experience** assist in developing a plan of care for James?

• When developing a plan of care what intellectual and professional **standards** were applied?

• What critical thinking **attitudes** might have been applied developing James' plan?

• How will Leah accomplish the goals?

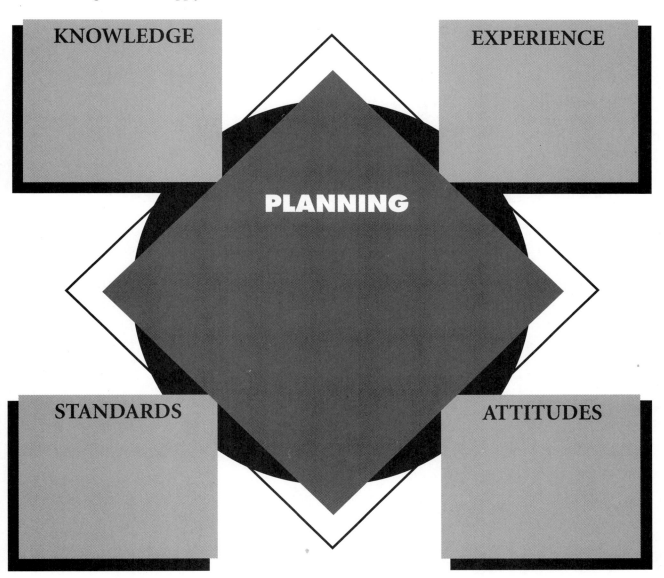

Chapter 28 *Synthesis Model for Nursing Care Plan for* **Spiritual Well-being.**

See answers on page 557.

Responding to Loss, Death, and Grieving

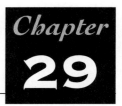

The nurse helps clients to understand and accept loss within the context of their culture so that life can continue.

PRELIMINARY READING
Chapter 29, pp. 612-642

COMPREHENSIVE UNDERSTANDING

GENERAL CONCEPTS OF THE GRIEVING PROCESS

LOSS

- Define *loss*: _____

- List and give an example of the five categories of loss.

    a. _____
    _____

    b. _____
    _____

    c. _____
    _____

    d. _____
    _____

    e. _____
    _____

GRIEF

- Describe the following types of *grief*.
    a. *Grief:* _____
    b. *Dysfunctional grief:* _____
    c. *Disenfranchised grief:* _____
    d. *Anticipatory grief:* _____

- Define the following types of losses.
  a. *Personal loss:* _____
  b. *Actual loss:* _____
  c. *Perceived loss:* _____
  d. *Maturational loss:* _____
  e. *Situational loss:* _____

COPING MECHANISMS IN GRIEF AND LOSS

- Summarize the following concepts related to coping mechanisms in grief and loss.
  a. *Hope:* _____
  _____
  _____
  _____
  _____

  b. *Mourning:* _____
  _____
  _____
  _____
  _____

  c. *Grief work:* _____
  _____
  _____
  _____
  _____

  c. *Closure:* _____
  _____
  _____
  _____
  _____

- Identify each of the following in the acronym (TEAR) that describes the tasks of grief work.
  a. T: _____
  b. E: _____
  c. A: _____
  d. R: _____

SCIENTIFIC KNOWLEDGE BASE

THEORIES OF THE GRIEVING PROCESS

- List the phases of the grieving process proposed by each of the theorists listed below.

Engle's Theory
  a. _____
  b. _____
  c. _____

Kübler-Ross's Stages of Dying
  a. _____
  b. _____
  c. _____
  d. _____
  e. _____

Rando's Phases of Grieving
  a. _____
  b. _____
  c. _____

- Summarize the psychosocial perspectives of loss and grief. _____
  _____
  _____
  _____

NURSING KNOWLEDGE BASE

DEATH AS A UNIQUE EXPERIENCE

- The nurse must learn many values, beliefs, cultural backgrounds, and attitudes about life, death, and loss to be able to deal with the dying client and the client or family experiencing a loss.

COMMUNICATION

- Communication is the basis for gathering accurate information regarding the perceptions and feelings of individualized clients. Give some examples of the following.
  a. Inappropriate communication: _____
  _____
  b. Therapeutic communication: _____
  _____

ETHICAL ISSUES

- List some of the moral and ethical issues of today. _____
  _____
  _____

THE NURSING PROCESS AND GRIEF

✒ ASSESSMENT

- The nurse should avoid assuming that a particular behavior indicates grief and allow persons to share what is happening in their own ways.

- Assessment of the client and family begins by exploring _____ _____.

- The nurse assesses how the client _____ reacting rather than how the client _____ reacting.

- The following factors influence the way any individual responds to loss. Briefly explain each one.
  a. Personal characteristics: _____
  _____
  _____

  b. Nature of relationships: _____
  _____
  _____

  c. Social support system: _____
  _____
  _____

  d. Nature of the loss: _____
  _____
  _____

  e. Cultural and spiritual beliefs: _____
  _____
  _____

  f. Loss of personal life goals: _____
  _____
  _____

✒ NURSING DIAGNOSIS

- List four nursing diagnoses for the following groups.
  a. The individual: _____
  _____
  _____
  _____

  b. The family: _____
  _____
  _____
  _____

  c. The community: _____
  _____
  _____
  _____

✒ PLANNING

- Grieving has a therapeutic value that enables people to work through their losses, recollect their thoughts and feelings, and resume life with new insights and direction.

- List five goals appropriate for a client dealing with loss.
  a. _____
  b. _____
  c. _____
  d. _____
  e. _____

- List the three most crucial needs of the dying client.
  a. _____
  b. _____
  c. _____

✒ IMPLEMENTATION

- To deliver the client's plan of care appropriately, the nurse must consider all levels of health. Briefly explain each of the following:
  a. Health promotion: _____
  _____
  _____

  b. Acute care: _____
  _____
  _____

- The nurse must schedule adequate private time with the client and family to promote open communication, accomplishing the following goals:
  a. _____
  b. _____
  c. _____

- Communication is blocked by

_____ ,

_____ ,

or _____ .

End-of-Life Care

- The nurse must take a special effort to stimulate all senses in a positive manner to maintain a sense of _____ ,

_____ , and _____ .

- When supporting the grieving client's family, the nurse must _____ ,

_____ , and _____

- List some suggestions for involving the family in the care of the dying client. _____

_____

_____

_____

_____

_____

_____

_____

_____

Hospice Care

- Identify the components of hospice care.

_____

_____

_____

_____

_____

_____

_____

_____

Care after Death

- Care after death includes caring for the body with dignity and sensitivity. Identify the physiological changes that take place after death and the appropriate nursing interventions.

_____

_____

_____

_____

_____

_____

_____

_____

_____

✍ EVALUATION

Client Care

- Grieving is an individual process, and resolution of loss does not follow a set schedule.

- The care of the dying client requires the nurse to evaluate the client's level of comfort with illness and the client's quality of life.

Client Expectations

- Client expectations evaluate care from the client perspective. The client expects individualization of care, including comfort, dignity, and cooperation, to maximize the client's quality of life.

REVIEW QUESTIONS

The student should select the appropriate answer and cite the rationale for choosing that particular answer.

1. Which statement about loss is accurate?
   a. Loss is only experienced when there is an actual absence of something valued.
   b. The more an individual has invested in what is lost, the less the feeling of loss.
   c. Loss may be maturational, situational, or both.
   d. The degree of stress experienced is unrelated to the type of loss.

Answer: _____   Rationale: _____

_____

_____

Chapter 29: Responding to Loss, Death, and Grieving 157

2. The developmental stage at which the child is first able to understand logical explanations about death is:
a. Toddlerhood
b. Preschool-age
c. School-age
d. Adolescence

Answer:_____ Rationale: _____
_____
_____

3. A hospice program emphasizes:
a. Curative treatment and alleviation of symptoms
b. Palliative treatment and control of symptoms
c. Hospital-based care
d. Prolongation of life

Answer:_____ Rationale: _____
_____
_____

4. Trying questionable and experimental forms of therapy is a behavior that is characteristic of which stage of dying?
a. Anger
b. Depression
c. Bargaining
d. Acceptance

Answer:_____ Rationale: _____
_____
_____

5. All of the following are crucial needs of the dying client *except:*
a. Control of pain
b. Preservation of dignity and self-worth
c. Love and belonging
d. Freedom from decision-making

Answer:_____ Rationale: _____
_____
_____

SYNTHESIS MODEL FOR NURSING CARE PLAN FOR GRIEF AND LOSS

Imagine that you are the student nurse, in the Care Plan on page 628 of your text. Complete the *Evaluation phase* of the synthesis model by writing your answers in the appropriate boxes of the model shown. Think about the following:

- In evaluating Mr. Miller's plan of care, what **knowledge** did you apply?

- In what way might your previous **experience** influence your evaluation of Mr. Miller's care?

- During evaluation, what intellectual and professional **standards** were applied to Mr. Miller's care?

- In what way does critical thinking **attitudes** play a role in how you approach evaluation of Mr. Miller's care?

- How might you adjust Mr. Miller's care?

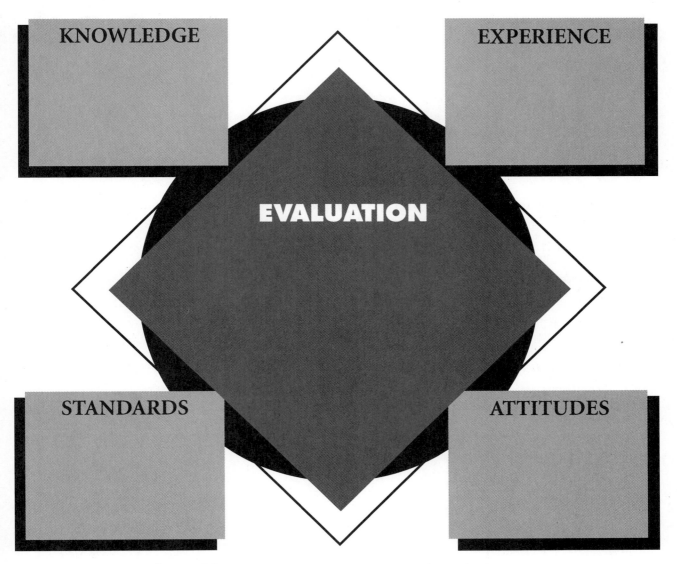

Chapter 29 *Synthesis Model for Nursing Care Plan for Grief and Loss.*

See answers on page 558.

Chapter 29: Responding to Loss, Death, and Grieving   159

Stress and Adaptation

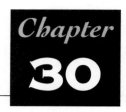

Chapter 30

Stress is a phenomenon that affects the social, psychological, developmental, spiritual, and physiological dimensions.

PRELIMINARY READING

Chapter 30, pp.643-667

COMPREHENSIVE UNDERSTANDING

SCIENTIFIC KNOWLEDGE BASE

STRESS AND STRESSORS

- *Stress* is: _____
- Stressors represent an _____
_____.

- Give an example of the following types of stressors.
  a. *Internal:* _____
  _____
  b. *External:* _____
  _____.

PHYSIOLOGICAL ADAPTATION

- *Physiological adaptation* is: _____

- Define *homeostasis*: _____

- Explain the three mechanisms of physiological adaptation.
  a. Medulla oblongata: _____
  _____
  _____
  b. Reticular formation: _____
  _____
  _____
  c. Pituitary gland: _____
  _____
  _____

- Briefly explain the limitations of physiological mechanisms of adaptation. _____
_____
_____

MODELS OF STRESS

- Stress models are used to identify the stressors for a particular individual and predict that person's responses to them. Summarize the following models.
  a. Response-based: _____
  _____
  _____
  b. Adaptation model: _____
  _____
  _____
  c. Transaction-based: _____
  _____
  _____
  d. Stimulus-based: _____
  _____
  _____

FACTORS INFLUENCING RESPONSE TO STRESSORS

- List the factors that influence the response to stressors.
  a. _____
  b. _____
  c. _____
  d. _____

- The greater the scope of a stressor, the greater the response of the client to it.

ADAPTATION TO STRESSORS

- *Adaptation* is: _____

- There are many forms of adaptation. Give some examples. _____
  _____
  _____

- List the four requirements for successful family adaptation.
  a. _____
  b. _____

c. _____
d. _____

- Stress can affect the _____, _____, _____, _____, and _____ dimensions.

RESPONSE TO STRESS

- When stress occurs, a person uses physiological and psychological energy to respond and adapt.

- The stress response is adaptive and protective, and the characteristics of this response are the result of integrated neuroendocrine responses.

- Identify the two physiological responses to stress.
  a. _____
  b. _____

- Describe the four common characteristics of the *local adaptation response (LAS)*.
  a. _____
  b. _____
  c. _____
  d. _____

- List (in sequence) and briefly describe the three stages of the *general adaptation syndrome (GAS)*.
  a. _____
  b. _____
  c. _____

NURSING KNOWLEDGE BASE

PSYCHOLOGICAL RESPONSE

- Psychological adaptive behaviors can be constructive or destructive. Give an example of each behavior.
  a. Constructive: _____
  _____
  _____
  b. Destructive: _____
  _____
  _____

- Physiological adaptive behaviors are referred to as _____ _____.

- Define each of the following:
  a. *Task-oriented behaviors:* _____
  _____
  b. *Ego-defense mechanisms:* _____
  _____

- Explain how the following factors can influence a client to deal with stress.
  a. Developmental: _____
  _____
  _____
  b. Intellectual: _____
  _____
  c. Emotional behavioral: _____
  _____
  d. Family: _____
  _____
  e. Lifestyle: _____
  _____
  f. Sociocultural: _____
  _____
  _____
  g. Spiritual: _____
  _____

NURSING PROCESS

ASSESSMENT

- A person's perception of a stressor is based on _____, _____, _____, _____, _____, _____, and _____.

- Stress response behaviors, both verbal and nonverbal, should be assessed.

- Identify six physical indicators of stress.
  a. _____
  b. _____
  c. _____
  d. _____
  e. _____
  f. _____

- Define the following stress situations:
  a. *Mild:* _____
  _____
  _____
  b. *Moderate:* _____
  _____
  _____
  c. *Severe:* _____
  _____
  _____

- Identify a psychological indicator of stress.
  _____
  _____

- Prolonged stress can affect the ability to complete developmental tasks. Identify one indicator for each developmental stage.
  a. Infancy: _____
  _____
  b. School-age: _____
  _____
  c. Adolescence: _____
  _____
  d. Young adult: _____
  _____
  e. Middle-age: _____
  _____
  f. Older adult: _____
  _____

- Identify three emotional indicators of stress.
  a. _____
  b. _____
  c. _____

- Identify four intellectual indicators of stress.
  a. _____
  b. _____
  c. _____
  d. _____

- Identify a family indicator of stress.

  _____

- Identify a lifestyle indicator of stress.

  _____

- Identify a sociocultural indicator of stress.

  _____

- Identify two spiritual indicators of stress.
  a. _____
  b. _____

🖎 NURSING DIAGNOSIS

- Stress can result in multiple diagnostic statements.

🖎 PLANNING

- The care plan is individualized to the client's perception of the stressor and response to stress.

- Stress-management techniques are designed to match the client's actual and potential stressors. General goals are: _____
  _____

🖎 IMPLEMENTATION

- Stress management may be seen as a health promotion activity or an intervention that modifies a response to illness.

Health Promotion
- Explain how the following methods reduce stressors.
  a. Time management: _____
  _____

  b. Regular exercise: _____
  _____

  c. Nutrition and diet: _____
  _____

  d. Rest: _____
  _____

  e. Support systems: _____
  _____

Acute Care
- *Crisis intervention* is: _____

- Crises occur _____.

- Clients and nurses are at risk for two types of crises. Describe them.
  a. *Situational crisis:* _____
  _____
  _____

  b. *Developmental crisis:* _____
  _____
  _____

Restorative care
- Explain how the following lifestyle choices are healthy and stress reducing.
  a. Humor: _____
  _____

  b. Enhancing self-esteem: _____
  _____

  c. Relaxation techniques: _____
  _____

  d. Spirituality: _____
  _____

  e. Stress management in workplace:
  _____
  _____

🖎 EVALUATION
- Briefly explain the client's care in relation to:
  a. Clients' perceptions of stress: _____
  _____

  b. Client's expectations: _____
  _____

REVIEW QUESTIONS

The student should select the appropriate answer and cite the rationale for choosing that particular answer.

1. Which definition does not characterize stress?
   a. Any situation in which a nonspecific demand requires an individual to respond or take action
   b. A phenomenon affecting social, psychological, developmental, spiritual, and physiological dimensions
   c. A condition eliciting an intellectual, behavioral, or metabolic response
   d. Efforts to maintain relative constancy within the internal environment

   Answer:_____   Rationale: _____
   _____
   _____

2. Which statement about homeostasis is inaccurate?
   a. Homeostatic mechanisms provide long-term and short-term control over the body's equilibrium.
   b. Homeostatic mechanisms are self-regulatory.
   c. Homestatic mechanisms function through negative feedback.
   d. Illness may inhibit normal homeostatic mechanisms.

   Answer:_____   Rationale: _____
   _____
   _____

3. Major homeostatic mechanisms are controlled by all of the following *except:*
   a. Thymus gland
   b. Medulla oblongata
   c. Reticular formation
   d. Pituitary gland

   Answer:_____   Rationale: _____
   _____
   _____

4. Which of the following is an example of the local adaptation syndrome?
   a. Alarm reaction
   b. Flight-or-fight response
   c. Ego-defense mechanisms
   d. Inflammatory response

   Answer:_____   Rationale: _____
   _____
   _____

5. The general adaptation syndrome consists of three stages. During which stage does the body stabilize and hormone levels return to normal?
   a. Exhaustion
   b. Regeneration
   c. Resistance
   d. Compensation

   Answer:_____   Rationale: _____
   _____
   _____

6. Crisis intervention is a specific measure used for helping a client resolve a particular, immediate, stress problem. This approach is based on:
   a. The ability of the nurse to solve the client's problems
   b. An in-depth analysis of a client's situation
   c. Teaching the client how to use ego-defense mechanisms
   d. Effective communication between the nurse and client

   Answer:_____   Rationale: _____
   _____
   _____

Synthesis Model for Nursing Care Plan for Care Giver Role Strain

Imagine that you are Janet, the nurse in the Care Plan on page 660 of your text. Complete the *Evaluation phase* of the synthesis model by writing your answers in the appropriate boxes of the model shown. Think about the following:

- In evaluating the care of Carl and Evelyn, what **knowledge** did Janet apply?

- In what way might Janet's previous **experience** influence the evaluation of Carl's care?

- During evaluation, what intellectual and professional **standards** were applied to Carl's care?

- In what way does critical thinking **attitudes** play a role in how Janet approaches the evaluation of Carl's care?

- How might Janet adjust Carl's care?

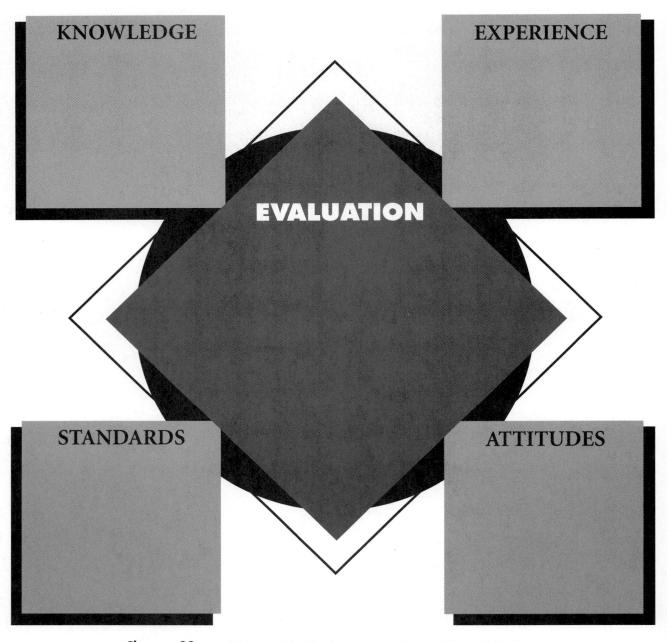

KNOWLEDGE

EXPERIENCE

EVALUATION

STANDARDS

ATTITUDES

Chapter 30 *Synthesis Model for Nursing Care Plan for* Care Giver Role Strain.

See answers on page 559

166   Chapter 30: Stress and Adaptation

Vital Signs

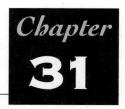
Chapter 31

> *As indicators of health status, vital signs demonstrate the effectiveness of the circulation, and of respiratory, neural, and endocrine body functions.*

PRELIMINARY READING
Chapter 31, pp. 668-723

COMPREHENSIVE UNDERSTANDING

GUIDELINES FOR TAKING VITAL SIGNS
• Identify the guidelines that assist the nurse to incorporate vital sign measurement into practice.

a. _____
b. _____
c. _____
d. _____
e. _____
f. _____
g. _____
h. _____
i. _____
j. _____
k. _____
l. _____

BODY TEMPERATURE

PHYSIOLOGY
• The body temperature is the difference between the _____ and the amount

_____.

• Define *core temperature*: _____

• Identify the sites of temperature measurement. _____

_____

_____

_____

• Average, normal temperatures vary depending on the measurement site.

- Measurement of the pulmonary artery temperature is the standard against which all other sites are judged for accuracy.

- Sites reflecting core temperatures are more reliable indicators of body temperature than sites reflecting surface temperatures.

- Define *thermoregulation*: _____

- Briefly summarize how neural and vascular mechanisms control body temperature.

  _____
  _____
  _____
  _____

- Define the following terms:
  a. *Vasodilation:* _____
     _____

  b. *Vasoconstriction:* _____
     _____

- List four sources, or mechanisms, for heat production.
  a. _____
  b. _____
  c. _____
  d. _____

- Explain the following mechanisms of body heat loss, and give an example of each.
  a. *Radiation:* _____

  b. *Conduction:* _____
     _____

  c. *Convection:* _____
     _____

  d. *Evaporation:* _____
     _____

  e. *Diaphoresis:* _____
     _____

Skin in Temperature Regulation

- Briefly explain the skin's role in temperature regulation.
  a. Insulation of the body: _____
     _____
     _____

  b. Vasoconstriction: _____
     _____
     _____

  c. Temperature sensation: _____
     _____
     _____

Behavioral Control

- Identify four factors that must be present for a person to control body temperature.
  a. _____
  b. _____
  c. _____
  d. _____

FACTORS AFFECTING BODY TEMPERATURE

- Changes in body temperature within the normal range occur when the relationship between heat production and heat loss is altered by physiological or behavioral variables. Summarize the following variables.
  a. Age: _____
     _____
     _____

  b. Exercise: _____
     _____
     _____

  c. Hormone level: _____
     _____
     _____

  d. Circadian rhythm: _____
     _____
     _____

  e. Stress: _____
     _____
     _____

  f. Environment: _____
     _____
     _____

- Temperature alterations can be related to _____, _____, _____, or any combination of these alterations.

- *Hyperpyrexia, or fever,* occurs because _____ _____

- Summarize the alteration in the hypothalamic set point that causes a true fever. _____ _____ _____

- Explain how a fever works as an important defense mechanism. _____ _____ _____

- Explain how a fever serves a diagnostic purpose. _____ _____ _____

- Explain how a fever affects metabolism. _____ _____ _____

- Define the following terms:
  a. *Hyperthermia:* _____ _____

  b. *Malignant hyperthermia:* _____ _____

- Define and explain the causes of *heat stroke.* _____ _____ _____

- Define and explain the causes of *heat exhaustion.* _____ _____ _____

- Define and explain the causes of *hypothermia.* _____ _____ _____

- *Frostbite* occurs when _____.

NURSING PROCESS AND THERMOREGULATION

- Independent measures can be implemented to increase or minimize heat loss, to promote heat conservation, and to increase comfort.

ASSESSMENT

- List at least five assessment sites for temperature measurement.
  a. _____
  b. _____
  c. _____
  d. _____
  e. _____

- State the formulas for the following conversions.
  a. Fahrenheit to centigrade: _____
  b. Centigrade to Fahrenheit: _____

- Identify the advantages and disadvantages of the types of thermometers.
  a. _____
  b. _____
  c. _____

NURSING DIAGNOSIS

- Identify three nursing diagnoses related to thermoregulation.
  a. _____
  b. _____
  c. _____

PLANNING

- The plan of care depends on the nurse's assessment of the client's perception and acceptance of the body temperature alteration.

- Care also depends on the extent to which the client's internal compensatory mechanisms and behaviors have adjusted to he temperature alteration.

IMPLEMENTATION

Health Promotion

- Health promotion for clients at risk of altered temperature is directed to _____ _____.

- Identify the risk factors. _____ _____

Acute Care

- The procedures used to intervene and treat an elevated temperature depend on the fever's cause, its adverse effects, and its strength, intensity, and duration.

- Explain the differences related to febrile states in each of the following.
  a. Children: _____

  b. Older adults: _____

  c. Physical condition: _____

  d. Hypersensitivities to drugs: _____

- Fever therapy reduces _____, increases _____, and prevents complications.

- Give three examples of each type of fever therapy.
  a. Pharmacological:
      1. _____
      2. _____
      3. _____
  b. Nonpharmacological:
      1. _____
      2. _____
      3. _____

- Identify an independent and a dependent nursing intervention to control shivering.
  _____
  _____
  _____

- First aid treatment for heatstroke is _____ _____.

- Summarize the treatment for hypothermia.
  _____
  _____

Restorative Care

- Summarize the client teaching in regard to the treatment of a fever. _____
  _____
  _____

EVALUATION

- After any intervention, the nurse measures the client's temperature to evaluate it for any change.

- Other evaluative measures are _____ and _____.

PULSE

- Define *pulse*: _____

PHYSIOLOGY AND REGULATION

- Define the following terms:
  a. *Stroke volume*: _____
  b. *Cardiac output*: _____

- _____, _____, and _____ factors regulate the strength of the heart's contractions and its stroke volume.

ASSESSMENT OF PULSE

- Identify the two most common peripheral pulse sites to assess.
  a. _____
  b. _____

Use of a Stethoscope

- Identify the five major parts of the stethoscope.
  a. _____
  b. _____
  c. _____
  d. _____
  e. _____

CHARACTER OF THE PULSE

- List four characteristics to identify during peripheral pulse assessment. By using an asterisk, specify the two characteristics to identify when assessing an apical pulse.
  a. _____
  b. _____
  c. _____
  d. _____

- Define the following:
  a. *Tachycardia*: _____
  b. *Bradycardia*: _____
  c. *Dysrhythmia*: _____
  d. *Pulse deficit*: _____

NURSING PROCESS AND PULSE DETERMINATION

- Pulse assessment determines the general state of cardiovascular health and the response to other system imbalances.

- The nurse evaluates client outcomes by assessing the pulse _____, _____, _____, and _____ following each intervention.

RESPIRATION

- Define the following:
  a. *Ventilation*: _____
  _____
  b. *Diffusion*: _____
  _____
  c. *Perfusion*: _____
  _____

- Identify some factors that can affect the character of respirations. _____
  _____
  _____

PHYSIOLOGICAL CONTROL

- Breathing is a _____ process. The respiratory center in the brainstem regulates the _____ control of respirations.

- Ventilation is controlled by levels of _____, _____, and _____ in the arterial blood.

- The most important factor in the control of ventilation is the level of _____.

- *Hypoxemia* is: _____

MECHANICS OF BREATHING

- Briefly summarize the process of inspiration.
  _____
  _____
  _____

- Define the following terms:
  a. *Tidal volume*: _____
  b. *Eupnea*: _____

ASSESSMENT OF RESPIRATIONS

- Accurate measurement requires _____ and _____ of the chest wall movement.

- List three objective measurements used in respiratory status assessment.
  a. _____
  b. _____
  c. _____

- Define the following alterations in breathing patterns.
  a. *Bradypnea*: _____
  b. *Tachypnea*: _____
  c. *Hyperpnea* : _____
  d. *Apnea*: _____
  e. *Hypoventilation/hyperventilation*: _____
  f. *Cheyne-Stokes*: _____
  g. *Kussmaul*: _____
  h. *Biot's*: _____

ASSESSMENT OF DIFFUSION AND PERFUSION

- The respiratory processes of diffusion and perfusion can be evaluated by measuring the oxygen saturation of the blood.

- The saturation of arterial blood is _____, and venous blood is _____.

- Explain the purpose of a pulse oximeter.
  _____
  _____
  _____

NURSING PROCESS AND RESPIRATORY VITAL SIGNS

- Vital sign measurement of respiratory rate, pattern, and depth, along with SvO_2, allows the nurse to assess ventilation, diffusion, and perfusion.

- The nurse evaluates client outcomes by assessing the _____, _____, _____, and _____ following each intervention.

BLOOD PRESSURE

- Define the following terms:
  a. *Blood pressure*: _____
  b. *Systolic*: _____
  c. *Diastolic*: _____

- The difference between the systolic and diastolic pressure is the _____.

PHYSIOLOGY OF ARTERIAL BLOOD PRESSURE

- Blood pressure is reflected by the following. Briefly explain each.
  a. Cardiac output: _____
  _____
  _____

  b. Peripheral resistance: _____
  _____
  _____

  c. Blood volume: _____
  _____
  _____

  d. Viscosity: _____
  _____
  _____

  e. Elasticity: _____
  _____
  _____

FACTORS INFLUENCING BLOOD PRESSURE

- List six factors that influence blood pressure.
  a. _____
  b. _____
  c. _____
  d. _____
  e. _____
  f. _____

HYPERTENSION

- Identify the criteria for the diagnosis of hypertension in an adult. _____
  _____
  _____

- Briefly summarize the physiology of hypertension. _____
  _____
  _____
  _____

- List five risk factors that are linked to hypertension.
  a. _____
  b. _____
  c. _____
  d. _____
  e. _____

HYPOTENSION

- Identify the criteria for the diagnosis of hypotension in an adult. _____
  _____
  _____

- Explain the physiology of hypotension and its causes. _____
  _____
  _____
  _____

- Orthostatic hypotension occurs when
  _____.

- Explain how you would assess a client for orthostatic hypotension. _____
_____
_____
_____

ASSESSMENT OF BLOOD PRESSURE

- Identify two methods for measuring blood pressure.
  - a. _____
  - b. _____

- Identify the two types of sphygmomanometers, and list their advantages and disadvantages.
  - a. _____
  - b. _____

- The sounds heard over an artery distal to the blood pressure cuff are Korotkoff sounds;
  - a. first _____
  - b. second _____
  - c. third _____
  - d. fourth _____
  - e. fifth _____

- During the initial assessment the nurse should obtain and record the blood pressure in _____ arms.

- Pressure differences between the arms greater than _____ indicate vascular problems.

- Identify five common mistakes in measurement.
  - a. _____
  - b. _____
  - c. _____
  - d. _____
  - e. _____

- Identify the four reasons why the measurement of blood pressure in infants and children is difficult.
  - a. _____
  - b. _____
  - c. _____
  - d. _____

- Explain the rationale for the use of an ultrasonic stethoscope. _____
_____
_____

- Identify the method the nurse may use to assess blood pressure when Korotkoff sounds are not audible with the standard stethoscope. _____
_____
_____

- Define *auscultatory gap*: _____

- Give an example as to when you would assess a clients blood pressure using his lower extremities. _____
_____

- Identify the advantage and disadvantage of using automatic blood pressure devices.
_____
_____
_____

- List the benefits of blood pressure self-measurement.
  - a. _____
  - b. _____
  - c. _____
  - d. _____

NURSING PROCESS AND BLOOD PRESSURE DETERMINATION

- The assessment of blood pressure along with pulse assessment is used to evaluate the general state of cardiovascular health and responses to other system imbalances.

- The nurse evaluates client outcomes by assessing the blood pressure following each intervention.

HEALTH PROMOTION AND VITAL SIGNS

- When teaching clients and their families the importance and significance of vital sign measurements, the client's age is an important factor.

- Identify some of the common variations in the older adult.
  a. Temperature: _____

  _____

  b. Pulse rate: _____

  _____

  c. Blood pressure: _____

  _____

  d. Respirations: _____

  _____

RECORDING VITAL SIGNS

- In addition to the actual vital sign values, the nurse records in the nurses' notes any accompanying or precipitating symptoms.

- The nurse needs to document any intervention initiated as a result of a vital sign measurement.

REVIEW QUESTIONS

The student should select the appropriate answer and cite the rationale for choosing that particular answer.

1. The skin plays a role in temperature regulation by:
   a. Insulating the body
   b. Constricting blood vessels
   c. Sensing external temperature variations
   d. All of the above

   Answer:_____   Rationale: _____

   _____

   _____

2. The nurse bathes the client who has a fever with cool water. The nurse does this to increase heat loss by means of:
   a. Radiation
   b. Convection
   c. Condensation
   d. Conduction

   Answer:_____   Rationale: _____

   _____

   _____

3. The nurse is assessing a client who she suspects has the nursing diagnosis: hyperthermia related to vigorous exercise in hot weather. In reviewing the data the nurse knows that the most important sign of heat stroke is:
   a. Confusion
   b. Hot, dry skin
   c. Excess thirst
   d. Muscle cramps

   Answer:_____   Rationale: _____

   _____

   _____

4. When the nurse takes the client's radial pulse, he notes a dysrhythmia. His most appropriate action is to:
   a. Inform the physician immediately
   b. Wait 5 minutes and retake the radial pulse
   c. Take the pulse apically for 1 full minute
   d. Check the client's record for the presence of a previous dysrhythmia

   Answer:_____   Rationale: _____

   _____

   _____

5. The nurse is auscultating Mrs. McKinnon's blood pressure. The nurse inflates the cuff to 180 mm Hg. At 156 mm Hg, the nurse hears the onset of a tapping sound. At 130 mm Hg the sound changes to a murmur or swishing. At 100 mm Hg the sound momentarily becomes sharper, and at 92 mm Hg it becomes muffled. At 88 mm Hg the sound disappears. Mr. McKinnon's blood pressure is:
   a. 180/92
   b. 180/130
   c. 156/88
   d. 130/88

   Answer:_____   Rationale: _____

   _____

   _____

Health Assessment and Physical Examination

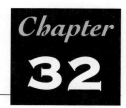
Chapter 32

The skills of physical assessment and examination provide nurses with powerful tools that they can use to detect subtle as well as obvious changes in a client's health.

PRELIMINARY READING
Chapter 32, pp. 724-833

COMPREHENSIVE UNDERSTANDING

PURPOSES OF PHYSICAL EXAMINATION
- List the five nursing purposes for performing a physical assessment.
  a. _____
  b. _____
  c. _____
  d. _____
  e. _____

GATHERING A HEALTH HISTORY
- The main objective of the nurse/client interaction is for the nurse to find out what is central to the client's concerns and to help them find solutions.

DEVELOPING NURSING DIAGNOSES AND A CARE PLAN
- After collecting a history, the nurse conducts a physical examination to _____, _____, or _____ the existing database.

- A complete assessment is needed to form a definitive diagnosis.

- The nurse learns to group significant findings into patterns of data that reveal actual or high-risk nursing diagnoses.

- The baseline is _____.

MANAGING CLIENT PROBLEMS
- The nurse's success in providing care depends on his or her ability to recognize a change in the client's status and to modify therapies so that the client gains the most desirable outcome.

- Physical assessment skills allow the nurse to _____ and _____.

EVALUATING NURSING CARE

- Physical assessment skills enhance the evaluation of nursing measures through monitoring _____ and _____ outcomes of care.

CULTURAL SENSITIVITY

- A client's culture will influence his or her willingness to assume responsibility for their health. Culture also influences a client's tendency to seek professional health care.

INTERGRATION OF PHYSICAL ASSESSMENT WITH NURSING CARE

- Whether a complete or partial physical assessment is performed, an examination should be integrated into routine care.

SKILLS OF PHYSICAL ASSESSMENT

INSPECTION

- Define *inspection:* _____

- List six principles to facilitate accurate inspection of body parts.
  a. _____
  b. _____
  c. _____
  d. _____
  e. _____
  f. _____

PALPATION

- Define *palpation:* _____

- Identify the parts of the hand used to assess each of the following.
  a. Temperature: _____
  b. Pulsations: _____
  c. Vibrations: _____
  d. Turgor: _____

- Briefly explain the following:
  a. Light palpation: _____
  _____
  b. Deep palpation: _____
  _____
  c. Percussion: _____
  _____

- Identify the information obtained through percussion. _____
  _____
  _____
  _____

- Explain the two types of percussion.
  a. Direct: _____
  _____
  b. Indirect: _____
  _____

- Percussion produces five types of sounds. Identify them.
  a. _____
  b. _____
  c. _____
  d. _____
  e. _____

AUSCULTATION

- Define *auscultation:* _____

- Briefly explain the following characteristics of sound.
  a. Frequency: _____
  b. Loudness: _____
  c. Quality: _____
  d. Duration: _____

OLFACTION

- Olfaction helps the nurse detect abnormalities that cannot be recognized by any other means.

PREPARATION FOR EXAMINATION

INFECTION CONTROL

• Examination techniques cause the nurse to contact body fluids and discharge. Standard precautions should be used throughout the examination.

ENVIRONMENT

• List at least three environmental factors that the nurse should attempt to control before performing a physical examination.

a. _____

b. _____

c. _____

EQUIPMENT

• Handwashing is done before equipment preparation and before the examination.

• All equipment should be checked to see that it functions properly.

PSYCHOLOGICAL PREPARATION OF THE CLIENT

• Briefly explain the following preparation before an examination.

a. Physical: _____

_____

_____

_____

b. Positioning: _____

_____

_____

_____

c. Psychological: _____

_____

_____

_____

ASSESSMENT OF AGE-GROUPS

• List at least six variations in the nurse's individual style that are appropriate when examining children.

a. _____

b. _____

c. _____

d. _____

e. _____

f. _____

• List at least five variations in the nurse's individual style that are appropriate when examining older adults.

a. _____

b. _____

c. _____

d. _____

e. _____

ORGANIZATION OF THE EXAMINATION

• List eight principles to follow for a well-organized examination.

a. _____

b. _____

c. _____

d. _____

e. _____

f. _____

g. _____

h. _____

GENERAL SURVEY

• List three assessment components of the general survey.

a. _____

b. _____

c. _____

GENERAL APPEARANCE AND BEHAVIOR

- Summarize the 14 specific observations of the client's general appearance and behavior.
  - a. _____
  - b. _____
  - c. _____
  - d. _____
  - e. _____
  - f. _____
  - g. _____
  - h. _____
  - i. _____
  - j. _____
  - k. _____
  - l. _____
  - m. _____
  - n. _____

VITAL SIGNS

- Assessment of vital signs is the first part of the physical assessment.

HEIGHT, WEIGHT, AND CIRCUMFERENCE

- A person's general level of health can be reflected in the ratio of height and weight.

- List three actions that should be taken to ensure accurate weight measurement of a hospitalized client.
  - a. _____
  - b. _____
  - c. _____

- In the infant a chest circumference can be compared with the head circumference to rule out problems in head or chest size.

SKIN, HAIR, AND NAILS

- The skin provides the body's _____ and _____ and acts as a sensory organ for _____, _____, _____, and _____.

- The physical assessment skills of _____, and _____ are used to assess the integument's function and integrity.

SKIN

- Assessment of the skin can reveal a variety of conditions including changes in _____, _____, _____, and _____.

- List at least four risks for skin lesions in the hospitalized client.
  - a. _____
  - b. _____
  - c. _____
  - d. _____

- Define the following terms:
  - a. *Melanoma:* _____
  - b. *Basal cell carcinoma* _____

- For each skin color variation, identify the mechanism that produces color change, common causes of the variation, and the optimal sites for assessment. (See the table at the top of next page.)

- Define *hyperpigmentation* and *hypopigmentation:* _____

- Define *moisture:* _____

- Excessive dryness can worsen skin conditions such as _____ and _____.

- The temperature of the skin depends on the amount of _____ circulating through the dermis.

- The character of the skin's surface and the feel of deeper portions are its _____.

- Define skin turgor and describe normal findings: _____

- *Petechiae* are: _____

Skin Color	Mechanisms	Causes	Assessment Sites
Cyanosis			
Pallor			
Jaundice			
Erythema			

- Identify the two causes of *edema*.
  a. _____
  b. _____

- Explain the following terms related to lesions.
  a. *Senile keratosis:* _____
  _____
  b. *Cherry angiomas:* _____
  _____

- When a lesion is detected, it is inspected for
  _____, _____,
  _____, _____,
  _____, _____,
  _____ and _____.

- Briefly describe the following primary skin lesions.
  a. Macule: _____
  b. Papule: _____
  c. Nodule: _____
  d. Tumor: _____
  e. Wheal: _____
  f. Vesicle: _____
  g. Pustule: _____
  h. Ulcer: _____
  i. Atrophy: _____

HAIR AND SCALP

- When inspecting the hair, the nurse notes the
  _____, _____,
  _____, _____,
  and _____.

- Define:
  a. *Alopecia:* _____
  b. *Hirsutism:* _____

- Name the three types of lice.
  a. _____
  b. _____
  c. _____

NAILS

- When inspecting the nail bed, the nurse notes the _____, _____,
  _____, _____,
  _____, and _____.

- The nurse palpates the nail base to determine
  _____
  _____.

Chapter 32: Health Assessment and Physical Examination   179

- Briefly describe the following abnormalities of the nail bed.
  a. *Clubbing:* _____
  b. *Beau's lines:* _____
  c. *Koilonychia:* _____
  d. *Splinter hemorrhages:* _____
  e. *Paronychia:* _____

HEAD AND NECK

HEAD

	Inspection	Palpation	Percussion	Auscultation
Head				

- Define the following head abnormalities:
  a. *Hydrocephalus:* _____
  b. *Aromegaly:* _____

EYES

	Inspection	Palpation	Percussion	Auscultation
Visual Acuity				
Visual Fields				
Extraocular Movements				
Visual Fields				

	Inspection	Palpation	Percussion	Auscultation
Eyebrows				
Eyelids				
Lacrimal Apparatus				
Conjunctivae and Sclerae				
Corneas, Pupils, and Irises				

- Define the following common eye and visual abnormalities.
  a. *Exophthalmos:* _____
  _____
  b. *Strabismus:* _____
  _____
  c. *Hyperopia:* _____
  _____
  d. *Myopia:* _____
  _____
  e. *Presbyopia:* _____
  _____
  f. *Astigmatism:* _____
  _____
  g. *Nystagmus:* _____
  _____

- Identify the six structures you would assess in the internal eye.
  a. _____
  b. _____
  c. _____
  d. _____
  e. _____
  f. _____

EARS

	Inspection	Palpation	Percussion	Auscultation
External Ear				
Middle Ear				
Inner Ear				

- Identify the mechanisms for sound transmission.
    - a. _____
    - b. _____
    - c. _____
    - d. _____
    - e. _____

- Identify the types of problems that affect the ear.
    - a. _____
    - b. _____
    - c. _____
    - d. _____

- The three types of hearing loss are _____, _____, and _____.

- Define *ototoxicity:* _____

- Briefly explain how a tuning fork works.
    _____
    _____

- Define *Weber's test:* _____
    _____

- Define *Rinne test:* _____
    _____

NOSE AND SINUSES

	Inspection	Palpation	Percussion	Auscultation
Nose				
Sinuses				

	Inspection	Palpation	Percussion	Auscultation
Lips				
Buccal Mucosa, Gums, and Teeth				
Tongue and Floor of Mouth				
Palate				
Pharynx				

- Define the following conditions of the mouth:
    a. *Caries:* _____
    b. *Leukoplakia:* _____
    c. *Varicosities:* _____
    d. *Exostosis:* _____

	Inspection	Palpation	Percussion	Auscultation
Neck Muscles				
Lymph Nodes				
Thyroid Gland				
Carotid Artery and Jugular Vein				
Trachea				

	Inspection	Palpation	Percussion	Auscultation
Posterior Thorax				
Lateral Thorax				
Anterior Thorax				

THORAX AND LUNGS

- Accurate physical assessment of the thorax and lungs requires review of the ventilatory and respiratory functions of the lung.

- Define *vocal* or *tactile fremitus:* _____
  _____

- Identify the normal breath sounds and where they are located. _____
  _____
  _____

- Complete the following table of adventitious breath sounds.

Sound	Auscultation Site	Cause	Character
Crackles			
Rhonchi			
Wheezes			
Pleural Friction Rub			

HEART

- Assessment of heart function involves a review of signs and symptoms from the nursing history, pulse assessment, and direct examination of the heart.

- Answer the following questions regarding the PMI.
  a. What is the *PMI*? _____
  b. Where is the PMI normally located in the infant and young child? _____
  _____
  c. Where is the PMI located in the older child and adult? _____
  _____
  d. What techniques may be used to locate the PMI? _____
  _____

- Define what occurs during the two phases of the cardiac cycle.
  a. Systole: _____
  _____
  b. Diastole: _____
  _____

- Define the following heart sounds:
  S_1: _____
  S_2: _____
  S_3: _____
  S_4: _____

- Define *dysrhythmia*: _____
  _____

- Define *murmur*: _____
  _____

- List the six factors to assess when a murmur is detected.
  a. _____
  b. _____
  c. _____
  d. _____
  e. _____
  f. _____

- Define *thrill*: _____
  _____

VASCULAR SYSTEM

- Examination of the vascular system includes measurement of the blood pressure and a thorough assessment of the integrity of the peripheral vascular system.

MOUTH AND PHARYNX

	Inspection	Palpation	Percussion	Auscultation
Carotid Arteries				
Jugular Veins				
Peripheral Arteries				
Peripheral Veins				
Lymphatic System				

- Explain the following conditions that are related to the vascular system:
  a. Syncope: _____
  b. Occlusion: _____
  c. Stenosis: _____
  d. Atherosclerosis: _____
  e. Bruit: _____

- Explain the steps the nurse would use to assess venous pressure.
  a. _____
  b. _____

  c. _____
  d. _____
  e. _____

- The *Allen's test* is used to _____.

- The 3 P's that characterize an occulsion are _____, _____, and _____.

- *Phlebitis* is _____.

BREASTS

- It is important to examine the breasts of female and male clients.

- The American Cancer Society (1998) recommends the following guidelines for early detection of breast cancer.
  a. _____
  b. _____
  c. _____
  d. _____
  e. _____

- Briefly explain the proper technique for palpating breast tissue. _____
  _____

- List seven characteristics that should be included when describing an abnormal breast mass.
  a. _____
  b. _____
  c. _____
  d. _____
  e. _____
  f. _____
  g. _____

- Define the following terms:
  a. *Metastasize:* _____
  _____
  b. *Fibrocystic breast disease:* _____
  _____

	Inspection	Palpation	Percussion	Auscultation
Breasts				

ABDOMEN

- The abdominal examination includes an assessment of the lower GI tract in addition to the liver, stomach, uterus, ovaries, kidneys, and bladder.

- Describe four techniques used to help the client relax during assessment of the abdomen.
  a. _____
  b. _____
  c. _____
  d. _____

	Inspection	Palpation	Percussion	Auscultation
Abdomen				
Liver				

- Define the following:
  a. *Hernias:* _____

  _____

  b. *Distention:* _____

  _____

  c. *Peristalsis:* _____

  _____

  d. *Paralytic ileus:* _____

  _____

  e. *Borborygmi:* _____

  _____

f. *Rebound tenderness:* _____

g. *Aneurysm:* _____

_____

FEMALE GENITALIA AND REPRODUCTIVE TRACT

- Briefly explain the preparation of a client for a complete examination of the genitalia and reproductive tract. _____

_____

_____

	Inspection	Palpation	Percussion	Auscultation
External Genitalia				
Cervix				
Vagina				

- Define the following terms:
  a. *Chancres:* _____

  _____

  b. *Cystocele:* _____

  _____

  c. *Rectocele:* _____

  _____

- Speculum examination of the internal genitalia includes _____ .

MALE GENITALIA

- An examination of the male genitalia includes assessment of the external genitalia and the inguinal ring and canal.

	Inspection	Palpation	Percussion	Auscultation
Penis				
Scrotum				
Inguinal Ring and Canal				
Rectum and Anus				

• Summarize how the nurse would assess sexual maturity. _____

RECTUM AND ANUS

• The purpose of digital palpation is _____.

	Inspection	Palpation	Percussion	Auscultation
Joint Motion				

MUSCULOSKELETAL SYSTEM

• The assessment of musculoskeletal function focuses on determining the range of joint motion, muscle strength and tone, and joint and muscle condition.

• Define:
a. *Hypertonicity:* _____
_____
b. *Hypotonicity:* _____
_____

c. *Kyphosis:* _____
_____
d. *Osteoporosis:* _____
_____
e. *Goniometer:* _____

NEUROLOGICAL SYSTEM

• The neurological system is responsible for many functions including _____
_____.

MENTAL AND EMOTIONAL STATUS

- There are five areas that Folstein's Mini-Mental State tool assesses. Name them.
  - a. _____
  - b. _____
  - c. _____
  - d. _____
  - e. _____

- An alteration in mental or emotional status may reflect a disturbance in cerebral functioning.

- List three factors that may change cerebral function.
  - a. _____
  - b. _____
  - c. _____

- Define *delirium* and list the clinical criteria for it. _____
  _____
  _____

- The level of consciousness exists along a continuum, from full awakening, alertness, and cooperation to unresponsiveness to any form of external stimuli.

- Identify the tool and the three factors to assess consciousness. _____
  _____

- Behavior, moods, hygiene, grooming, and choice of dress reveal pertinent information about mental status.
- Explain the function of the cerebral cortex in language. _____
  _____

- Intellectual function includes the following. Briefly explain how each is assessed.
  a. Abstract thinking: _____
  _____

  b. Judgment: _____
  _____

  c. Memory: _____
  _____

  d. Knowledge: _____
  _____

- There are two types of *aphasia*. Describe each one.
  - a. _____
  - b. _____

CRANIAL NERVE FUNCTION

- Identify the 12 cranial nerves:
  - a. _____
  - b. _____
  - c. _____
  - d. _____
  - e. _____
  - f. _____
  - g. _____
  - h. _____
  - i. _____
  - j. _____
  - k. _____
  - l. _____

SENSORY FUNCTION

- The sensory pathways of the central nervous system conduct sensations of _____, _____, _____, _____, and _____.

- Summarize how a nurse would assess the client's sensory function. _____
  _____
  _____

MOTOR FUNCTION

- Identify the functions of the cerebellum.
  _____
  _____

- Describe the maneuvers used to assess balance and gross motor function.
  - a. _____
  - b. _____
  - c. _____

REFLEXES

- Eliciting reflex reactions allows the nurse to assess the integrity of sensory and motor pathways of the reflex arc and specific spinal cord segments.

- Briefly explain the two categories of normal reflexes. _____
_____
_____

REVIEW QUESTIONS

The student should select the appropriate answer and cite the rationale for choosing that particular answer.

1. The component that should receive the highest priority before a physical examination is:
   a. Preparation of the environment
   b. Preparation of the equipment
   c. Physical preparation of the client
   d. Psychological preparation of the client

   Answer:_____ Rationale: _____
   _____
   _____

2. The nurse assesses the skin turgor of the client by:
   a. Grasping a fold of skin on the back of the forearm and releasing
   b. Palpating the skin with the dorsum of the hand
   c. Pressing the skin for 5 seconds, releasing, and noting each centimeter of depth
   d. Inspecting the buccal mucosa with a penlight

   Answer:_____ Rationale: _____
   _____
   _____

3. While examining Mr. Parker, the nurse notes a circumscribed elevation of skin filled with serous fluid on his upper lip. The lesion is 0.4 cm in diameter. This type of lesion is called a:
   a. Macule
   b. Nodule
   c. Vesicle
   d. Pustule

   Answer:_____ Rationale: _____
   _____
   _____

4. When assessing the client's thorax, the nurse should:
   a. Complete the left side and then the right side
   b. Change the position of the stethoscope between inspiration and expiration
   c. Compare symmetrical areas from side to side
   d. Begin with the posterior lobes on the right side

   Answer:_____ Rationale: _____
   _____
   _____

5. In a client with pneumonia, the nurse hears high-pitched, continuous musical sounds over the bronchi on expiration. These sounds are called:
   a. Crackles
   b. Rhonchi
   c. Wheezes
   d. Friction rubs

   Answer:_____ Rationale: _____
   _____
   _____

6. The second heart (S_2) sound occurs when:
   a. The mitral and tricuspid valves close
   b. There is rapid ventricular filling
   c. Systole begins
   d. The aortic and pulmonic valves close

   Answer:_____ Rationale: _____
   _____
   _____

Infection Control

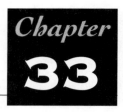

Practices or techniques that control or prevent transmission of infection help to protect clients and health care workers from disease.

PRELIMINARY READING
Chapter 33, pp. 834-883

COMPREHENSIVE UNDERSTANDING

NATURE OF INFECTION

• An *infection* is an _____.

• Define *asymptomatic*: _____

CHAIN OF INFECTION

• Development of an infection occurs in a cycle that depends on the following elements.
   a. _____
   b. _____
   c. _____
   d. _____
   e. _____
   f. _____

• Microorganisms include _____, _____, and
   _____.

• Define:
   a. *Resident organisms:* _____
   b. *Transient microorganisms:* _____

• The potential for microorganisms or parasites to cause disease depends on four factors. Name them.
   a. _____
   b. _____
   c. _____
   d. _____

- Define *reservoir*: _____
  _____

- Define *carriers*: _____
  _____

- To thrive, organisms require the following. Briefly explain each one.
  a. Food: _____
  _____

  b. Oxygen: _____
  _____

  c. Water: _____
  _____

  d. Temperature: _____
  _____

  e. pH: _____
  _____

  f. Light: _____
  _____

- Microorganisms can exit through a variety of sites. Briefly explain each one.
  a. Skin and mucous membranes: _____
  _____
  _____

  b. Respiratory tract: _____
  _____
  _____

  c. Urinary tract: _____
  _____
  _____

  d. Gastrointestinal tract: _____
  _____
  _____

  e. Reproductive tract: _____
  _____
  _____

  f. Blood: _____
  _____
  _____

- List the six routes through which microorganisms are transmitted from the reservoir to the host.
  a. _____
  b. _____
  c. _____

  d. _____
  e. _____
  f. _____

- List the four common modes of infection transmission and identify the one that is the most common.
  a. _____
  b. _____
  c. _____
  d. _____

- Organisms can enter the body through
  _____.

- Define *susceptibility*: _____

- Define *virulent*: _____

THE INFECTION PROCESS
- The severity of the client's illness depends on the _____, the _____, and _____.

- Describe the two types of infections.
  a. *Localized*: _____
  b. *Systemic*: _____

DEFENSES AGAINST INFECTION

- The *inflammatory response* is _____
  _____.

- Explain the normal body defenses against infection.
  a. Normal flora: _____
  _____
  _____

  b. Body system defenses: _____
  _____
  _____

  c. Inflammation: _____
  _____
  _____

- For each body system or organ, identify at least one defense mechanism and the primary action to prevent infection. Complete the grid.

System/Organ	Defense Mechanism	Action
Skin		
Mouth		
Respiratory Tract		
Urinary Tract		
Gastrointestinal Tract		

- The inflammatory response includes the following. Explain each briefly.
  a. Vascular and cellular responses: _____
  _____
  _____
  b. Inflammatory exudate: _____
  _____
  _____
  c. Tissue repair: _____
  _____
  _____

- Define *immune response:* _____

- After an antigen enters the body, it travels in the blood or lymph and initiates the following responses. Briefly explain each.
  a. Cell-mediated immunity: _____
  _____
  _____
  b. Humoral immunity: _____
  _____
  _____

- Define the following terms:
  a. *Antibodies:* _____
  _____
  b. *Immunoglobulins:* _____
  _____
  c. *Natural immunity:* _____
  d. *Passive immunity:* _____
  _____

- Define *complement:* _____

- Define *interferon:* _____

NOSOCOMIAL INFECTIONS

- Define *nosocomial infections:* _____
  _____

- Define the following types of nosocomial infections:
  a. *Iatrogenic:* _____
  _____
  b. *Exogenous:* _____
  _____
  c. *Endogenous:* _____
  _____

- Identify at least three factors that increase a hospitalized client's risk of acquiring a nosocomial infection.
  a. _____
  b. _____
  c. _____

- Identify the major sites for nosocomial infection. _____
  _____
  _____

THE NURSING PROCESS IN INFECTION CONTROL

ASSESSMENT
- The nurse assesses the client's _____, _____, and _____.

- Knowing the factors that increase the client's susceptibility or risk for infection, the nurse is better able to plan preventive therapy that includes aseptic technique.

- Any reduction in the body's primary or secondary defenses against infection places a client at risk. List at least four risk factors of each.
  a. Inadequate primary defenses: _____
  _____
  b. Inadequate secondary sources: _____
  _____

- The following factors influence client susceptibility. Explain each one.
  a. Age: _____
  _____
  _____
  b. Nutritional status: _____
  _____
  _____
  c. Stress: _____
  _____
  _____
  d. Heredity: _____
  _____
  _____

  e. Disease process: _____
  _____
  _____

  f. Medical therapy: _____
  _____
  _____

Clinical Appearance
- Describe the clinical appearance of each type of infection.
  a. *Local:* _____
  _____
  b. *Systemic:* _____
  _____

- Describe how an infection is manifested in an older adult. _____
  _____

Laboratory Data
- List at least five laboratory values that may indicate infection:
  a. _____
  b. _____
  c. _____
  d. _____
  e. _____

Clients with Infection
- The ways in which infection can affect the client's and family's needs may be _____, _____, _____, or _____.

NURSING DIAGNOSIS
- The nurse may diagnose a risk for infection or make diagnoses that result from the effects of infection on health status.

PLANNING
- List four common goals for the client with an actual or potential risk for infection.
  a. _____
  b. _____
  c. _____
  d. _____

IMPLEMENTATION

Health Promotion

- List five ways a nurse may prevent an infection from developing or spreading.

    a. _____

    b. _____

    c. _____

    d. _____

    e. _____

- List preventive interventions to protect a client from invasion by pathogens:

    _____

    _____

    _____

Acute Care Measures

- The nurse follows certain principles and procedures to prevent infection and to control its spread. Briefly explain each one.

    a. Concept of asepsis: _____

    _____

    b. Medical asepsis: _____

    _____

- Explain the following methods of controlling or eliminating of infectious agents.

    a. Proper cleansing: _____

    _____

    b. Disinfection: _____

    _____

    c. Sterilization of objects: _____

    _____

    d. Control or elimination of reservoirs:

    _____

    _____

    e. Control of portals of exit: _____

    _____

    f. Control of transmission (handwashing):

    _____

    _____

- Nurses should wash their hands in the following situations.

    a. _____

    b. _____

    c. _____

    d. _____

    e. _____

- Many measures that control the exit of microorganisms also control the entrance of pathogens. Give at least five examples.

    a. _____

    b. _____

    c. _____

    d. _____

    e. _____

- A client's resistance to infection improves as the nurse protects the body's normal defenses against infection. Explain. _____

    _____

    _____

- Isolation or barrier precautiuons include the appropriate use of _____,

    _____, _____,

    _____, and _____.

- Barrier protection is indicated for use with _____ clients. Explain.

    _____

- The CDC's new isolation guidelines (1996) contain a two-tiered approach. Explain.

    a. Standard Precautions (Tier one): _____

    _____

    _____

    _____

    b. Transmission Categories (Tier 2): _____

    _____

    _____

    _____

- Regardless of the type of isolation system, the nurse must follow the following basic principles. _____ _____ _____

- Briefly summarize the psychological implications of isolation: _____ _____ _____

- Explain the two types of private rooms used for isolation:
  a. Negative-pressure airflow: _____ _____ _____

  b. Positive-pressure airflow: _____ _____ _____

- Place an X under the barriers required to maintain protective asepsis for each category-specific isolation technique:

Type of Isolation	Room	Gown	Gloves	Mask
Strict				
Content				
Respiratory				
Enteric Precautions				
Tuberculosis Isolation				
Drainage and Decretion Precautions				
Universal Blood and Body Fluid Precautions				
Care of the Severly Compromised Client				

- Explain the techniques for collecting specimens from the client with a suspected infection:
  a. Wound: _____ _____

  b. Blood: _____ _____

  c. Stool: _____ _____

  d. Urine: _____ _____

- Explain the CDC recommendations for bagging trash or linen. _____ _____ _____

- Describe how you would transport a client. _____

Role of the Infection Control Professional
- List eight responsibilities of the infection control professional.
  a. _____
  b. _____
  c. _____
  d. _____
  e. _____
  f. _____
  g. _____
  h. _____

Infection Prevention and Control for Hospital Personnel
- List the OSHA guidelines that were established to protect employees.
  a. _____
  b. _____
  c. _____
  d. _____
  e. _____

Client Education

- List six topics the nurse needs to discuss with the client in relation to infection-control practices.
  a. _____
  b. _____
  c. _____
  d. _____
  e. _____
  f. _____

Surgical Asepsis

- List three teaching points that reduce the risk of client-associated contamination during sterile procedures or treatments.
  a. _____
  b. _____
  c. _____

- List the seven principles of surgical asepsis.
  a. _____
  b. _____
  c. _____
  d. _____
  e. _____
  f. _____
  g. _____

- List and briefly explain the nine steps of a sterile procedure.
  a. _____
  b. _____
  c. _____
  d. _____
  e. _____
  f. _____
  g. _____
  h. _____
  i. _____

≈ EVALUATION

- The success of infection-control techniques is measured by determining whether the goals for reducing or preventing infection are achieved.

- Two important skills in evaluation are ability to correctly assess wounds for healing and the ability to conduct a physical assessment of body systems.

- A clear description of any signs and symptoms of systemic or local infection is necessary to give all nurses a baseline for comparative evaluation.

- List three expected outcomes for clients with a risk for infection:
  a. _____
  b. _____
  c. _____

REVIEW QUESTIONS

The student should select the appropriate answer and cite the rationale for choosing that particular answer.

1. Of the following, which is not an element in the development or chain of infection?
   a. Infectious agent or pathogen
   b. Reservoir for pathogen growth
   c. Means of transmission
   d. Formation of immunoglobulin

Answer:_____   Rationale: _____
_____
_____

2. Pathogenic organisms include all of the following *except:*
   a. Bacteria
   b. Leukocytes
   c. Viruses
   d. Fungi

Answer:_____   Rationale: _____
_____
_____

3. The severity of a client's illness will depend on all of the following *except:*
   a. Extent of infection
   b. Pathogenicity of the microorganism
   c. Susceptibility of the host
   d. Incubation period

Answer:_____   Rationale: _____
_____
_____

4. Which of the following best describes an iatrogenic infection?
   a. It results from a diagnostic or therapeutic procedure.
   b. It occurs when clients are infected with their own organisms as a result of immunodeficiency.
   c. It involves an incubation period of 3 to 4 weeks before it can be detected.
   d. It results from an extended infection of the urinary tract.

Answer:_____   Rationale: _____
_____
_____

5. The nurse sets up a nonbarrier sterile field on the client's overbed table. In which of the following instances is the field contaminated?
   a. The nurse keeps the top of the table above his or her waist.
   b. Sterile saline solution is spilled on the field.
   c. Sterile objects are kept within a 1-inch border of the field.
   d. The nurse, who has a cold, wears a double mask.

Answer:_____   Rationale: _____
_____
_____

6. When a client on respiratory isolation must be transported to another part of the hospital, the nurse:
   a. Places a mask on the client before leaving the room.
   b. Obtains a physician's order to prohibit the client from being transported.
   c. Advises other health team members to wear masks and gowns when coming in contact with the client.
   d. Instructs the client to cover her mouth and nose with a tissue when coughing or sneezing.

Answer:_____   Rationale: _____
_____
_____

Medication Administration

The nurse is responsible for evaluating the effects of medications on the client's health status, teaching clients about their medications and the side effects of those medications, ensuring client compliance with the medication regimen, and evaluating the client's technique in self-administration.

PRELIMINARY READING
Chapter 34, pp. 884-966

COMPREHENSIVE UNDERSTANDING

SCIENTIFIC KNOWLEDGE BASE
• The medications administered to clients are used to prevent, diagnose, or treat disease.

• *Pharmacokinetics* is _____

PHARMACOLOGICAL CONCEPTS
• A single medication may have three different names. Define each one.
  a. *Chemical name:* _____
  b. *Generic name:* _____
  c. *Trade name:* _____

• A medication classification indicates _____.

• The form of the medication determines its _____

MEDICATION LEGISLATION, AND STANDARDS
• Briefly summarize the role of the federal government in regulation. _____
_____

• Explain the Pure Food and Drug Act of 1906. _____
_____

• The Food and Drug Administration (FDA) is responsible for _____
_____.

• The USP and the National Formulary set standards for _____
_____.

- Summarize the role of state and local regulation. _____

  _____

- Summarize the role of health care institutions. _____

  _____

- *Nurse Practice Acts* are responsible for

  _____

  _____

PHARMACOKINETICS AS THE BASIS OF MEDICATION

ABSORPTION

- Define *absorption:* _____

  _____

- Briefly explain the following factors that influence drug absorption.
  a. Route of administration: _____

  _____

  b. Ability of a medication to dissolve:

  _____

  _____

  _____

  c. Blood flow to the area of absorption:

  _____

  _____

  _____

  d. Body surface area: _____

  _____

  _____

  e. Lipid solubility of a medication: _____

  _____

  _____

DISTRIBUTION

- The rate and extent of distribution depend on the physical and chemical properties of the drug and on the physiological makeup of the person taking the drug.

- Explain how each of the following affect the rate and extent of medication distribution.
  a. Circulation: _____

  _____

  _____

  b. Membrane permeability: _____

  _____

  c. Protein binding: _____

  _____

  _____

METABOLISM

- Define *biotransformation* and identify where it occurs. _____

  _____

EXCRETION

- After drugs are metabolized, they exit the body through the _____,

  _____, _____,

  _____, and _____.

- Identify the primary organ for drug excretion and explain what happens if this organ function declines. _____

  _____

TYPES OF MEDICATION ACTION

- Define the following predicted or unintended effects of drugs:
  a. *Therapeutic effects:* _____

  _____

  _____

  b. *Side effects:* _____

  _____

  _____

  c. *Adverse effects:* _____

  _____

  _____

  d. *Toxic effects:* _____

  _____

  _____

  e. *Idiosyncratic reactions:* _____

  _____

  _____

f. *Allergic reactions:* _____

_____

_____

g. *Anaphylactic reactions:* _____

_____

_____

- A *medication interaction* is: _____

- A *synergistic effect* is: _____

MEDICATION DOSE RESPONSES

- When a medication is prescribed, the goal is to achieve a constant blood level within a safe therapeutic range.

- Repeated doses are required to achieve a constant therapeutic concentration of a medication because a portion of a drug is always being excreted.
- Define:
  a. *Serum concentration:* _____

  _____

  b. *Serum half-life:* _____

  _____

- Explain the following time intervals of medication actions:
  a. Onset of drug action: _____

  _____

  b. Peak action:_____

  _____

  c. Trough: _____

  _____

  d. Duration of action: _____

  _____

  e. Plateau: _____

  _____

- Identify the route that is ideal for achieving a constant therapeutic drug level. _____

  _____

ROUTES OF ADMINISTRATION

- The route prescribed for a drug's administration depends on its properties, the desired effect, and the client's physical and mental condition.

ORAL ROUTES

- The oral route is the easiest and the most commonly used route.

- Identify the types of oral routes; explain how the oral routes are used; and identify the effects of using these routes. _____

  _____

  _____

  _____

PARENTERAL ROUTES

- The *parenteral* route involves administering a drug through injection into body tissues.

- List the four major types of parenteral injections.
  a. _____
  b. _____
  c. _____
  d. _____

- Define the following advanced techniques of medication administration.
  a. *Epidural:* _____
  b. *Intrathecal:* _____
  c. *Intraosseous:* _____
  d. *Intraperitoneal:* _____
  e. *Intrapleural:* _____
  f. *Intraarterial:* _____

TOPICAL ADMINISTRATION

- Medications that are applied to the skin and mucous membranes principally have local effects.

- Identify five methods for applying medications to mucous membranes.
  a. _____
  b. _____
  c. _____
  d. _____
  e. _____

INHALATION ROUTE

- Explain the following types of inhalations.
  a. Nasal: _____
  b. Oral: _____
  c. Endotracheal or tracheal: _____

INTRAOCULAR ROUTE

- *Intraocular* administration involves inserting a medication disk, similar to contact lens, into the client's eye.

SYSTEMS OF MEDICATION MEASUREMENT

- The following are measurements used in drug therapy. Briefly explain their basic units.
  a. Metric ystem: _____
  b. Apothecary system: _____
  c. Household measurements: _____

SOLUTIONS

- A *solution* is: _____

CLINICAL CALCULATIONS

CONVERSIONS WITHIN ONE SYSTEM

- Indicate which direction the decimal point is moved for the following mathematical calculations in the metric system.
  a. Division: _____
  b. Multiplication: _____

CONVERSION BETWEEN SYSTEMS

- To make actual drug calculations, it is necessary to work with units in the same measurement system.

- Before making a conversion, the nurse compares the measurement system available with that ordered.

- Complete the following measurement equivalents:

Metric	Apothecary	Household
1 ml	_____ minims	_____ drops
_____ ml	_____ fluid drams	1 tablespoon
30 ml	_____ fluid ounce(s)	_____ tablespoon
_____ ml	_____ fluid ounce(s)	1 cup
_____ ml	1 pint	_____ pint
_____ ml	_____ quart	1 quart

- Complete the following conversions:
  a. 100 mg = _____ g
  b. 2.5 L = _____ ml
  c. 500 ml = _____ L
  d. 15 mg = _____ gr
  e. 30 gtt = _____ ml
  f. gr 1/6 = _____ mg

DOSAGE CALCULATIONS

- Write out the formula used to determine the correct dose when preparing solid or liquid forms of medications.

- Define the following:
  a. *Dose ordered:* _____
  b. *Dose on hand:* _____
  c. *Amount on hand:* _____

PEDIATRIC DOSAGES

- Write out the formula applied to accurately calculate pediatric dosages.

ADMINISTERING MEDICATIONS

- The nurse who is administering the medications is accountable for: _____
  _____.

PRESCRIBER'S ROLE

- Identify the primary responsibilities of the prescriber in giving medications to clients.
  _____
  _____

Types of Orders in Acute Care Agencies

- Briefly explain the four common types of medication orders.
  a. Standing: _____
  b. PRN: _____
  c. Single (one-time): _____
  d. STAT: _____

- List the five parts of a prescription.
  a. _____
  b. _____
  c. _____
  d. _____
  e. _____

- Identify the primary responsibility of the pharmacist in the administration of medications.
  _____
  _____

- List the three medication distribution systems and identify the advantages and disadvantages of each.
  a. _____
  b. _____
  c. _____

- Summarize the nurse's primary responsibilities when administering medications.
  _____
  _____
  _____

CRITICAL THINKING IN MEDICATION ADMINISTRATION

- Summarize the knowledge needed from other disciplines to safely administer medications. _____
  _____
  _____

- Psychomotor skills, the client's attitudes, knowledge, physical and mental status, and responses can make medication administration a complex experience.

- Accountability for the nurse in administering medications is _____
  _____.

- A *medication error* is _____

STANDARDS

- List the "five rights" of medication administration:
  a. _____
  b. _____
  c. _____
  d. _____
  e. _____

Maintaining Client's Rights

- Briefly summarize the *Patient's Bill of Rights* related to drug administration. _____
  _____
  _____
  _____

NURSING PROCESS AND MEDICATION ADMINISTRATION

ASSESSMENT

- Explain the following factors to assess.
  a. History: _____
  _____

  b. History of allergies: _____
  _____

  c. Medication data: _____
  _____

  d. Diet history: _____
  _____

  e. Client's perceptual or coordination problems: _____
  _____

  f. Client's current condition: _____
  _____

  g. Client's attitude about medication use: _____
  _____
  _____

  h. Client's knowledge and understanding of medication therapy: _____
  _____

  i. Client's learning needs: _____
  _____

NURSING DIAGNOSIS

- Assessment provides data on the client's condition, his or her ability to self-administer medications, and medication use patterns; this information can be used to determine actual or potential problems with medication therapy.

PLANNING

- The nurse organizes care activities to ensure the safe administration of medications.

- Identify the four goals that the nurse or client needs to meet before administration of medications.
  a. _____
  b. _____
  c. _____
  d. _____

IMPLEMENTATION

Health Promotion

- Identify factors that can influence the client's compliance with the medication regimen.
  _____

- Explain information that needs to be taught to the client and family in relation to medications. _____
  _____

Acute Care

- Explain why the following interventions are essential for safe and effective medication administration.
  a. Receiving medication orders: _____
  _____
  _____

  b. Correct transcription and communication of orders: _____
  _____
  _____

  c. Accurate dose calculation and measurement: _____
  _____
  _____

  d. Correct administration: _____
  _____
  _____

  e. Recording medication administration: _____
  _____
  _____

Restorative Care

- Regardless of the type of medication activity, the nurse is responsible for _____
  _____.

Special Considerations for Administering Medications to Specific Age-Groups

Infants and Children
- Identify the appropriate nursing action used in administering medications to an infant or child. _____
  _____

- List the five behavioral patterns of medication use characteristic of the older adult and briefly explain each one.
  a. _____
  b. _____
  c. _____
  d. _____
  e. _____

EVALUATION

- The nurse must know the therapeutic action and common side effects of each medication in order to monitor a client's response to that medication.

- Many different evaluation measures can be used in the context of medication administration. Name some of them. _____
  _____

- The most common type of measurement is
  _____ .

ORAL ADMINISTRATION

- The easiest and most desirable way to administer medications is by mouth.

- The primary contraindication to giving oral medications is _____
  _____ .

- To protect the client against possible aspiration, the nurse _____
  _____

TOPICAL MEDICATION APPLICATIONS

- Topical medications are applied most often to intact skin. They can also be applied to mucous membranes.

SKIN APPLICATIONS

- Explain the procedure for administering the following skin applications.
  a. Ointment: _____
  b. Lotion: _____
  c. Powder: _____

NASAL INSTILLATION

- Summarize the rationale for nasal instillations. _____
  _____

EYE INSTILLATION

- List four principles for administering eye instillations.
  a. _____
  b. _____
  c. _____
  d. _____

Intraocular Administration

- Explain the rationale for intraocular administration. _____
  _____

EAR INSTILLATION

- Explain the procedure for administering ear instillations.
  a. Adult: _____
  _____
  b. Children: _____
  _____

VAGINAL INSTILLATION

- Vaginal medications are available as
  _____, _____,
  _____, or _____.

RECTAL INSTILLATION

- Explain the differences between vaginal and rectal suppositories and the reason for these differences. _____
  _____ .

ADMINISTERING MEDICATIONS BY INHALATION

- To maximize the effect of metered dose inhalers, the nurse advises the client to
  _____
  _____
  _____ .

ADIMINISTERING MEDICATIONS BY IRRIGATIONS

- Identify the principles the nurse follows when performing irrigations. _____
_____

PARENTERAL ADMINISTRATION OF MEDICATIONS

- Each type of injection requires certain skills to ensure that the drug reaches the proper location.

- When medications are administered parenterally, it is an invasive procedure that must be performed using aseptic techniques.

EQUIPMENT

- Identify the three major types of syringes.
  a. _____
  b. _____
  c. _____

- Identify three factors that must be considered when selecting a needle for an injection.
  a. _____
  b. _____
  c. _____

- Identify the advantages of using the Tubex or Carpuject injection systems. _____
_____

PREPARING AN INJECTION FROM AN AMPULE

- An *ampule* is: _____

- The procedure for withdrawing medications from ampules is outlined in Procedure 34-7.

PREPARING AN INJECTION FROM A VIAL

- A *vial* is a _____.

- The vial is a closed system, and air must be injected into it to permit easy withdrawal of the solution.

- The procedure for withdrawal of medications from vials is outlined in Procedure 34-7.

MIXING MEDICATIONS

- It is possible to mix two drugs together into one injection if the total dosage is within accepted limits.

- List the three principles to follow when mixing medications from two vials:
  a. _____
  b. _____
  c. _____

- When mixing medications from an ampule and a vial, which medication should be prepared first?

INSULIN PREPARATION

- *Insulin* is: _____

- Explain why insulin must be administered by injection. _____

- Insulin is classified by _____.

- _____ is the only insulin used for sliding scales.

- Identify the simple guidelines for mixing two kinds of insulin in the same syringe.
_____
_____

ADMINISTERING INJECTIONS

- The characteristics of the tissues injected influence the _____
_____.

- List the techniques used to minimize client discomfort that is associated with injections.
  a. _____
  b. _____
  c. _____
  d. _____
  e. _____
  f. _____
  g. _____

Chapter 34: Medication Administration   207

Subcutaneous Injections

- Subcutaneous injections involve placing the medications into the loose connective tissue under the dermis.

- Explain the differences in absorption between a subcutaneous and an intramuscular injection. _____

  _____

- The best sites for SQ injections include _____, _____, and _____.

- The site most frequently recommended for heparin injection is _____.

- The site chosen should be free of _____, _____, and _____.

- Identify the maximum amount of water-soluble medication given by the SQ route. _____

  _____

- State the rule that may be followed to determine if a SQ injection should be given at a 90- or 45-degree angle. _____

  _____

Intramuscular Injections

- Identify the major risk of using the IM route: _____

  _____

- The angle of insertion for an IM injection is _____ degrees.

- Indicate the maximum volume of medication for IM injection in each of the following groups.
  a. Well-developed adult: _____
  b. Older children, older adults, or thin adults: _____
  c. Older infants and small children:

  _____

Sites

- List the assessment criteria for selecting an IM site.
  a. _____
  b. _____
  c. _____
  d. _____

- Describe the advantages and disadvantages of the following injection sites.
  a. Vastus lateralis: _____

  _____

  b. Ventrogluteal: _____

  _____

  c. Dorsogluteal: _____

  _____

  d. Deltoid: _____

  _____

Special Techniques in IM Injections

- Explain the rationale for administering an intramuscular injection using the air-lock technique. _____

  _____

- Explain the rationale for using the Z-track method of injection. _____

  _____

Intradermal Injections

- Explain the rationale for administering an intradermal injection. _____

  _____

Safety in Administering Medications by Injection

- Explain the rationale for each of the following.
  a. Needleless device: _____

  _____

  b. One-handed needle recapping technique:

  _____

  _____

INTRAVENOUS ADMINISTRATION

- The nurse administers medications intravenously by the following methods. _____

  _____

  _____

- Identify the advantage and disadvantage of the large-volume infusion method. _____
_____

- Explain the advantage and disadvantage of the IV bolus route of administration. _____
_____

- List the advantages of using volume-controlled infusions.
  a. _____
  b. _____
  c. _____

- Piggyback sets are _____ .

- A tandem setup is _____ .

- Volume-control administration sets are
_____ .

- A miniinfusor pump is _____ .

- List the three advantages of using intermittent venous access devices.
  a. _____
  b. _____
  c. _____

ADMINISTRATION OF INTRAVENOUS THERAPY IN THE HOME

- When receiving home intravenous therapy, client education should include _____
_____

REVIEW QUESTIONS

The student should select the appropriate answer and cite the rationale for choosing that particular answer.

1. The study of how drugs enter the body, reach their sites of action, are metabolized, and exit from the body is called:
   a. Pharmacology
   b. Pharmacokinetics
   c. Pharmacopeia
   d. Biopharmaceutica

   Answer:_____   Rationale: _____
   _____
   _____

2. Which statement correctly characterizes drug absorption?
   a. Most drugs must enter the systemic circulation to have a therapeutic effect.
   b. Mucous membranes are relatively impermeable to chemicals, making absorption slow.
   c. Oral medications are absorbed more quickly when administered with meals.
   d. Drugs administered subcutaneously are absorbed more quickly than those injected intramuscularly.

   Answer:_____   Rationale: _____
   _____
   _____

3. The onset of drug action is the time it takes for a drug to:
   a. Produce a response
   b. Accelerate the cellular process
   c. Reach its highest effective concentration
   d. Produce blood serum concentration and maintenance

   Answer:_____   Rationale: _____
   _____
   _____

4. Which of the following is not a parenteral route of administration?
   a. Buccal
   b. Subcutaneous
   c. Intramuscular
   d. Intradermal

Answer:_____   Rationale: _____
_____
_____

5. Using the body surface area formula, what dose of drug X should a child who weighs 12 kg (body surface area = 0.54 m²) receive if the normal adult dose of drug X is 300 mg?
   a. 50 mg
   b. 90 mg
   c. 100 mg
   d. 200 mg

Answer:_____   Rationale: _____
_____
_____

6. The nurse is preparing an insulin injection in which both regular and modified insulin will be mixed. Into which vial should the nurse inject air first?
   a. The vial of modified insulin
   b. The vial of regular insulin
   c. Either vial, as long as modified insulin is drawn up first
   d. Neither vial; it is not necessary to put air into vials before withdrawing medication

Answer:_____   Rationale: _____
_____
_____

Complementary and Alternative Therapies

Chapter 35

Complementary and alternative therapies can be the same, depending on whether the therapy is prescribed in addition to or in place of the Western (primary) treatment.

PRELIMINARY READING
Chapter 35, pp. 967-988

COMPREHENSIVE UNDERSTANDING
- Describe the difference between the following terms.
  a. *Complementary therapies:* _____

  _____

  b. *Alternative therapies:* _____

  _____

- Give an example of the following types of therapies:
  a. Traditional: _____

  _____

  b. Bioelectromagnetic: _____

  _____

  c. Diet: _____

  _____

  d. Herbal: _____

  _____

  e. Manual: _____

  _____

  f. Biobehavioral: _____

  _____

  g. Pharmacological: _____

  _____

- Describe integrative medical programs: _____

  _____

BIOBEHAVIORAL THERAPIES
- Biobehavioral therapy is designed to _____

  _____.

RELAXATION THERAPIES

- Define *stress response*: _____

- *Chronic stress* is _____
  _____.

- *Relaxation* is _____

- Progressive relaxation training helps to
  _____
  _____

- Passive relaxation involves teaching _____
  _____.

- Relaxation techniques are effective in
  _____, _____,
  _____, and _____.

- The type of relaxation intervention should be
  matched to _____
  _____.

- Identify the limitations of relaxation therapy.
  _____
  _____

IMAGERY

- *Imagery* is _____
  _____

- *Creative visualization* is _____
  _____

- Identify the clinical applications of imagery.
  _____
  _____
  _____

- Identify the limitations of imagery. _____
  _____
  _____

BIOFEEDBACK

- *Biofeedback* is _____
  _____

- Identify the clinical applications of biofeedback. _____
  _____
  _____

- Identify the limitations of biofeedback.
  _____
  _____

HYPNOTHERAPY

- *Hypnotherapy* is _____
  _____

- Explain the three levels of a hypnotic trance.
  a. Light: _____

  b. Medium: _____
  _____

  c. Deep: _____
  _____

- Identify the clinical applications of hypnosis.
  _____
  _____
  _____

- Identify the limitations of hypnosis. _____
  _____

MEDITATION

- *Meditation* is _____
  _____

- Identify the clinical applications of meditation. _____
  _____
  _____

- Identify the limitations of meditation. _____
  _____
  _____

MANUAL HEALING THERAPIES

- Manual healing therapies are based on _____
  _____
  _____.

THERAPEUTIC TOUCH

- *Therapeutic touch* is _____
  _____

- Therapeutic touch consists of five phases. Explain each one.
  a. Centering: _____

  b. Assessment: _____

  c. Unruffling: _____

  d. Treatment: _____

  e. Evaluation: _____

- Identify the physiological indicators of energy imbalance. _____

- Identify the clinical applications for therapeutic touch. _____
  _____

- Identify the limitations of therapeutic touch.
  _____
  _____

CHIROPRACTIC THERAPY

- *Chiropractic therapy* is _____
  _____

- Describe the clinical applications of chiropractic therapy. _____
  _____

- Identify the limitations of chiropractic therapy. _____

TRADITIONAL AND ETHOMEDICINE THERAPIES

TRADITIONAL CHINESE MEDICINE

- *Traditional Chinese Medicine (TCM)* is _____
  _____
  _____

- Explain the concept of Yin and Yang. _____
  _____
  _____

- *Qi* is _____
  _____

- Traditional Chinese medicine classifies disease into 3 categories, state the influences of each:
  a. External causes: _____

  b. Internal causes: _____

  c. Nonexternal causes: _____
  _____

- Define *meridian*s: _____
  _____

ACUPUNCTURE

- *Acupuncture* is _____
  _____

- Describe the clinical applications of acupuncture. _____
  _____
  _____

- Identify the limitations of acupuncture. _____
  _____
  _____

HERBAL THERAPIES

- *Herbal therapy* is _____
  _____

- The goal of herbal therapy is _____
  _____.

Chapter 35: Complementary and Alternative Therapies   213

- Describe the clinical applications of herbal therapy. _____
  _____

- Identify the limitations of herbal therapy.
  _____
  _____

- Herbal products should be used cautiously with_____
  _____

NURSING ROLE IN COMPLEMENTARY AND ALTERNATIVE THERAPIES

- Summarize the role of the nurse in relation to providing recommendations regarding complementary and alternative medicine therapies. _____
  _____
  _____

REVIEW QUESTIONS

The student should select the appropriate answer and cite the rationale for choosing that particular answer.

1. Patients choose to use unconventional therapy because
   a. They are willing to pay more to feel better
   b. It is now widely accepted by the Food and Drug Administration
   c. They are dissatisfied with conventional medicine
   d. They want religious approval for the remedies they use.

   Answer:_____   Rationale: _____
   _____
   _____

2. The Dietary Supplement and Health Education Act states that
   a. Herbs, vitamins, and minerals may be sold with their therapeutic advantages listed on the label
   b. The Food and Drug Administration must evaluate all herbal therapies
   c. Herbs, vitamins, and minerals may be sold as long as no therapeutic claims are made on the label.
   d. In conjunction with the Food and Drug Administration, all supplements are considered safe for use.

   Answer:_____   Rationale: _____
   _____
   _____

3. Nurses can best assess their patient's use of alternative therapies by:
   a. Asking the patient true/false questions about their health
   b. Asking for a thorough medical history
   c. Reviewing laboratory studies that assess levels of certain herbs.
   d. Asking open-ended questions on alternative therapies

   Answer:_____   Rationale: _____
   _____
   _____

4. Which of the following steps should nurses take to be better informed about alternative therapies?
   a. Read current books and magazines on alternative therapies
   b. Familiarize themselves with recent case studies on alternative therapies.
   c. Familiarize themselves with general principles of pytotherapy.
   d. Review herb manufacturer's literature on specific herbs.

   Answer:_____   Rationale: _____
   _____
   _____

Activity and Exercise

Chapter 36

 Activity and exercise are important to all individuals' well-being.

PRELIMINARY READING
Chapter 36, pp. 989-1017

COMPREHENSIVE UNDERSTANDING

SCIENTIFIC KNOWLEDGE BASE

• *Body mechanics* include: _____.

OVERVIEW OF BODY MECHANICS, EXERCISE, AND ACTIVITY

• The coordinated efforts of the musculoskeletal and nervous systems maintain _____, _____, and _____ during lifting, bending, moving, and performing _____ provide the foundation for body mechanics.

• Define *body alignment:* _____

• Body balance is achieved when a _____, _____, and _____.

• Proper body alignment and posture are maintained by using two simple techniques. Name them.
   a. _____
   b. _____

• Coordinated body movement is the result of _____, _____, and _____.

• Define *center of gravity:* _____

• Define *friction:* _____

• List two techniques that minimize friction.
   a. _____
   b. _____

• *Activity tolerance* is: _____

- There are three categories of exercises. Briefly explain each one and give an example of each.
  a. *Isotonic contraction:* _____

  _____

  _____

  b. *Isometric contraction:* _____

  _____

  _____

  c. *Resistive isometric:* _____

  _____

  _____

REGULATION OF MOVEMENT

- List three systems responsible for coordinating body movements.
  a. _____
  b. _____
  c. _____

- List five functions of the skeletal system.
  a. _____
  b. _____
  c. _____
  d. _____
  e. _____

- Describe the following:
  a. *Joints:* _____

  _____

  b. *Cartilaginous joint:* _____

  _____

  c. *Fibrous joint:* _____

  _____

  d. *Synovial joint:* _____

  _____

  e. *Ligaments:* _____

  _____

  f. *Cartilage:* _____

  _____

  g. *Tendons:* _____

  _____

- Briefly describe how skeletal muscles affect movement. _____

  _____

- Briefly explain the muscles concerned with:
  a. Movement: _____

  b. Posture: _____

  _____

- Coordination and regulation of different muscle groups depend on the following. Briefly explain each.
  a. Antagonistic muscles: _____

  _____

  b. Synergistic muscles: _____

  _____

  c. Antigravity muscles: _____

  _____

- Briefly describe how movement and posture are regulated by the nervous system. _____

  _____

- Define *proprioception:* _____

  _____

- Balance is the ability to _____

PRINCIPLES OF BODY MECHANICS

- Identify the physiological and pathological influences on body alignment and mobility. _____

  _____

  _____

  _____

Pathological Influences on Body Mechanics

- Briefly explain how the following pathological conditions affect body alignment and mobility.
  a. Congenital defects: _____

  _____

  b. Disorders of bones, joints, and muscles: _____

  _____

  _____

c. Damage to the central nervous system:

_____
_____
_____

d. Direct trauma to the musculoskeletal system: _____

_____
_____

NURSING KNOWLEDGE BASE

- _____, _____,
  _____, _____,
  and _____ are important
  aspects of an individual and must be incorporated into the plan.

DEVELOPMENTAL CHANGES

- The greatest change and impact on the maturational process is observed in _____
  and _____.

- Identify the descriptive characteristics of body alignment and mobility related to the following developmental changes.
  a. Infants: _____
  _____
  _____

  b. Toddlers: _____
  _____
  _____

  c. Preschool through adolescence: _____
  _____
  _____

  d. Young to middle adults: _____
  _____
  _____

  e. Older adults: _____
  _____
  _____

BEHAVIORAL ASPECTS

- Nurses need to take into consideration the client's _____, _____,
  and _____.

- Clients are more open to developing an exercise program if they are at the stage of readiness to change their behavior.

ENVIRONMENTAL ISSUES

- Explain the following related sites.
  a. Worksite: _____
  _____

  b. Schools: _____
  _____

  c. Community: _____
  _____

CULTURAL AND ETHNIC INFLUENCES

- The nurse must consider what motivates and what is deemed appropriate and enjoyable when developing a physical fitness program for culturally diverse populations.

FAMILY AND SOCIAL SUPPORT

- Briefly explain how a family be a motivational tool in regard to physical fitness.
  _____

NURSING PROCESS

ASSESSMENT

- Throughout the assessment, the nurse will be able to determine _____,
  _____, and _____.

- Briefly explain how assessment of body alignment and posture is carried out.
  a. Standing: _____
  _____

  b. Sitting: _____
  _____

  c. Recumbent: _____
  _____

- There are three components to assess in regard to mobility. Explain each.
  a. Range of motion: _____
  _____

  b. Gait: _____
  _____

  c. Exercise: _____
  _____

Chapter 36: Activity and Exercise   217

- Identify some factors that affect *activity tolerance.* _____

  _____

- Assessment of the _____,

  _____, _____,

  and _____ provides clusters of data or defining characterisitics that lead the nurse to identify nursing diagnoses. Give five examples.

  a. _____
  b. _____
  c. _____
  d. _____
  e. _____

🐍 **PLANNING**

- The plan should include consideration of:

  a. _____
  b. _____
  c. _____
  d. _____
  e. _____

🐍 **IMPLEMENTATION**

Health Promotion Activities

- List the five recommendations for exercise.

  a. _____
  b. _____
  c. _____
  d. _____
  e. _____

- Explain how to calculate the client's Maximum Heart Rate (MHR). _____

  _____

- An exercise program can consist of the following. Explain each one.
  a. Aerobic exercise: _____

  _____

  _____

  b. Stretching and flexibility exercises:

  _____

  _____

  _____

  c. Resistance training: _____

  _____

  _____

- The most common back injury is:

  _____.

Body mechanics

- Briefly explain proper lifting techniques.

  _____

  _____

Acute Care

- The musculoskeletal system can be maintained by encouraging the use of stretching and isometric type exercises.

- Explain the isometric exercises for each of the following and describe its benefits.
  a. *Quadriceps:* _____

  _____

  b. *Gluteal muscle:* _____

  _____

  c. *Abdominal muscle:* _____

  _____

  d. *Foot muscle:* _____

  _____

  e. *Hand muscle:* _____

  _____

  f. *Biceps:* _____

  _____

  g. *Triceps:* _____

  _____

- Explain how the nurse would maintain or improve joint mobility. _____

  _____

- Identify six approaches that help older adults to use body mechanics and prevent injury.
  a. _____
  b. _____
  c. _____
  d. _____
  e. _____
  f. _____

- Identify the general guidelines that apply to the use of range-of-motion exercises.
  a. _____
  b. _____
  c. _____
  d. _____
  e. _____
  f. _____
  g. _____

- Explain how walking affects joint mobility.
  _____
  _____

- Explain how the nurse would assist the client to walk. _____
  _____
  _____

Restorative and Continuing Care
- The nurse, in collaboration with others, promotes activity and exercise by teaching the use of assistive devices most appropriate for a client's condition. Briefly explain.
  a. *Canes:* _____
  _____
  b. *Crutches:* _____
  _____
  c. *Crutch gait:* _____
  _____

- Explain the following gaits.
  a. Four-point: _____
  _____
  b. Three-point: _____
  _____
  c. Two-point: _____
  _____
  d. Swing-through: _____
  _____

- Explain how the nurse would instruct the client in each of the following.
  a. Crutch walking on stairs: _____
  _____
  _____
  b. Sitting in the chair with crutches: _____
  _____
  _____

- Explain how the nurse would implement a plan of care to increase activity and exercise in the following specific disease conditions:
  a. Coronary heart disease (CHD): _____
  _____
  b. Hypertension: _____
  _____
  c. Chronic obstructive pulmonary disease:
  _____
  _____
  _____
  d. Diabetes mellitus: _____
  _____
  _____

⁂ EVALUATION

Client Care
- This phase of the nursing process evaluates the actual care delivered by the health team based on the expected outcomes.

- Comparisons are made with baseline measures that include pulse, blood pressure, strength, endurance, and physical well being.

Client Expectations
- The nurse needs to know the client's expectations concerning activity and exercise.

REVIEW QUESTIONS

The student should select the appropriate answer and cite the rationale for choosing that particular answer.

1. Which of the following is true of body mechanics?
   a. The narrower the base of support, the greater the stability of the nurse.
   b. The higher the center of gravity, the greater the stability of the nurse.
   c. When friction is reduced between the object to be moved and the surface on which it is moved, less force is required to move it.
   d. Rolling, turning, or pivoting requires more work than lifting.

   Answer:_____ Rationale: _____
   _____
   _____

2. White, shiny, flexible bands of fibrous tissue binding joints together and connecting various bones and cartilage types are known as:
   a. Muscles
   b. Ligaments
   c. Joints
   d. Tendons

   Answer:_____ Rationale: _____
   _____
   _____

3. The nurse would expect all of the following physiological effects of exercise on the body systems *except:*
   a. Decreased cardiac output
   b. Increased respiratory rate and depth
   c. Increased muscle tone, size, and strength
   d. Change in metabolic rate

   Answer:_____ Rationale: _____
   _____
   _____

4. Which of the following is not appropriate in performing a three-person carry to transfer a client from bed to a stretcher?
   a. Use three nurses of a similar height.
   b. Place the stretcher parallel to the bed.
   c. Nurses roll client to their chests.
   d. One nurse assumes the leadership role and directs the other two.

   Answer:_____ Rationale: _____
   _____
   _____

5. Movements of the hip include all of the following *except:*
   a. Flexion
   b. Hyperextension
   c. Circumduction
   d. Opposition

   Answer:_____ Rationale: _____
   _____
   _____

SYNTHESIS MODEL FOR NURSING CARE PLAN FOR ACTIVITY INTOLERANCE

Imagine that you are Mary, the nurse in the Care Plan on page 1002 of your text. Complete the *Planning phase* of the synthesis model by writing your answers in the appropriate boxes of the model shown. Think about the following:

• In developing Mrs. Swain's plan of care, what **knowledge** did Mary apply?

• In what way might Mary's previous **experience** assist in developing a plan of care for Mrs. Swain?

• When developing a plan of care, what intellectual or professional **standards** were applied to Mrs. Swain?

• What critical thinking **attitudes** might have been applied developing Mrs. Swain plan?

• How will Mary accomplish her goals?

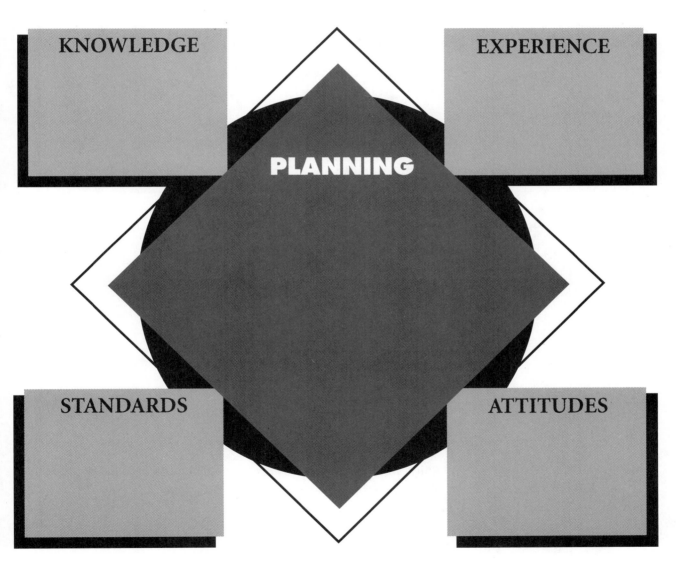

Chapter 36 *Synthesis Model for Nursing Care Plan for* Activity Intolerance.

See answers on page 560

Safety

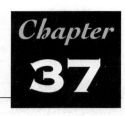

Safety, often defined as freedom from psychological and physical injury, is a basic human need that must be met.

PRELIMINARY READING
Chapter 37, pp. 1019-1053

COMPREHENSIVE UNDERSTANDING

SCIENTIFIC KNOWLEDGE BASE

ENVIRONMENTAL SAFETY

• A client's *environment* includes _____.

• List the five characteristics of a safe environment.
   a. _____
   b. _____
   c. _____
   d. _____
   e. _____

• Give an example of the four basic physiological needs that influence a person's safety.
   a. Oxygen: _____
   _____

   b. Nutrition: _____
   _____

   c. Temperature: _____
   _____

   d. Humidity: _____
   _____

• Physical hazards in the community and health care settings place clients at risk for accidental injury and death. List the four physical hazards that contribute to falls.
   a _____
   b. _____
   c. _____
   d. _____

• Define *pathogen*: _____

- Identify the most effective method for limiting the transmission of pathogens.
  _____
  _____

- Define *immunization:* _____
  _____

- Describe the two types of immunity.
  a. Active: _____
  b. Passive: _____

- Describe how the human immunodeficiency virus (HIV) is transmitted and who is at risk. _____
  _____

- A healthy environment is free of pollution. A *pollutant* is _____
  _____.

- Define the following types of pollution.
  a. Air: _____
  b. Land: _____
  c. Water: _____
  d. Noise: _____

NURSING KNOWLEDGE BASE

- In addition to being knowledgeable about the environment, nurses must be familiar with:
  a. _____
  b. _____
  c. _____
  d. _____
  e. _____

RISKS AT DEVELOPMENTAL STAGES

- Identify at least three threats to safety in the following developmental stages.
  a. Infant, toddler, preschooler: _____
  _____

  b. School-age: _____
  _____

  c. Adolescents: _____
  _____

  d. Adult: _____
  _____

  e. Older adult: _____
  _____

INDIVIDUAL RISK FACTORS

- Explain how the following risk factors can increase safety risks.
  a. Lifestyle: _____
  _____

  b. Mobility: _____

  c. Sensory impairment: _____
  _____

  d. Safety awareness: _____
  _____

RISKS IN THE HEALTH CARE AGENCY

- List the four major risks to client safety in the health care environment.
  a. _____
  b. _____
  c. _____

NURSING PROCESS

ASSESSMENT

- In order to conduct a thorough client assessment, the nurse will consider possible threats to the client's safety, including the client's immediate environment, as well as any individual risk factors.

- Identify the specific assessments a nurse needs to do in the following settings.
  a. Caring for a client in the home: _____
  _____
  _____

  b. Caring for a client in the health care facility: _____
  _____
  _____

NURSING DIAGNOSIS

- Identify four actual or potential nursing diagnoses for safety risks.
  a. _____
  b. _____
  c. _____
  d. _____

PLANNING

- Identify common goals that focus on the client's need for safety.
  a. _____
  b. _____
  c. _____

IMPLEMENTATION

Health Promotion

- In order to promote an individual's health it is necessary for the individual to be in a safe environment and to practice a lifestyle that minimizes risk of injury.

- Identify at least four interventions for each of the following developmental age groups.
  a. Infant, toddler, preschooler: _____

  b. School-age: _____

  c. Adolescents: _____

  d. Adult: _____

  e. Older adult: _____

- Nursing interventions directed at eliminating environmental threats include _____, _____, _____, and _____.

- Define *medical asepsis:* _____

- Specific safety concerns in the environment consist of _____, _____, _____, and _____.

- List eight measures to prevent falls in the health care setting.
  a. _____
  b. _____
  c. _____
  d. _____
  e. _____
  f. _____
  g. _____
  h. _____

- A physical *restraint* is _____

- The immobility imposed by restraining a client can lead to:
  a. Physical: _____

  b. Psychological: _____

- OBRA (1987) defines the reasons/guidelines for the use of restraints. Explain. _____

- Use of restraints must meet the following objectives.
  a. _____
  b. _____
  c. _____
  d. _____

- List eight alternatives to the use of restraints.
  a. _____
  b. _____
  c. _____
  d. _____
  e. _____
  f. _____
  g. _____
  h. _____

- Explain why an *Ambularm* is used. _____

- Explain the use for siderails. _____

- Describe four fire containment guidelines.
  a. _____
  b. _____
  c. _____
  d. _____

- A *poison* is _____

224   Chapter 37: Safety

- List five teaching strategies for prevention of electrical hazards.
  a. _____
  b. _____
  c. _____
  d. _____
  e. _____

- A *seizure* is: _____
  _____.

- Identify the measures with which the nurse must be familiar to reduce exposure to radiation. _____
  _____
  _____

EVALUATION

Client Care
- The nurse continually assesses the client and family's need for additional support services such as _____, _____, _____, and _____.

Client Expectations
- The expected outcomes include a _____, _____, and _____.

REVIEW QUESTIONS

The student should select the appropriate answer and cite the rationale for choosing that particular answer.

1. Which of the following would most threaten an individual's safety?
   a. 70% humidity
   b. Carbon dioxide
   c. Unrefrigerated fresh vegetables
   d. Lack of water supply

   Answer: _____ Rationale: _____
   _____
   _____

2. The developmental stage that carries the highest risk of an injury from a fall is:
   a. Preschool
   b. School-age
   c. Adulthood
   d. Older adulthood

   Answer: _____ Rationale: _____
   _____

3. Mrs. Field falls asleep while smoking in bed and drops the burning cigarette on her blanket. When she awakens, her bed is on fire, and she quickly calls the nurse. On observing the fire, the nurse should immediately:
   a. Report the fire
   b. Attempt to extinguish the fire
   c. Assist Mrs. Fields to a safe place
   d. Close all windows and doors to contain the fire

   Answer: _____ Rationale: _____
   _____
   _____

4. Sixteen-year-old Jimmy is admitted to an adolescent unit with a diagnosis of substance abuse. The nurse examines Jimmy and finds that he has bloodshot eyes, slurred speech, and an unstable gait. He smells of alcohol and is unable to answer questions appropriately. The appropriate nursing diagnosis would be:
   a. Self-care deficit related to alcohol abuse
   b. Altered thought processes related to sensory overload
   c. Knowledge deficit related to alcohol abuse
   d. High risk for injury related to impaired sensory perception

   Answer: _____ Rationale: _____
   _____
   _____

5. If a client receives an electric shock, the nurse's first action should be to:
   a. Assess the client's pulse
   b. Assess the client for thermal injury
   c. Notify the physician
   d. Notify the maintenance department

Answer: _____ Rationale: _____
_____
_____

SYNTHESIS MODEL FOR NURSING CARE PLAN FOR RISK FOR INJURY

Imagine that you are Mr. Key, the nurse in the Care Plan on page 1031 of your text. Complete the *Assessment phase* of the synthesis model by writing your answers in the appropriate boxes of the model shown. Think about the following:

- In developing Ms. Cohen's plan of care, what **knowledge** did Mr. Key apply?

- In what way might Mr. Key's previous **experience** assist in this case?

- What intellectual or professional **standards** were applied to Ms. Cohen?

- What critical thinking **attitudes** might have been applied in this case?

- As you review your **assessment** what key areas did you cover?

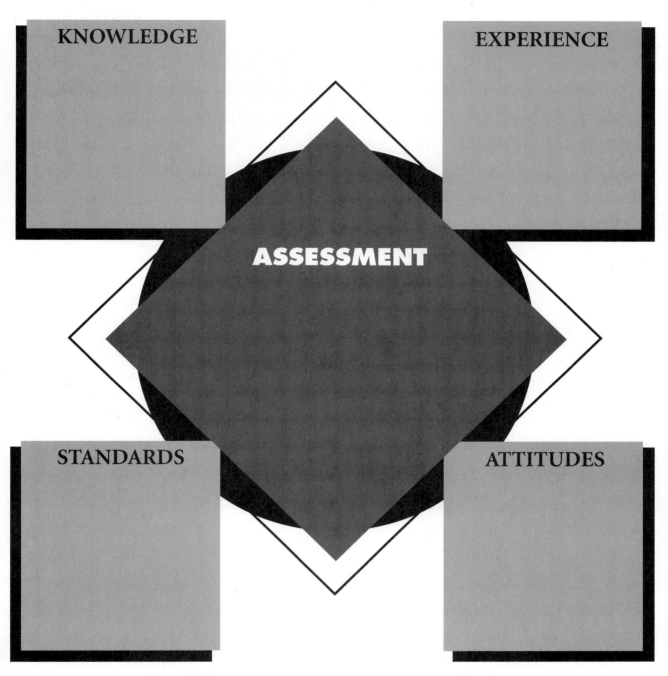

KNOWLEDGE

EXPERIENCE

ASSESSMENT

STANDARDS

ATTITUDES

Chapter 37 *Synthesis Model for Nursing Care Plan for* Risk for Injury.

See answers on page 561.

Hygiene

 Maintenance of personal hygiene is necessary for an individual's comfort, safety, and well-being.

PRELIMINARY READING
Chapter 38, pp. 1054-1123

COMPREHENSIVE UNDERSTANDING

SCIENTIFIC KNOWLEDGE BASE
- Proper hygienic care requires an understanding of the anatomy and physiology of the integument, oral cavity, eyes, ears, and nose.

THE SKIN
- Define the following terms:
    - a. *Epidermis:* _____
    - b. *Dermis:* _____
    - c. *Eccrine glands:* _____
    - d. *Apocrine glands:* _____
    - e. *Cerumen:* _____

- Identify the functions of the skin. _____
  _____

THE FEET, HANDS, AND NAILS
- The structure of the foot is similar to that of the hand, with certain differences that adapt it for supporting weight.

- Define the following terms:
    - a. *Cuticle:* _____
    - b. *Lunula:* _____

THE ORAL CAVITY
- There are three pairs of salivary glands that secrete about 1 liter of saliva a day.

- The *buccal glands* are _____

- Teeth are responsible for _____.

- Regular oral hygiene is necessary to maintain the integrity of tooth surfaces and to prevent _____.

THE HAIR

- Identify the factors that can affect the hair's characteristics. _____
_____

THE EYES, EARS, AND NOSE

- Cleansing of the sensitive sensory tissues should be done so as to prevent injury and client discomfort.

NURSING KNOWLEDGE BASE

- It is important to understand that numerous sociocultural, economic, and developmental factors affect a client's hygiene.

- Briefly explain each of the following.
  a. Social practices: _____
  _____
  _____

  b. Personal preferences: _____
  _____
  _____

  c. Body image: _____
  _____
  _____

  d. Socioeconomic status: _____
  _____
  _____

  e. Health beliefs and motivation: _____
  _____
  _____

  f. Cultural variables: _____
  _____
  _____

  g. Physical condition: _____
  _____
  _____

THE NURSING PROCESS

ASSESSMENT

Skin

- The nurse uses the skills of inspection and palpation to look for alterations in the integrity and function of tissues.

- When inspecting the skin the nurse examines _____, _____, _____, _____, _____, and _____.

- Common skin problems can affect how hygiene is administered. Describe the hygiene provided for the following.
  a. Dry skin: _____
  _____

  b. Acne: _____
  _____

  c. Skin rashes: _____
  _____

  d. Hirsutism: _____
  _____

  e. Contact dermatitis: _____
  _____

  f. Abrasion: _____
  _____

- Briefly explain the six conditions that place clients at risk for impaired skin integrity.
  a. Immobilization: _____
  _____

  b. Reduced sensation: _____
  _____

  c. Nutrition and hydration: _____
  _____

  d. Secretions and excretions: _____
  _____

  e. Vascular insufficiency: _____
  _____

  f. External devices: _____
  _____

Feet and Nails
- Assessment of the feet involves a thorough examination of all skin surfaces, including the soles of the feet and the areas between the toes.

- Inspection of the feet for lesions includes _____.

- *Neuropathy* is _____. Describe how the nurse would assess for this. _____

- Identify the characteristics of the following foot and nail problems.
  a. Callus: _____
  _____
  b. Corns: _____
  _____
  c. Plantar warts: _____
  _____
  d. Tinea pedis: _____
  _____
  e. Ingrown nails: _____
  _____
  f. Ram's horn nails: _____
  _____
  g. Paronychia: _____
  _____
  h. Foot odors: _____
  _____

Oral Cavity
- The nurse inspects all areas of the oral cavity for _____, _____, _____, and _____.

- _____ is a common symptom of gum disease and certain tooth disorders.

Hair
- Identify the characterisitics of the following hair and scalp conditions.
  a. Dandruff: _____
  _____
  b. Ticks: _____
  _____
  c. Pediculosis: _____
  _____

  d. Pediculosis capitis: _____
  _____
  e. Pediculosis corporis: _____
  _____
  f. Pediculosis pubis: _____
  _____
  g. Alopecia: _____

Eyes, Ears, and Nose
- Identify the normal assessment findings for the following.
  a. Eyes: _____
  _____
  b. Nose: _____
  _____
  c. Ears: _____
  _____

DEVELOPMENTAL CHANGES

Skin
- For each developmental stage, briefly describe normal conditions that create a high risk for impaired skin integrity.
  a. Neonate: _____
  _____
  _____
  b. Toddler: _____
  _____
  _____
  c. Adolescent: _____
  _____
  _____
  d. Older adult: _____
  _____
  _____

Feet and Nails
- Identify the changes that occur with the feet and nails through the developmental stages:
  a. Infants: _____
  _____
  b. Children: _____
  _____
  c. Adult: _____
  _____

- Identify the common foot problems of the older adult. _____

_____

The Mouth

- Complete the grid in relation to the physiological development of the oral cavity.

Hair

- Throughout life, changes in the growth, distribution, and condition of hair influence hygiene. Explain each stage.

  a. Infancy: _____

  _____

  b. Childhood: _____

  _____

  c. Puberty: _____

  _____

  d. Adolescence: _____

  _____

  e. Adulthood: _____

  _____

  f. Older adult: _____

  _____

PHYSIOLOGIC DEVELOPMENT OF THE ORAL CAVITY

Development Level	Changes
Infant	
18 months to 6 years	
6 to 12 years	
12 to 18 years	
Pregnancy	
40 to 65 years	
65 years and over	

SELF-CARE ABILITY

- Identify the factors that are assessed to determine a client's ability to perform routine hygiene. _____
  _____
  _____
  _____

HYGIENIC PRACTICES

- To assess the client's routine hygienic practices the nurse would _____
  _____.

CULTURAL FACTORS

- Culture plays a role in _____
  and _____.

CLIENTS AT RISK FOR HYGIENE PROBLEMS

- Give examples of clients at risk for the following.
  a. Oral problems: _____
     _____
  b. Skin problems: _____
     _____
  c. Foot problems: _____
     _____
  d. Eye care problems: _____
     _____

SPECIAL CONSIDERATIONS IN HYGIENE ASSESSMENT

- Explain briefly how footwear may predispose a client to foot and nail problems.
  _____
  _____
  _____

NURSING DIAGNOSIS

- List five possible nursing diagnoses that apply to clients in need of hygienic care.
  a. _____
  b. _____
  c. _____
  d. _____
  e. _____

PLANNING

- Identify some factors to consider when planning care. _____
  _____
  _____

IMPLEMENTATION

HEALTH PROMOTION

- The nurse educates clients about hygiene by _____
  _____.

- Summarize the goals for *Healthy People 2000.*
  _____
  _____
  _____

ACUTE AND RESTORATIVE CARE

Bathing and Skin Care

- A *complete bed bath* is _____

- A *partial bed bath* involves _____

- Identify guidelines the nurse should follow when assisting or providing a client with any type of bath. _____
  _____
  _____

- Explain bag baths and identify the advantages of this method. _____
  _____

- Define *perineal care* and identify the clients at risk for skin breakdown in the perineal area.
  _____
  _____

- A back rub promotes _____,
  _____, _____,
  and _____,

- Provide the rationale for each action included in bathing an infant.
  a. Keeping the infant covered as much as possible: _____

  b. Using plain water (no soaps) for bathing: _____

  c. Avoiding the use of lotions and oils: _____

  d. Eliminating the use of cotton-tipped swabs for cleansing the ears or nares: _____

  e. Applying alcohol or triple dye to the umbilical cord: _____

  f. Drying gently but thoroughly: _____

Foot and Nail Care
- Routine care involves _____,
  _____, _____,
  and _____.

- List 16 guidelines to include when advising clients with peripheral neuropathy or vascular insufficiency about foot care.
  a. _____
  b. _____
  c. _____
  d. _____
  e. _____
  f. _____
  g. _____
  h. _____
  i. _____
  j. _____
  k. _____
  l. _____
  m. _____
  n. _____
  o. _____
  p. _____

Oral Hygiene
- Oral hygiene helps maintain:
  _____.

- Briefly explain the following interventions in relation to oral hygiene.
  a. Diet: _____

  b. Brushing: _____

  c. Flossing: _____

  d. Denture care: _____

- The following clients require special oral hygiene methods because of their level of dependence on the nurse or the presence of oral mucosa problems. Explain.
  a. Unconscious clients: _____

  b. Clients at risk for stomatitis: _____

  c. Clients with diabetes: _____

  d. Clients with oral infections: _____

Hair and Scalp Care
- Briefly describe the rationale for the following interventions.
  a. Brushing and combing: _____

  b. Shampooing: _____

  c. Shaving: _____

  d. Mustache and beard care: _____

Care of the Eyes, Ears, and Nose
- Care focuses on preventing infection and maintaining normal sensory function.

- Describe basic eye care for an unconscious client. _____

- Describe the correct procedure for cleaning eyeglasses. _____
_____
_____

- List the common problems for contact lens wearers and identify the cause of each.
  a. _____
  b. _____
  c. _____
  d. _____
  e. _____

- Describe each of the following techniques necessary in caring for an artificial eye.
  a. Removal: _____
  _____
  b. Cleansing: _____
  _____
  c. Reinsertion: _____
  _____
  d. Storage: _____
  _____

Ear Care

- Describe the procedure for removing cerumen from the ear. _____
_____

- Describe the following types of hearing aids.
  a. In-the-canal (ITC): _____
  _____
  b. In-the-ear (ITE): _____
  _____
  c. Behind-the-ear (BTE): _____
  _____

Nasal Care

- Describe three interventions used to remove secretions from the nose.
  a. _____
  b. _____
  c. _____

Maintaining Comfort

- Identify four factors the nurse can control to create a more comfortable environment.
  a. _____
  b. _____
  c. _____
  d. _____

Room Equipment

- A typical hospital room contains the following basic pieces of furniture: _____, _____, _____, _____, and _____.

- Draw a simple stick figure to illustrate each of the following common bed positions:
  a. Fowler's:

  b. Semi-Fowler's:

  c. Trendelenburg's:

  d. Reverse Trendelenburg's:

- Identify the points the nurse should remember when making a client's bed: _____
_____

Client Care

- Client care evaluates the actual care delivered by the health care team based on the expected outcomes.

- The standards for evaluation are the expected outcomes established in the planning stage of the client's care.

Client Expectations

- A client expectation evaluates care from the client's perspective.

- The client's expectations are important guidelines in determining client satisfaction.

REVIEW QUESTIONS

The student should select the appropriate answer and cite the rationale for choosing that particular answer.

1. Mr. Gray is a 19-year-old client in the rehabilitation unit. He is completely paralyzed below the neck. The most appropriate bath for Mr. Gray is a:
   a. Partial bed bath
   b. Complete bed bath
   c. Sitz bath
   d. Tepid bath

   Answer:_____   Rationale: _____
   _____
   _____

2. All of the following will help maintain skin integrity in the older adult *except:*
   a. Environmental air that is cold and dry
   b. Use of warm water and mild cleansing agents for bathing
   c. Bathing every other day
   d. Drinking 8 to 10 glasses of water a day

   Answer:_____   Rationale: _____
   _____
   _____

3. When preparing to give complete AM care to a client, what would the nurse do first?
   a. Gather the necessary equipment and supplies.
   b. Remove the client's gown or pajamas, while maintaining privacy.
   c. Assess the client's preferences for bathing practices.
   d. Lower the side rails and assist the client to assume a comfortable position.

   Answer:_____   Rationale: _____
   _____
   _____

4. Mrs. Veech is a diabetic. Which intervention should be included in her teaching plan regarding foot care?
   a. Use a pumice stone to smooth corns and calluses
   b. File toenails straight across and square
   c. Apply powder to dry areas along the feet and between the toes
   d. Wear elastic stockings to improve circulation

   Answer:_____   Rationale: _____
   _____
   _____

5. Assessment of the hair and scalp reveals that John has head lice. An appropriate intervention would be:
   a. Shave hair off the affected area
   b. Place oil on the hair and scalp until all of the lice are dead
   c. Shampoo with Kwell and repeat 12 to 24 hours later
   d. Shampoo with regular shampoo and dry with hairdryer set at the hottest setting

   Answer:_____   Rationale: _____
   _____
   _____

SYNTHESIS MODEL FOR NURSING CARE PLAN FOR SELF-CARE DEFICIT, BATHING/HYGIENE

Imagine that you are Jeanette, the nurse in the Care Plan on page 1073 of your text. Complete the *Planning phase* of the synthesis model by writing your answers in the appropriate boxes of the model shown. Think about the following:

- In developing Mrs. Wyatt's plan of care, what **knowledge** did Jeanette apply?

- In what way might Jeanette's previous **experience** assist in developing a plan of care for Mrs. Wyatt?

- When developing a plan of care, what intellectual and professional **standards** were applied?

- What critical thinking **attitudes** might have been applied developing Mrs. Wyatts' plan of care?

- How will Jeanette accomplish the goals?

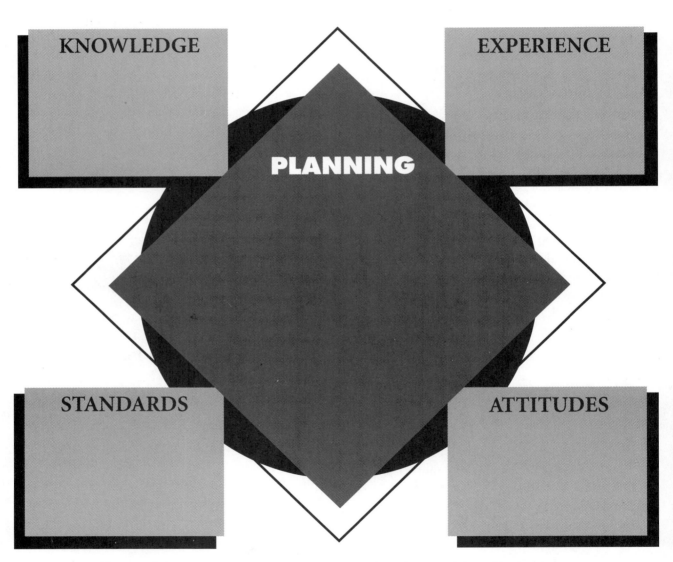

Chapter 38 *Synthesis Model for Nursing Care Plan for* Self-Care Deficit, Bathing/Hygiene.

See answers on page 562.

Oxygenation

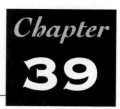

Chapter 39

 The cardiac and respiratory systems function to supply the body's oxygen demands.

PRELIMINARY READING

Chapter 39, pp. 1124-1192

COMPREHENSIVE UNDERSTANDING

SCIENTIFIC KNOWLEDGE BASE

• The cardiopulmonary physiology involves _____ and
_____.

CARDIOVASCULAR PHYSIOLOGY

• The function of the cardiac system is to deliver _____, _____,
and other _____ and to remove the _____ through the
_____, _____, and the _____.

• The right ventricle pumps blood through the _____ while the left ventricle
pumps blood to the _____, supplying oxygen and nutrients to the tissues and
removing wastes from the body.

• The chambers of the heart fill during _____ and empty during _____.

• Describe the Frank-Starling law of the heart. _____
_____

• Briefly describe the flow of blood through the heart. _____
_____
_____

• Describe the following types of circulation.
   a. Coronary artery: _____
   _____
   _____

   b. Systemic: _____
   _____
   _____

- Describe the following terms related to blood flow regulation.

   a. *Cardiac output:* _____
   _____
   _____
   _____

   b. *Cardiac index:* _____
   _____
   _____
   _____

   c. *Stroke volume:* _____
   _____
   _____
   _____

   d. *Preload:* _____
   _____
   _____
   _____

   e. *Afterload:* _____
   _____
   _____
   _____

   f. *Myocardial contractility:* _____
   _____
   _____
   _____

- The autonomic nervous system influences the rate of impulse generation as well as the speed of transmission through the conductive pathway and the strength of atrial and ventricular contractions.

- Describe how the following affect the conduction system of the heart.

   a. Sympathetic nerve fibers: _____
   _____
   _____
   _____

   b. Parasympathetic nerve fibers: _____
   _____
   _____
   _____

- Diagram and label the electrical conduction system of the heart.

- Diagram and label the components of the ECG waveform for normal sinus rhythm (NSR).

RESPIRATORY PHYSIOLOGY

- The three steps in the process of oxygenation are _____, _____, and _____.

- The _____, _____, _____, and _____ are essential for ventilation, perfusion, and exchange of respiratory gases.

- Define *ventilation:* _____
  _____

- Define the following terms related to the work of breathing.
  a. *Compliance:* _____
  _____
  _____
  _____

  b. *Surfactant:* _____
  _____
  _____
  _____

  c. *Airway resistance:* _____
  _____
  _____
  _____

  d. *Accessory muscles:* _____
  _____
  _____
  _____

- Spirometry is used to _____
  _____.

- Variations in lung volumes may be associated with health states such as _____,
  _____, _____,
  or _____.

- The amount of _____,
  _____, and _____
  can affect pressures and volumes within the lungs.

- The total lung capacity is _____
  _____
  _____
  _____.

- Gases are moved into and out of the lungs through pressure changes. Describe the changes that must occur to facilitate air into the lungs. _____
  _____
  _____
  _____

- Briefly describe the pulmonary circulation.
  _____
  _____
  _____
  _____

- Identify the normal distribution of pressures within the pulmonary circulation. _____
  _____
  _____
  _____

- Respiratory gases are exchanged in the _____ and the _____

- Define *diffusion:* _____
  _____

- The rate of diffusion can be affected by
  _____
  _____.

- List four factors required for oxygen transport and delivery.
  a. _____
  _____
  b. _____
  _____
  c. _____
  _____
  d. _____
  _____

- Describe the breakdown of carbon dioxide as it is diffused into the red blood cells.
  _____
  _____
  _____
  _____
  _____
  _____
  _____

- Regulation of respiration is necessary to ensure _____ and _____.

- Explain the two regulators that control the process of respiration.
  a. Neural: _____
  _____

  b. Chemical: _____
  _____

FACTORS AFFECTING OXYGENATION

- List the four factors that influence oxygenation.
  a. _____
  _____

  b. _____
  _____

  c. _____
  _____

  d. _____
  _____

- Explain the physiological process and give an example of each that affect a client's oxygenation.
  a. Decreased carrying capacity: _____
  _____
  _____

  b. Decreased inspired oxygen concentration:
  _____
  _____
  _____
  _____

  c. Hypovolemia: _____
  _____
  _____

  d. Increased metabolic rate: _____
  _____
  _____
  _____

- Explain how the following conditions affect chest wall movement.
  a. Pregnancy: _____

  b. Obesity: _____
  _____

  c. Musculoskeletal abnormalities:
  _____

  d. Trauma: _____

  e. Neuromuscular diseases: _____

  f. Central nervous system alterations:
  _____

  g. Influences of chronic disease: _____
  _____

ALTERATIONS IN CARDIAC FUNCTIONING

- Alterations in cardiac functioning are caused by illnesses and conditions that affect _____, _____, _____, and _____.

- Define *dysrhythmias:* _____
  _____

- Briefly describe the following dysrhythmias.
  a. Sinus tachycardia: _____
  _____
  _____

  b. Sinus bradycardia: _____
  _____
  _____

  c. Sinus dysrhythmia: _____
  _____
  _____

  d. PSVT: _____
  _____
  _____

  e. PVCs: _____
  _____

  f. Ventricular tachycardia: _____
  _____
  _____
  _____

- Failure of the myocardium to eject sufficient volume to the systemic and pulmonary circulations can result in left-sided and right-sided heart failure. Complete the grid below.

Type of Failure	Clinical Findings
Left-sided	
Right-sided	

- Define each of the following.

  a. *Valvular heart disease:* _____

  _____

  b. *Stenosis:* _____

  _____

  c. *Regurgitation:* _____

  _____

  d. *Myocardial ischemia:* _____

  _____

  e. *Angina pectoris:* _____

  _____

  f. *Myocardial infarction:* _____

  _____

- Describe the chest pain associated with myocardial infarction. _____

  _____

  _____

  _____

ALTERATIONS IN RESPIRATORY FUNCTIONING

- The three primary alterations in respiratory function are _____, _____, and _____.

- Complete the grid on the next page.

- Define the following terms:

  a. *Atelectasis:* _____

  _____

  b. *Cyanosis:* _____

  _____

NURSING KNOWLEDGE BASE

DEVELOPMENTAL FACTORS

- Identify at least one physiological factor influencing tissue oxygenation for each developmental level listed.

  a. Premature infant and toddlers: _____

  _____

  _____

  _____

  b. School-age children and adolescents: ____

  _____

  _____

  _____

  c. Young and middle-age adults: _____

  _____

  _____

  _____

  d. Older adults: _____

  _____

  _____

  _____

Alterations	Causes	Signs and Symptoms
Hyperventilation		
Hypoventilation		
Hypoxia		

LIFESTYLE FACTORS

- Briefly describe how the following lifestyle factors influence respiratory function.

    a. Nutrition: _____

    _____

    _____

    _____

    b. Exercise: _____

    _____

    _____

    _____

    c. Cigarette smoking: _____

    _____

    _____

    _____

    d. Substance abuse: _____

    _____

    _____

    _____

ENVIRONMENTAL FACTORS

- List four occupational pollutants.

    a. _____

    _____

    b. _____

    _____

    c. _____

    _____

    d. _____

    _____

STRESS/ANXIETY

- Explain how stress and anxiety increase the oxygen demand. _____

    _____

    _____

    _____

NURSING PROCESS

ASSESSMENT

- The nursing assessment of a client's cardiopulmonary functioning should include data from the following areas. Briefly explain each.

    a. Nursing history: _____

    _____

    _____

    _____

    _____

    _____

    b. Physical examination: _____

    _____

    _____

    _____

    _____

    c. Laboratory and diagnostic tests: _____

    _____

    _____

    _____

    _____

    _____

- The nursing history for cardiac function includes:

  a. _____
  _____

  b. _____
  _____

  c. _____
  _____

  d. _____
  _____

  e. _____
  _____

  f. _____
  _____

- The nursing history for respiratory function includes:

  a. _____
  _____

  b. _____
  _____

  c. _____
  _____

  d. _____
  _____

  e. _____
  _____

  f. _____
  _____

  g. _____
  _____

  h. _____
  _____

  i. _____
  _____

  j. _____
  _____

- Define the following terms:

  a. *Fatigue:* _____
  _____

  b. *Dyspnea:* _____
  _____

  c. *Orthopnea:* _____
  _____

  d. *Cough:* _____
  _____

- e. *Productive cough:* _____
  _____

- f. *Hemoptysis:* _____
  _____

- g. *Wheezing:* _____
  _____

- List the major characteristics to be included in a description of sputum.

  a. _____
  _____

  b. _____
  _____

  c. _____
  _____

  d. _____
  _____

- Describe the following types of chest pain:

  a. Cardiac: _____
  _____

  b. Pleuritic: _____
  _____

  c. Musculoskeletal: _____
  _____

- List the three most common types of environmental exposures in the home.

  a. _____
  _____

  b. _____
  _____

  c. _____
  _____

- List the familial and environmental risk factors. _____
  _____
  _____
  _____

- List three common drugs that may affect cardiopulmonary functioning.

  a. _____
  _____

  b. _____
  _____

  c. _____
  _____

- Briefly explain the following techniques used during the physical examination to assess tissue oxygenation.
  a. Inspection: _____
  _____
  _____
  _____

  b. Palpation: _____
  _____
  _____
  _____

  c. Percussion: _____
  _____
  _____
  _____

  d. Auscultation: _____
  _____
  _____
  _____

- Describe the following diagnostic tests used to determine the adequacy of the cardiac conduction system.
  a. Electrocardiogram: _____
  _____
  _____
  _____

  b. Holter monitor: _____
  _____
  _____
  _____

  c. Exercise stress test: _____
  _____
  _____
  _____

  d. Thallium stress test: _____
  _____
  _____
  _____

  e. Electrophysiological studies (EPS): _____
  _____
  _____
  _____

- Describe the following tests that determine myocardial contraction and blood flow.
  a. Echocardiography: _____
  _____
  _____
  _____

  b. Scintigraphy: _____
  _____
  _____
  _____

  c. Cardiac catheterization and angiography:
  _____
  _____
  _____
  _____

- Describe the following tests used to measure the adequacy of ventilation and oxygenation.
  a. Pulmonary function tests: _____
  _____
  _____
  _____

  b. Peak expiratory flow rate (PEFR):
  _____
  _____
  _____
  _____

  c. Arterial blood gases: _____
  _____
  _____
  _____

  d. Oximetry: _____
  _____
  _____
  _____

  e. Complete blood count: _____
  _____
  _____
  _____

  f. Cardiac enzymes: _____
  _____
  _____
  _____

g. Serum electrolytes _____

_____

_____

_____

h. Cholesterol: _____

_____

_____

_____

- Describe the following tests used to visualize structures of the respiratory system.
  a. Chest x-ray: _____

  _____

  _____

  _____

  b. Bronchoscopy: _____

  _____

  _____

  _____

  c. Lung scan: _____

  _____

  _____

  _____

- Describe the following tests used to determine abnormal cells or infection in the respiratory tract.
  a. Throat cultures: _____

  _____

  _____

  _____

  b. Sputum specimens: _____

  _____

  _____

  _____

  c. Skin testing: _____

  _____

  _____

  _____

  d. Thoracentesis: _____

  _____

  _____

  _____

NURSING DIAGNOSIS

- Clients with an altered level of oxygenation can have nursing diagnoses that are primarily of a cardiovascular or pulmonary origin.

PLANNING

- List six goals appropriate for a client with actual or potential oxygenation needs.
  a. _____

  _____

  b. _____

  _____

  c. _____

  _____

  d. _____

  _____

  e. _____

  _____

  f. _____

  _____

IMPLEMENTATION

- Briefly explain the following types of nursing interventions for promoting and maintaining adequate oxygenation.
  a. Dependent nursing actions: _____

  _____

  _____

  _____

  b. Interdependent-dependent nursing actions:

  _____

  _____

  _____

  _____

Health Promotion

- Describe the purpose of the influenza and pneumococcal vaccine and explain for whom the vaccines are recommended.

  _____

  _____

  _____

  _____

- Avoiding exposure to secondhand smoke is essential to maintaining optimal cardiopulmonary function.

- Identify some healthy lifestyle behaviors that decrease the risk of cardiopulmonary disease. _____
  _____
  _____
  _____
  _____
  _____
  _____

Acute Care

- Nursing interventions for the client with acute pulmonary illnesses are directed toward _____, _____, and _____.

- List five treatment modalities appropriate for a client with dyspnea.
  a. _____
    _____
  b. _____
    _____
  c. _____
    _____
  d. _____
    _____
  e. _____
    _____

Airway Maintenance

- Describe selected nursing interventions used to promote and maintain adequate oxygenation by completing the grid below. Include the purpose of the intervention.

Nursing Interventions	Purpose
Cascade cough	
Huff cough	
Quad cough	
Oropharyngeal and nasopharyngeal suctioning	
Tracheal suctioning	
Oral airway	
Tracheal airway	

Mobilization of Pulmonary Secretions

- Nursing interventions that promote mobilization of pulmonary secretions include the following. Briefly explain each one.
  a. Hydration: _____
  _____
  _____
  _____

  b. *Humidification:* _____
  _____
  _____
  _____

  c. *Nebulization:* _____
  _____
  _____
  _____

  d. *Chest physiotherapy (CPT):* _____
  _____
  _____
  _____

- Briefly describe the three activities involved in CPT.
  a. *Postural drainage:* _____
  _____

  b. *Chest percussion:* _____
  _____

  c. *Vibration:* _____
  _____

- Nursing interventions that maintain or promote lung expansion include the following noninvasive techniques. Briefly explain each one.
  a. Positioning: _____
  _____

  b. *Incentive spirometry:* _____
  _____

- Identify the three reasons for inserting chest tubes.
  a. _____
  _____

  b. _____
  _____

  c. _____
  _____

- Define the following:
  a. *Hemothorax:* _____
  _____

  b. *Pneumothorax:* _____
  _____

- List the four types of drainage systems used with chest tubes.
  a. _____
  _____

  b. _____
  _____

  c. _____
  _____

  d. _____
  _____

- Identify five special considerations the nurse needs to address when dealing with chest tubes.
  a. _____
  _____

  b. _____
  _____

  c. _____
  _____

  d. _____
  _____

  e. _____
  _____

- Promotion of lung expansion, mobilization of secretions, and maintenance of a patent airway assist the client in meeting oxygenation needs.

- Identify the goals of oxygen therapy.
  _____
  _____
  _____
  _____

- List four safety measures to institute when a client receives oxygen administration.
  a. _____
  _____

  b. _____
  _____

c. _____

_____

d. _____

_____

- Describe the following methods of oxygen delivery and identify the usual flow rates.
  a. *Nasal cannula*: _____

  b. Nasal catheter: _____

  c. *Transtracheal oxygen*: _____

  d. Face mask: _____

  e. Venturi mask: _____

- Identify the indications for a client to receive home oxygen therapy. _____

_____

_____

_____

- Identify the teaching required by the client for use of home oxygen therapy. _____

_____

_____

_____

_____

- List the three goals of cardiopulmonary resuscitation (CPR).
  a. _____

  _____

  b. _____

  _____

  c. _____

  _____

Restorative Care

- *Cardiopulmonary rehabilitation* is: _____

_____

_____

- Respiratory muscle training improves muscle strength and endurance resulting in improved activity tolerance. Briefly explain *ISRBD (incentive spirometer resistive breathing device)*. _____

_____

_____

_____

_____

- Briefly explain the following breathing exercises used to improve ventilation and oxygenation.
  a. Pursed-lip breathing: _____

  _____

  _____

  _____

  b. Diaphragmatic breathing: _____

  _____

  _____

  _____

✍ EVALUATION

Client Care

- Evaluates the actual care provided the client by the health care team based on the expected outcomes.

- The client is the only one that can evaluate their degree of breathlessness.

- Evaluation of _____,

_____, _____,

_____, and _____

provide the nurse with object measurements of the success of therapies and treatments.

Client Expectations

- Evaluate the care from the client's perspective.

- Working closely with the client will enable the nurse to redefine those client expectations that can be realistically met within the limitations of the client's condition and treatment.

- List three evaluative criteria for a client with alterations in oxygenation.

  a. _____
  _____

  b. _____
  _____

  c. _____
  _____

REVIEW QUESTIONS

The student should select the appropriate answer and cite the rationale for choosing that particular answer.

1. Ventilation, perfusion, and exchange of gases are the major purposes of:
   a. Respiration
   b. Circulation
   c. Aerobic metabolism
   d. Anaerobic metabolism

   Answer:_____   Rationale: _____
   _____

2. Afterload refers to:
   a. The amount of blood ejected from the left ventricle each minute
   b. The amount of blood ejected from the left ventricle with each contraction
   c. The resistance to left ventricle ejection
   d. The amount of blood in the left ventricle at the end of diastole

   Answer:_____   Rationale: _____
   _____

3. The movement of gases into and out of the lungs depends on the:
   a. 50% Oxygen content in the atmospheric air
   b. Pressure gradient between the atmosphere and the alveoli
   c. Use of accessory muscles of respiration during expiration
   d. Amount of carbon dioxide dissolved in the fluid of the alveoli

   Answer:_____   Rationale: _____
   _____

4. The client's ECG shows an abnormal rhythm that slows during inspiration and increases with expiration. The rate is 70 to 80 beats per minute. The P-wave, PR interval, and QRS complex are normal. This is referred to as:
   a. Sinus tachycardia
   b. Sinus dysrhythmia
   c. Supraventricular tachycardia
   d. Premature ventricular contractions

   Answer:_____   Rationale: _____
   _____

5. Mr. Issac comes to the ER complaining of difficulty breathing. An objective finding associated with his dyspnea might include:
   a. Statements about a sense of impending doom
   b. Complaints of shortness of breath
   c. Feelings of heaviness in the chest
   d. Use of accessory muscles of respiration

   Answer:_____   Rationale: _____
   _____

6. The use of chest physiotherapy to mobilize pulmonary secretions involves the use of:
   a. Hydration
   b. Percussion
   c. Nebulization
   d. Humidification

   Answer:_____   Rationale: _____
   _____

SYNTHESIS MODEL FOR NURSING CARE PLAN FOR INEFFECTIVE AIRWAY CLEARANCE

Imagine that you are the student nurse, in the Care Plan on page 1157 of your text. Complete the *Assessment phase* of the synthesis model by writing your answers in the appropriate boxes of the model shown. Think about the following:

- What **knowledge** base was applied to Mr. Edwards?

- In what way might your previous **experience** apply in this case?

- What intellectual or professional **standards** were applied to Mr. Edwards?

- What critical thinking **attitudes** did you use in assessing Mr. Edwards?

- As you review your **assessment** what key areas did you cover?

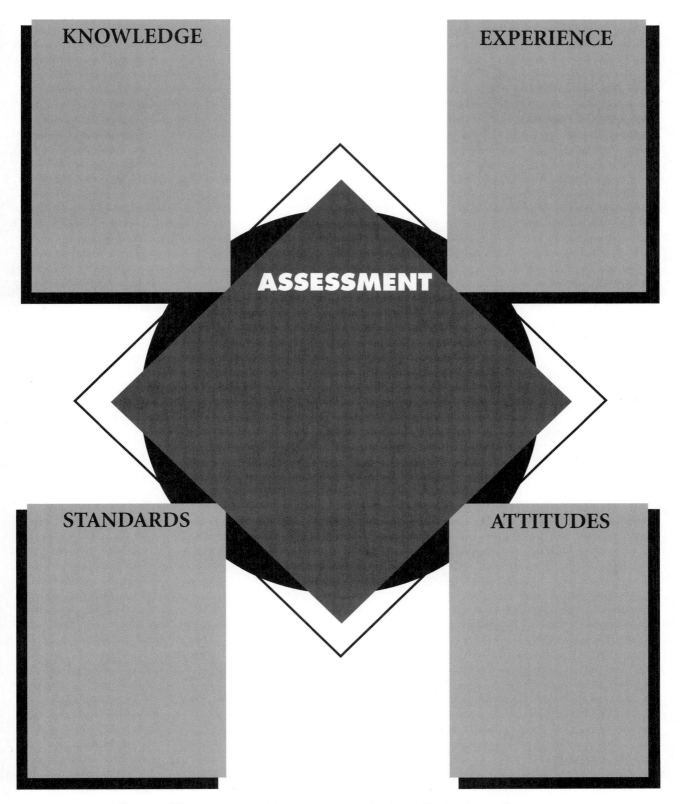

KNOWLEDGE

EXPERIENCE

ASSESSMENT

STANDARDS

ATTITUDES

Chapter 39   *Synthesis Model for Nursing Care Plan for* **Ineffective Airway Clearance.**

See answers on page 563.

Fluid, Electrolyte, and Acid-Base Balances

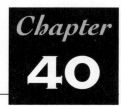
Chapter 40

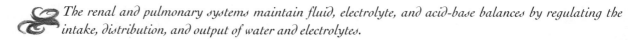
The renal and pulmonary systems maintain fluid, electrolyte, and acid-base balances by regulating the intake, distribution, and output of water and electrolytes.

PRELIMINARY READING
Chapter 40, pp. 1193-1249

COMPREHENSIVE UNDERSTANDING

SCIENTIFIC KNOWLEDGE BASE
- _____ is the largest single component of the body; 60% of the average adult's weight is _____.

DISTRIBUTION OF BODY FLUIDS
- Body fluids are distributed in two distinct compartments. Briefly explain each one.
  a. Extracellular: _____
  _____
  b. Intracellular: _____
  _____

- Extracellular fluids (ECF) are divided into two smaller compartments. Explain each one.
  a. Interstitial: _____
  b. Intravascular: _____

COMPOSITION OF BODY FLUIDS
- Define *electrolyte:* _____

- Define the following terms related to the composition of body fluids.
  a. *Cations:* _____
  b. *Anions:* _____
  c. *mEq/L:* _____
  d. *Solute:* _____
  e. *Solvent:* _____
  f. *Minerals:* _____
  g. *Cells:* _____

MOVEMENT OF BODY FLUIDS

- Fluids and electrolytes shift from compartment to compartment to facilitate body processes.

- List and briefly describe the four factors responsible for movement of body fluids.

  a. _____

  _____

  b. _____

  _____

  c. _____

  _____

  d. _____

  _____

- Define the following terms related to osmosis.

  a. *Osmotic pressure:* _____

  _____

  b. *Isotonic:* _____

  _____

  c. *Hypotonic:* _____

  _____

  d. *Hypertonic:* _____

  _____

- Define *hydrostatic pressure:* _____

  _____

REGULATION OF BODY FLUIDS

- Body fluids are regulated by _____,
  _____, and _____.
  This balance is termed _____.

- Briefly describe the physiological stimuli triggering the thirst mechanism. _____

  _____

  _____

  _____

  _____

  _____

- For each hormone, identify the stimuli for its release and its influence on fluid and electrolyte balance in the grid below.

Hormone	Stimuli	Action
ADH		
Aldosterone		
Glucocorticoids		

- Fluid output occurs through four organs. List and explain each one.

  a. _____

  _____

  b. _____

  _____

  c. _____

  _____

  d. _____

  _____

- Define:

  a. *Insensible water loss:* _____

  _____

  b. *Sensible water loss:* _____

  _____

REGULATION OF ELECTROLYTES

- The major cations are _____,
  _____, _____,
  and _____. They are located
  in the _____ and _____
  fluid.

Chapter 40: Fluid, Electrolyte, and Acid-Base Balances   253

- The major anions are _____,
  _____, and _____.

- Give the normal values, function, and regulatory mechanisms for the major body electrolytes in the grid below.

Electrolyte	Values	Function	Regulatory Mechanism
Sodium			
Potassium			
Calcium			
Magnesium			
Chloride			
Bicarbonate			
Phosphate			

REGULATION OF ACID-BASE BALANCE

- Acid-base balance exists when the _____ _____ _____.

- The concentration of hydrogen ions in a body fluid is expressed as _____ _____.

- A pH value of _____ is neutral. Below _____ is acid, and above _____ is alkaline.

- A *buffer* is _____ _____.

- Identify and describe the acid-base regulatory mechanisms for each of the following buffering systems.

a. Chemical regulation: _____
_____
_____
_____
_____

b. Biological regulation: _____
_____
_____
_____
_____

c. Physiological regulation: _____
_____
_____
_____
_____

- Describe the physiological mechanism through which the lungs regulate hydrogen ion concentration. _____
_____
_____
_____
_____

- List three ways in which the kidneys can regulate hydrogen concentration.

  a. _____
  _____

  b. _____
  _____
  _____

  c. _____
  _____

DISTURBANCES IN ELECTROLYTE, FLUID, AND ACID-BASE BALANCES

  a. _____
  _____

  b. _____
  _____

c. _____
_____

d. _____
_____

- For each electrolyte disturbance, identify the diagnostic laboratory finding, and list at least four characteristic signs and symptoms in the grid below.

- The basic types of fluid imbalances are _____ and _____.

- Isotonic deficit and excess exist when _____
_____.

- *Osmolar imbalances* are _____
_____.

- Complete the grid below giving the causes, signs, and symptoms of the listed fluid disturbances.

Fluid Disturbances	Causes	Signs and Symptoms
Fluid volume deficit (FVD)		
Fluid volume deficit (FVE)		
Third-space syndrome		
Hyperosmolar imbalance		
Hypoosmolar imbalance		

Imbalance	Lab Finding	Signs and Symptoms
Hyponatremia		
Hypernatremia		
Hypokalemia		
Hyperkalemia		
Hypocalcemia		
Hypercalcemia		
Hypomagnesemia		
Hypermagnesemia		

- Briefly explain the following components of the acid-base balance.
  a. pH: _____
  _____

  b. $PaCO_2$: _____
  _____

  c. PaO_2: _____
  _____

  d. Oxygen saturation: _____
  _____

  e. Base excess: _____
  _____

  f. Bicarbonate: _____
  _____

- The four primary types of acid-base imbalances are listed in the grid below. For each acid-base imbalance, identify the diagnostic laboratory finding and list the characteristic signs and symptoms.

Acid-Base Imbalance	Lab Findngs	Signs and Symptoms
Respiratory acidosis		
Respiratory alkalosis		
Metabolic acidosis		
Metabolic alkalosis		

NURSING KNOWLEDGE BASE

- List the five major risk factors that can affect fluid and electrolyte imbalances. Give two examples of each.
  a. _____
  _____

  b. _____
  _____

  c. _____
  _____

  d. _____
  _____

  e. _____
  _____

NURSING PROCESS

ASSESSMENT

- Briefly describe the fluid changes that are associated with aging and development.
  a. Infants: _____
  _____
  _____

  b. Children: _____
  _____
  _____

  c. Adolescents: _____
  _____
  _____

  d. Older adults: _____
  _____
  _____
  _____

- Explain how the following acute illnesses affect fluid, electrolyte, and acid-base balances.
  a. Surgery: _____
  _____
  _____

  b. Burns: _____
  _____
  _____
  _____

  c. Respiratory disorders: _____
  _____
  _____

  d. Head injury: _____
  _____
  _____
  _____

- Describe how the following chronic illnesses affect fluid, electrolyte, and acid-base imbalances.
  a. Cancer: _____
  _____
  _____
  _____

  b. Cardiovascular disease: _____
  _____
  _____
  _____

  c. Renal disorders: _____
  _____
  _____

  d. Gastrointestinal disturbances: _____
  _____
  _____
  _____

- Briefly explain how the following affect fluid, electrolyte, and acid-base imbalance.
  a. Diet: _____
  _____
  _____
  _____
  _____

  b. Lifestyle factors _____
  _____
  _____

  c. Medication _____
  _____
  _____

- Indicate the possible fluid, electrolyte, or acid-base imbalances associated with each physical finding.
  a. Weight loss of 6% to 9%: _____
  _____

  b. Irritability: _____
  _____

  c. Lethargy: _____
  _____

  d. Bulging fontanels (infant): _____
  _____

  e. Periorbital edema: _____
  _____

  f. Sticky, dry mucous membranes: _____
  _____

  g. Chvostek's sign: _____
  _____

  h. Distended neck veins: _____
  _____

  i. Dysrhythmias: _____
  _____

  j. Weak pulse: _____
  _____

  k. Low blood pressure: _____
  _____

  l. Third heart sound : _____
  _____

  m. Increased respiratory rate: _____
  _____

  n. Crackles: _____
  _____

  o. Anorexia: _____
  _____

  p. Abdominal cramps: _____
  _____

  q. Poor skin turgor: _____
  _____

  r. Oliguria or anuria: _____
  _____

s. Increased specific gravity: _____

_____

t. Muscle cramps, tetany: _____

_____

u. Hypertonicity of muscles on palpation:

_____

_____

v. Decreased or absent deep tendon reflexes:

_____

_____

w. Increased temperature: _____

_____

x. Distended abdomen: _____

_____

y. Cold, clammy skin: _____

_____

z. 2+ edema: _____

_____

- Recording I & O is essential for obtaining an accurate database. This information helps maintain an ongoing evaluation of hydration status to prevent severe imbalances.

- Explain the rationale for each of the following laboratory tests.
  a. Serum electrolytes: _____

  _____

  b. CBC: _____

  _____

  c. Creatinine: _____

  _____

  d. BUN: _____

  _____

  e. Serum osmolality: _____

  _____

  f. Urine specific gravity: _____

  _____

- Arterial blood gas levels (ABG) provide information on the status of acid-base balance. Give the normals for each.
  a. pH: _____

  _____

  b. $PaCO_2$: _____

  _____

c. PaO_2: _____

_____

d. SaO_2: _____

_____

e. HCO_3: _____

_____

🐍 NURSING DIAGNOSIS

- List five potential or actual nursing diagnoses for a client with fluid, electrolyte, or acid-base imbalances.
  a. _____

  _____

  b. _____

  _____

  c. _____

  _____

  d. _____

  _____

  e. _____

  _____

🐍 PLANNING

- List three goals that are appropriate for a client with altered fluid, electrolyte, or acid-base imbalances.
  a. _____

  _____

  b. _____

  _____

  c. _____

  _____

🐍 IMPLEMENTATION

Health Promotion

- Identify some common risk factors for imbalances for which the caregiver may implement appropriate preventive measures. _____

  _____

  _____

  _____

Chapter 40: Fluid, Electrolyte, and Acid-Base Balances   259

Acute Care

- When implementing specific measures to increase or decrease fluid, two interventions are necessary. Explain each one.

  a. Daily weights: _____

  _____

  b. Intake and output: _____

  _____

- List and briefly describe the enteral replacements of fluids.

  a. _____

  _____

  b. _____

  _____

- Briefly explain the need for a restricted fluid intake and how the nurse would implement the restriction. _____

  _____

  _____

  _____

  _____

- List the three methods of parenteral replacement.

  a. _____

  _____

  b. _____

  _____

  c. _____

  _____

- *Vascular assist devices* are _____

  _____

- *Total parenteral nutrition (TPN)* is _____

  _____

  _____

- Identify the primary goal of IV fluid replacement. _____

  _____

- Define the following types of electrolyte solutions.

  a. *Isotonic:* _____

  _____

  b. *Hypotonic:* _____

  _____

  c. *Hypertonic:* _____

  _____

- List two major purposes of infusion pumps.

  a. _____

  _____

  b. _____

  _____

- List three groups of clients in whom venipunctures may be difficult.

  a. _____

  _____

  b. _____

  _____

  c. _____

  _____

- List four factors that may affect IV flow rates.

- List four interventions that can reduce the risk of infusion-related infections.

  a. _____

  _____

  b. _____

  _____

  c. _____

  _____

  d. _____

  _____

- Indicate the sequence to be followed when changing the gown of a client with an IV line.

  a. _____

  _____

  b. _____

  _____

  c. _____

  _____

  d. _____

  _____

  e. _____

  _____

  f. _____

  _____

- Complete the grid below describing complications of IV therapy.

Complication	Assessment Finding	Nursing Action
Infiltration		
Phlebitis		
Fluid overload		
Bleeding		

- Briefly summarize the procedure for discontinuing intravenous infusions.

  _____

  _____

  _____

  _____

  _____

  _____

- List three objectives for blood transfusion.

  a. _____

  _____

  b. _____

  _____

  c. _____

- Complete the grid below describing the major blood groups.

	A	B	O	AB
Antigens present				
Antibodies present				

Chapter 40: Fluid, Electrolyte, and Acid-Base Balances   261

- Define *autotransfusion:* _____
_____

- Identify the five nursing interventions associated with blood transfusions and give the rationale for each.
  a. _____
  _____
  b. _____
  _____
  c. _____
  _____
  d. _____
  _____
  e. _____
  _____

- Define *transfusion reaction* and identify its cause. _____
  _____
  _____
  _____

- List the five signs and symptoms most commonly associated with transfusion reactions.
  a. _____
  _____
  b. _____
  _____
  c. _____
  _____
  d. _____
  _____
  e. _____
  _____

- Define the following risks associated with blood transfusions.
  a. Hyperkalemia: _____

  b. Hypocalcemia: _____

  c. Iron overload (hemosiderosis): _____

  d. Circulatory overload: _____
  _____

- List the nine steps the nurse should follow if a transfusion reaction is suspected.
  a. _____
  _____
  b. _____
  _____
  c. _____
  _____
  d. _____
  _____
  e. _____
  f. _____
  _____
  g. _____
  _____
  h. _____
  _____
  i. _____
  _____

- Identify three nursing interventions to correct acid-base imbalances and give the rationale for each.
  a. _____
  _____
  b. _____
  _____
  c. _____
  _____

Restorative Care
- Older adults and the chronically ill require special considerations to prevent complications from developing.

- Briefly summarize the following.
  a. Home intravenous therapy: _____
  _____
  _____
  b. Nutritional support: _____
  _____
  _____
  c. Medication safety: _____
  _____
  _____
  _____

Client Care

- Evaluates the actual care delivered by the health care team based on the expected outcomes.

- The nurse integrates what he or she knows about the health alterations, the effects of medications and fluids, and the client's presenting clinical status.

Client Expectations

- Evaluation of care from the client's perspective.

- Often the client's level of satisfaction with care also depends on the nurse's success in involving friends and family.

REVIEW QUESTIONS

The student should select the appropriate answer and cite the rationale for choosing that particular answer.

1. The body fluids comprising the interstitial fluid and blood plasma are:
   a. Intracellular
   b. Extracellular
   c. Hypotonic
   d. Hypertonic

   Answer:＿＿＿＿ Rationale: ＿＿＿＿＿＿＿
   ＿＿＿＿＿＿＿＿＿＿＿＿＿＿＿＿＿＿＿＿＿＿＿

2. Which of the following statements is true with regard to the lungs' regulation of acid-base balance?
   a. The lungs serve a minor role in the physiological buffering of H ions.
   b. It takes several days for the lungs to restore pH to a normal level.
   c. The lungs correct imbalances by alternating the rate and depth of respiration.
   d. The lungs maintain normal pH by either retaining or excreting bicarbonate.

   Answer:＿＿＿＿ Rationale: ＿＿＿＿＿＿＿
   ＿＿＿＿＿＿＿＿＿＿＿＿＿＿＿＿＿＿＿＿＿＿＿

3. Mrs. Green's arterial blood gas results are as follows: pH, 7.32; $PaCO_2$, 52; PaO_2, 78; HCO_3, 24. Mrs. Green has:
   a. Respiratory acidoses
   b. Respiratory alkalosis
   c. Metabolic acidosis
   d. Metabolic alkalosis

   Answer:＿＿＿＿ Rationale: ＿＿＿＿＿＿＿
   ＿＿＿＿＿＿＿＿＿＿＿＿＿＿＿＿＿＿＿＿＿＿＿

4. Mr. Frank is an 82-year-old client who has had a 3-day history of vomiting and diarrhea. Which symptom would you expect to find on a physical examination?
   a. Neck vein distention
   b. Crackles in the lungs
   c. Tachycardia
   d. Hypertension

   Answer:＿＿＿＿ Rationale: ＿＿＿＿＿＿＿
   ＿＿＿＿＿＿＿＿＿＿＿＿＿＿＿＿＿＿＿＿＿＿＿

5. Which of the following is most likely to result in respiratory alkalosis?
   a. Fad dieting
   b. Hyperventilation
   c. Chronic alcoholism
   d. Steroid use

Answer:_____   Rationale: _____
_____

6. Ten minutes after her blood transfusion started, Ms. White began experiencing fever, chills, and difficulty breathing. The nurse should:
   a. Realize that this is a harmless reaction and continue to monitor the blood transfusion
   b. Slow the transfusion rate
   c. Turn off the blood, and turn on the normal saline on the Y-tubing infusion set
   d. Turn off the blood and "piggyback" 0.9% saline into the IV line

Answer:_____   Rationale: _____
_____

SYNTHESIS MODEL FOR INEFFECTIVE AIRWAY CLEARANCE/RISK FOR FLUID VOLUME DEFICIT

Imagine that you are the student nurse in the Care Plan on page 1217 of your text. Complete the *Planning phase* of the synthesis model by writing your answers in the appropriate boxes of the model shown. Think about the following:

- In developing Mrs. Bottomly's plan of care, what **knowledge** did you apply?

- In what way might your previous **experience** assist you in developing a plan of care for Mrs. Bottomly?

- When developing a plan of care what intellectual and professional **standards** were applied?

- What critical thinking **attitudes** might have been applied to developing Mrs. Bottomly's care?

- How will you accomplish your goals?

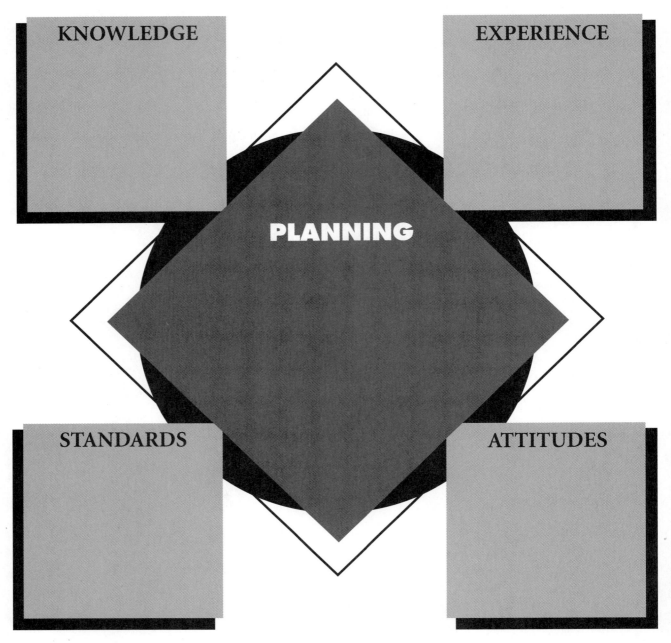

KNOWLEDGE

EXPERIENCE

PLANNING

STANDARDS

ATTITUDES

Chapter 40 *Synthesis Model for* Ineffective Airway Clearance/Risk for Fluid Volume Deficit.

See answers on page 564.

Sleep

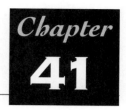

Chapter 41

Achieving the best possible sleep quality is important in promoting good health as well as recovering from illness.

PRELIMINARY READING

Chapter 41, pp. 1250-1280

COMPREHENSIVE UNDERSTANDING

SCIENTIFIC KNOWLEDGE BASE

PHYSIOLOGY OF SLEEP

• Define *sleep:* _____

• Define the following terms related to sleep:
   a. *Circadian rhythm:* _____
   _____

   b. *Biological clocks:* _____
   _____

• Sleep involves a sequence of physiological states maintained by highly integrated central nervous system activity that is associated with changes in the _____, _____, _____, and _____ systems.

• The control and regulation of sleep depends on the interrelationship between two cerebral mechanisms that intermittently active and suppress the brain's higher centers to control sleep and wakefulness.

• Summarize the function of the reticular activating system (RAS). _____
_____

• The area of the brain called the bulbar synchronizing region (BSR) is responsible for _____
_____

- Explain the two phases of sleep.
  a. *NREM:* _____
  _____
  _____
  _____

  b. *REM:* _____
  _____
  _____
  _____

- Describe the characteristics of the following stages of sleep.
  a. Stage 1: _____
  _____

  b. Stage 2: _____
  _____

  c. Stage 3: _____
  _____

  d. Stage 4: _____
  _____

  e. REM: _____
  _____

- Dreams occur mostly during _____ sleep. They can be influenced by _____
  _____.

PHYSICAL ILLNESS

- Explain how the following conditions affect sleep.
  a. Discomfort: _____
  _____

  b. Respiratory disease: _____

  c. Coronary artery disease: _____

  d. Hypertension: _____
  _____

  e. Hypothyroidism: _____
  _____

  f. Hyperthyroidism: _____
  _____

  g. Nocturia: _____

  h. Restless legs syndrome: _____
  _____

  i. Peptic ulcer disease: _____
  _____

SLEEP DISORDERS

- Briefly describe the four major categories of sleep disorders.
  a. *Dyssomnias:* _____
  _____
  _____
  _____

  b. *Parasomnias:* _____
  _____
  _____
  _____

  c. Associated with medical-psychiatric disorders: _____
  _____
  _____
  _____

  d. Proposed sleep disorders _____
  _____
  _____

- Define *insomnia:* _____
  _____

- List two conditions that are associated with insomnia.
  a. _____
  _____

  b. _____
  _____

- Define *sleep apnea:* _____
  _____

- Define the following types of apnea:
  a. *Central apnea:* _____

  b. *Obstructive apnea:* _____
  _____

- Identify treatment modalities for a client with sleep apnea. _____
  _____
  _____
  _____

- Define *narcolepsy:* _____
  _____

- Define the following terms related to narcolepsy.
  a. *Cataplexy:* _____

  _____
  b. *Hypnagogic hallucinations:* _____

  _____

- Identify the developmental stage in which narcolepsy symptoms first develop. _____

  _____

- Identify the treatment modalities for a client with narcolepsy. _____

  _____

- *Sleep deprivation* is _____

  _____

- List the physiological and psychological manifestations of sleep deprivation in the grid below.

Physiological Symptoms	Psychological Symptoms

- Explain the following parasomnias.
  a. Somnambulism: _____

  _____
  b. Nocturnal enuresis: _____

  _____
  c. Bruxism: _____

  _____

NURSING KNOWLEDGE BASE

SLEEP AND REST

- Define:
  a. *Rest:* _____

  _____
  b. *Sleep:* _____

  _____

NORMAL SLEEP REQUIREMENTS AND PATTERNS

- Complete the grid listing the normal sleep patterns and rituals for the following developmental stages.

FACTORS AFFECTING SLEEP

- A number of factors affect the quantity and quality of sleep.

Developmental Stage	Sleep Patterns	Usual Rituals
Neonates		
Infants		
Toddlers		
Preschoolers		
School-age children		
Adolescents		
Young adults		
Middle adults		
Older adults		

- Sleepiness and sleep deprivations are common side effects of medications. Describe how each of the following affects sleep.
  a. Hypnotics: _____

  _____

  b. Diuretics: _____

  _____

  c. Antidepressants: _____

  _____

  d. Alcohol: _____

  _____

  e. Caffeine: _____

  _____

  f. Beta-blockers: _____

  _____

  g. Benzodiazepines: _____

  _____

  h. Narcotics: _____

  _____

  i. Anticonvulsants: _____

  _____

- List four alterations in routine that can disrupt sleep patterns.
  a. _____

  _____

  b. _____

  _____

  c. _____

  _____

  d. _____

  _____

- *Excessive daytime sleepiness (EDS)* often results in _____, _____, _____, and _____.

- Explain how emotional stress affects sleep.

  _____

  _____

  _____

  _____

- List and briefly describe three environmental factors that affect sleep.
  a. _____

  _____

  b. _____

  _____

  c. _____

  _____

- Explain how exercise promotes sleep.

  _____

  _____

  _____

  _____

- List and briefly describe five foods that affect sleep.
  a. _____

  _____

  b. _____

  _____

  c. _____

  _____

  d. _____

  _____

  e. _____

  _____

NURSING PROCESS

ASSESSMENT

- Sleep is a subjective experience.

- Assessment is aimed at understanding the characteristics of any sleep problem and the client's usual sleep habits so that ways for promoting sleep can be incorporated into the nursing care.

- Identify three sources for sleep assessment.
  a. _____

  _____

  b. _____

  _____

  c. _____

  _____

- List the ten components of a sleep history.
  a. _____
  _____

  b. _____
  _____

  c. _____
  _____

  d. _____
  _____

  e. _____
  _____

  f. _____
  _____

  g. _____
  _____

  h. _____
  _____

  i. _____
  _____

  j. _____
  _____

- List and briefly describe the six areas to assess with a client who has a sleeping problem.
  a. _____
  _____

  b. _____
  _____

  c. _____
  _____

  d. _____
  _____

  e. _____
  _____

  f. _____
  _____

- Give an example of three questions to ask clients with the following sleep disorders.
  a. Insomnia
    1. _____
    _____

    2. _____
    _____

    3. _____
    _____

  b. Sleep apnea
    1. _____
    _____

    2. _____
    _____

    3. _____
    _____

  c. Narcolepsy
    1. _____
    _____

    2. _____
    _____

    3. _____
    _____

- Identify the questions a nurse would ask to determined the client's usual sleep pattern.
  _____
  _____
  _____
  _____
  _____
  _____

- Briefly explain how the following factors interfere with sleep.
  a. Physical illness: _____
  _____
  _____
  _____

  b. Current life events: _____
  _____
  _____

  c. Emotional and mental status: _____
  _____
  _____
  _____

  d. Bedtime routines: _____
  _____
  _____
  _____

  e. Bedtime environment: _____
  _____
  _____

- List four behaviors a client may manifest with sleep deprivation.

  a _____
  _____

  b. _____
  _____

  c. _____
  _____

  d. _____
  _____

NURSING DIAGNOSIS

- If a sleep pattern disturbance is identified, the nurse specifies the specific condition.

- Assessment should also identify the related factor or probable cause of the sleep disturbance.

PLANNING

- It is important for the plan of care to include strategies that are appropriate for the client's environment and lifestyle.

- List four goals appropriate for a client needing rest or sleep.

  a. _____
  _____

  b. _____
  _____

  c. _____
  _____

  d. _____
  _____

IMPLEMENTATION

- Nursing interventions designed to improve the quality of a person's sleep are largely focused on health promotion.

Health Promotion

- Many factors affect the ability to gain adequate rest and sleep. Briefly give examples of each of the following.

  a. Environmental control: _____
  _____
  _____

  b. Promoting bedtime rituals: _____
  _____
  _____

  c. Comfort: _____
  _____
  _____

  d. Periods of rest and sleep: _____
  _____
  _____

  e. Stress reduction: _____
  _____
  _____
  _____

  f. Bedtime snacks: _____
  _____
  _____
  _____

  g. Pharmacological approaches: _____
  _____
  _____

Acute Care

- For each of the following situations, give two examples of nursing measures that will promote sleep.

  a. Environmental control:

    1. _____
    _____

    2. _____
    _____

  b. Promoting comfort:

    1 _____
    _____

    2. _____
    _____

c. Establishing periods of rest and sleep:

1. _____

   _____

2. _____

   _____

d. Stress reduction:

1. _____

   _____

2. _____

   _____

Restorative or Continuing Care

- Give an example of the following interventions that are implemented in restorative environment.

  a. Promoting comfort: _____

  _____

  _____

  _____

  b. Controlling physiological disturbances:

  _____

  _____

  _____

  _____

  c. Pharmacological approaches: _____

  _____

  _____

  _____

- Briefly describe the effect of benzodiazepines in promoting sleep.

- Identify three types of clients that should not use benzodiazepines and explain why.

  a. _____

  _____

  b. _____

  _____

  c. _____

  _____

- The regular use of sleeping medication can lead to _____

  _____.

Client Care

- With regard to sleep disturbances, the client is the source for outcomes evaluation. List three outcomes for a client with a sleep disturbance.

  a. _____

  _____

  b. _____

  _____

  c. _____

  _____

Client Expectations

- Client expectations evaluate care from the client's perspective. Identify some subtle behaviors a client may exhibit that indicate their satisfaction. _____

  _____

  _____

  _____

REVIEW QUESTIONS

The student should select the appropriate answer and cite the rationale for choosing that particular answer.

1. The 24-hour day-night cycle is known as:
   a. Circadian rhythm
   b. Infradium rhythm
   c. Ultradian rhythm
   d. NonREM rhythm

Answer: _____   Rationale: _____

_____

_____

2. Which of the following substances will promote normal sleep patterns?
   a. L-tryptophan
   b. Beta-blockers
   c. Alcohol
   d. Narcotics

Answer:_____   Rationale: _____
_____
_____

3. All of the following are symptoms of sleep deprivation *except:*
   a. Hyperactivity
   b. Irritability
   c. Rise in body temperature
   d. Decreased motivation

Answer:_____   Rationale: _____
_____
_____

4. Mrs. Peterson complains of difficulty falling asleep, awakening earlier than desired, and not feeling rested. She attributes these problems to leg pain that is secondary to her arthritis. What would be the appropriate nursing diagnosis for her?
   a. Sleep pattern disturbances related to arthritis
   b. Fatigue related to leg pain
   c. Knowledge deficit regarding sleep hygiene measures
   d. Sleep pattern disturbances related to chronic leg pain

Answer:_____   Rationale: _____
_____
_____

5. A nursing care plan for a client with sleep problems has been implemented. All of the following would be expected outcomes *except:*
   a. Client reports no episodes of awakening during the night.
   b. Client falls asleep within 1 hour of going to bed.
   c. Client reports satisfaction with amount of sleep.
   d. Client rates sleep as an 8 or above on the visual analog scale.

Answer:_____   Rationale: _____
_____
_____

SYNTHESIS MODEL FOR NURSING CARE PLAN FOR SLEEP PATTERN DISTURBANCE

Imagine that you are the nurse in the Care Plan on page 1270 of your text. Complete the *Evaluation phase* of the synthesis model by writing your answers in the appropriate boxes of the model shown. Think about the following:

- What **knowledge** did you apply in evaluating Julie's care?

- In what way might your previous **experience** influence your evaluation of Julie's care?

- During evaluation, what intellectual and professional **standards** were applied to Julie's care?

- In what way does critical thinking **attitudes** play a role in how you approach the evaluation of Julie's plan?

- How might you **evaluate** Julie's plan of care?

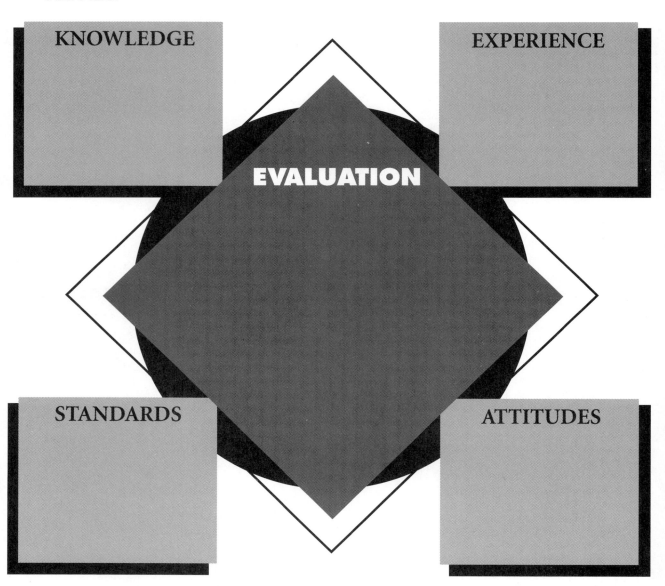

Chapter 41 *Synthesis Model for Nursing Care Plan for* Sleep Pattern Disturbance.

See answers on page 565.

Comfort

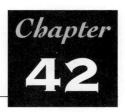

Chapter
42

Pain is subjective. No two persons experience pain in the same way, and no two painful events create identical responses or feelings for one person.

PRELIMINARY READING
Chapter 42, pp. 1281-1322

COMPREHENSIVE UNDERSTANDING
- The concept of comfort is as subjective as that of pain.

- Each individual brings _____, _____, _____, _____, and _____, characterisitics that influence how comfort is interpreted and experienced.

- Define *comfort,* as described by Yolcaba (1992): _____

- Effective pain management not only reduces _____ but promotes earlier _____, _____, _____, and _____.

SCIENTIFIC KNOWLEDGE BASE

NATURE OF PAIN
- Define *pain,* as described by Mahon (1994): _____

- _____ knows whether pain is present and what the experience is like.

- Explain how pain is a protective physiological mechanism. _____

PHYSIOLOGY OF PAIN
- The three types of pain are _____, _____, and _____.

- The classification of pain by inferred pathology is _____.

- Explain the four processes of nociceptive pain.
  a. *Transduction:* _____
  _____
  _____

  b. *Transmission:* _____
  _____
  _____
  _____

  c. *Perception:* _____
  _____
  _____
  _____

  d. *Modulation:* _____
  _____
  _____
  _____
  _____

- *Neuroregulators* are _____
  _____

- Explain the two types of neuroregulators.
  a. *Neurotransmitters:* _____
  _____
  _____
  _____

  b. Neuromodulators: _____
  _____
  _____
  _____
  _____

- Identify the neurophysiological function of the following neuroregulators.
  a. Substance P: _____
  _____
  _____
  _____

  b. *Prostaglandins:* _____
  _____
  _____
  _____

  c. Serotonin: _____
  _____
  _____
  _____

d. Endorphins: _____
_____
_____
_____

e. Bradykinin: _____
_____
_____
_____

- Describe the basic concept underlying the gate-control theory of pain. _____
  _____
  _____
  _____

- *Perception* is the point at which _____
  _____

- Stimulation of the autonomic nervous system results in physiological responses to pain. Give five examples of each and their effect.
  a. Sympathetic stimulation:
  1. _____
  _____
  2. _____
  _____
  3. _____
  _____
  4. _____
  _____
  5. _____
  _____

  b. Parasympathetic stimulation
  1. _____
  _____
  2. _____
  _____
  3. _____
  _____
  4. _____
  _____
  5. _____
  _____

- Identify four behavioral changes that reflect a client experiencing pain.

  a. _____
  _____

  b. _____
  _____

  c. _____
  _____

  d. _____
  _____

- Define *pain tolerance:* _____
  _____

TYPES OF PAIN

- List four characteristics of *acute pain*.

  a. _____
  _____

  b. _____
  _____

  c. _____
  _____

  d. _____
  _____

- List four symptoms associated with chronic pain.

  a. _____
  _____

  b. _____
  _____

  c. _____
  _____

  d. _____
  _____

- Identify the characteristics of *cancer pain*.

  _____
  _____
  _____
  _____

NURSING KNOWLEDGE BASE

KNOWLEDGE, ATTITUDES, AND BELIEFS

- The medical model of illness describes pain as _____
  _____
  _____
  _____.

- Identify common bias and misconceptions about pain. _____
  _____
  _____
  _____
  _____
  _____
  _____
  _____
  _____
  _____
  _____

FACTORS INFLUENCING PAIN

- Explain the developmental differences of client's reaction to pain.

  a. Young children: _____
  _____
  _____
  _____

  b. Toddlers and preschoolers: _____
  _____
  _____
  _____

  c. Older adults: _____
  _____
  _____
  _____

- Identify five reasons why older clients may not report pain.

  a. _____
  _____

  b. _____
  _____

  c. _____
  _____

  d. _____
  _____

  e. _____
  _____

Chapter 42: Comfort   279

- Describe the cultural influences on gender in relation to expressing pain. _____
  _____
  _____
  _____

- Cultural beliefs and values affect how individuals deal with pain. Individuals learn what is expected and accepted by their culture; this includes how to react to pain.

- Explain how the meaning of pain is a factor.
  _____
  _____
  _____
  _____

- The degree to which a client focuses attention on pain can influence pain perception. Explain. _____
  _____
  _____
  _____
  _____
  _____

- Anxiety _____ the perception of pain, but pain may cause feelings of anxiety.

- Fatigue heightens the perception of pain. Explain. _____
  _____
  _____
  _____

- Briefly explain how the following factors influence pain.
  a. Previous experience: _____
  _____
  _____
  _____

  b. Internal loci of control: _____
  _____
  _____
  _____

c. External loci of control: _____
_____
_____
_____

d. Family and social support: _____
_____
_____
_____

NURSING PROCESS AND PAIN

- Pain management extends beyond pain relief, encompassing the client's _____, _____, and _____.

ASSESSMENT

- For clients with acute pain, the nurse primarily assesses _____, _____, and _____.

- For clients with chronic pain, assessment should be focused on _____, _____, and _____ dimensions of the pain experience and on its history and context.

- Pain assessment and management "ABCDE"
  A: _____
  B: _____
  _____
  C: _____
  _____
  D: _____
  _____
  E: _____
  _____

- Identify examples of nonverbal expressions of pain. _____
  _____
  _____
  _____
  _____

- Cognitively impaired clients require simple assessment approaches involving close observation of behavior changes.

- Briefly explain the common characteristics of pain.
  a. Onset and duration: _____
  _____
  _____
  _____

  b. Location: _____
  _____
  _____
  _____

  c. Intensity: _____
  _____

- Describe the following descriptive scales for measuring the severity of pain.
  a. Verbal descriptor scale (VDS): _____
  _____
  _____
  _____

  b. Visual analog scale (VAS) _____
  _____
  _____
  _____

  c. Faces scale: _____
  _____
  _____
  _____

- Identify some terms a client can use to describe the quality of pain. _____
  _____
  _____
  _____

- Identify some relief measures a client may use to relieve pain. _____
  _____
  _____
  _____

- Identify some concomitant symptoms that occur with pain. _____
  _____
  _____
  _____

- Summarize how pain affects the psychological well-being of the client. _____
  _____
  _____
  _____
  _____
  _____

- Give examples of the following behavioral indicators of pain.
  a. Vocalizations: _____
  _____

  b. Facial expressions: _____
  _____

  c. Body movement: _____
  _____

  d. Social interaction: _____
  _____

- Explain how pain can influence activities of daily living in regard to the following:
  a. Sleep: _____
  _____
  _____
  _____

  b. Hygiene: _____
  _____
  _____
  _____

  c. Sexual relations: _____
  _____
  _____
  _____

  d. Employment: _____
  _____
  _____
  _____

  e. Social activities: _____
  _____
  _____
  _____

NURSING DIAGNOSIS

- The nursing diagnosis should focus on the specific nature of the pain to help the nurse identify the most useful types of interventions for alleviating pain and minimizing its effect on the client's lifestyle and function.

- List five potential or actual nursing diagnoses related to a client in pain.

    a. _____
    _____
    b. _____
    _____
    c. _____
    _____
    d. _____
    _____
    e. _____
    _____

PLANNING

- An intervention that works for one client will not work for all clients.

- When developing a plan of care, the nurse selects priorities based on the client's level of pain and its effect on the client's condition.

- List the client outcomes appropriate for the client experiencing pain.

    a. _____
    _____
    b. _____
    _____
    c. _____
    _____
    d. _____
    _____
    e. _____
    _____

IMPLEMENTATION

Health Promotion

- Teaching clients about the pain experience reduces anxiety and helps clients achieve a sense of control.

- Describe how you would teach a child about a painful procedure. _____
    _____
    _____
    _____

- Define the *holistic health approach to pain control:* _____
    _____
    _____
    _____

- The AHCPR guidelines for acute pain management cite nonpharmacological interventions to be appropriate for clients who meet certain criteria. List those criteria.

    a. _____
    _____
    b. _____
    _____
    c. _____
    _____
    d. _____
    _____
    e. _____
    _____

- There are many nonpharmacological interventions that lesson pain. Briefly explain each one.
    a. *Acupressure:* _____
    _____
    _____
    _____

    b. Relaxation and *guided imagery:* _____
    _____
    _____
    _____

- Briefly explain how the nurse would lead a client through *guided imagery.* _____
    _____
    _____
    _____

- Briefly explain how the nurse would guide a client through progressive relaxation exercises. _____

  _____

  _____

  _____

  _____

- Define *distraction*, and list one disadvantage and advantage of using distraction. _____

  _____

  _____

  _____

- Describe the effects of using music as a distraction to control pain. _____

  _____

  _____

  _____

  _____

- Define the following pain-relief measures and the rationale for their use.
  a. *Biofeedback:* _____

  _____

  _____

  b. Self-hypnosis: _____

  _____

  _____

  c. Reducing pain perception: _____

  _____

  _____

  d. Cutaneous stimulation: _____

  _____

  _____

  _____

- What is *TENS*, and how is it believed to reduce pain? _____

  _____

  _____

  _____

  _____

Acute Care

Pharmacological Pain-Relief Interventions
- *Analgesics* are the most common method of pain relief.

- Identify the three types of analgesics and explain the conditions for which they are generally prescribed.
  a. _____

  _____

  b. _____

  _____

  c. _____

  _____

- List the seven characteristics of an ideal analgesic.
  a. _____

  _____

  b. _____

  _____

  c. _____

  _____

  d. _____

  _____

  e. _____

  _____

  f. _____

  _____

  g. _____

  _____

- Describe four major principles for analgesic administration.
  a. _____

  _____

  b. _____

  _____

  c. _____

  _____

  d. _____

  _____

- Explain the benefits of *Patient-Controlled Analgesia (PCA).* _____

  _____

  _____

  _____

Chapter 42: Comfort   283

- Describe what a *local anesthetic* is and give its physiological properties. _____
  _____
  _____

- Identify four types of local anesthetics and the level of anesthesia they provide.
  a. _____
  _____
  b. _____
  _____
  c. _____
  _____
  d. _____
  _____

- List the seven advantages of an epidural analgesia.
  a. _____
  _____
  b. _____
  _____
  c. _____
  _____
  d. _____
  _____
  e. _____
  _____
  f. _____
  _____
  g. _____
  _____

- List four goals for the care of a client with epidural infusions. Describe one action for each goal.
  a. _____
  _____
  b. _____
  _____
  c. _____
  _____
  d. _____
  _____

- Explain the following surgical measures used to relieve pain:
  a. Dorsal rhizotomy: _____
  _____
  _____
  _____
  b. Chordotomy: _____
  _____
  _____
  _____

- Identify the three-step approach to cancer pain management recommended by the World Health Organization (1990).
  a. _____
  _____
  b. _____
  _____
  c. _____
  _____

- Identify clients who are candidates for continuous infusions.
  a. _____
  _____
  b. _____
  _____
  c. _____
  _____
  d. _____
  _____

- List four guidelines for safe administration of morphine sulfate via ambulatory infusion pumps.
  a. _____
  _____
  b. _____
  _____
  c. _____
  _____
  d. _____
  _____

Restorative Care

- Explain hospice programs. _____
_____
_____
_____

🐍 EVALUATION

Client Care

- Client care evaluates the actual care delivered by the health care team based on the expected outcomes.

- The nurse needs to know what responses to anticipate on the basis of the type of pain, the intervention, the timing of the intervention, the physiological nature of the injury or disease, and the client's previous responses.

Client Expectations

- The client, if able, is the best resource for evaluating the effectiveness of pain-relief measures.

- The family often is another valuable resource, particularly in the case of the client with cancer who may not be able to express discomfort during the latter stages of terminal illness.

REVIEW QUESTIONS

The student should select the appropriate answer and cite the rationale for choosing that particular answer.

1. Pain is a protective mechanism warning of tissue injury and is largely a(an):
   a. Symptom of a severe illness or disease
   b. Subjective experience
   c. Objective experience
   d. Acute symptom of short duration

   Answer:_____ Rationale: _____
   _____
   _____

2. A substance that can cause analgesia when it attaches to opiate receptors in the brain is:
   a. Substance P
   b. Serotonin
   c. Prostaglandin
   d. Endorphin

   Answer:_____ Rationale: _____
   _____
   _____

3. To adequately assess the quality of a client's pain, which question would be appropriate?
   a. "Tell me what your pain feels like."
   b. "Is your pain a crushing sensation?"
   c. "How long have you had this pain?"
   d. "Is it a sharp pain or a dull pain?"

   Answer:_____ Rationale: _____
   _____
   _____

4. The use of client distraction in pain control is based on the principle that:
   a. Small C fibers transmit impulses via the spinothalamic tract
   b. The reticular formation can send inhibitory signals to gating mechanisms
   c. Large A fibers compete with pain impulses to close gates to painful stimuli
   d. Transmission of pain impulses from the spinal cord to the cerebral cortex can be inhibited

   Answer:_____ Rationale: _____
   _____
   _____

5. Teaching a child about painful procedures is best achieved by:
   a. Early warnings of the anticipated pain
   b. Storytelling about the upcoming procedure
   c. Relevant play directed toward procedure activities
   d. Avoiding explanations until the pain is experienced

   Answer:_____ Rationale: _____
   _____
   _____

Synthesis Model for Nursing Care Plan for Acute Pain

Imagine that you are the student nurse in the Care Plan on page 1304 of your text. Complete the *Assessment phase* of the synthesis model by writing your answers in the appropriate boxes of the model shown. Think about the following:

- What **knowledge** base was applied to Mrs. Mays?

- In what way might previous **experience** assist you in this case?

- What intellectual or professional **standards** were applied to the care of Mrs. Mays?

- What critical thinking **attitudes** did you use in assessing Mrs. Mays?

- As you review your **assessment** what key areas did you cover?

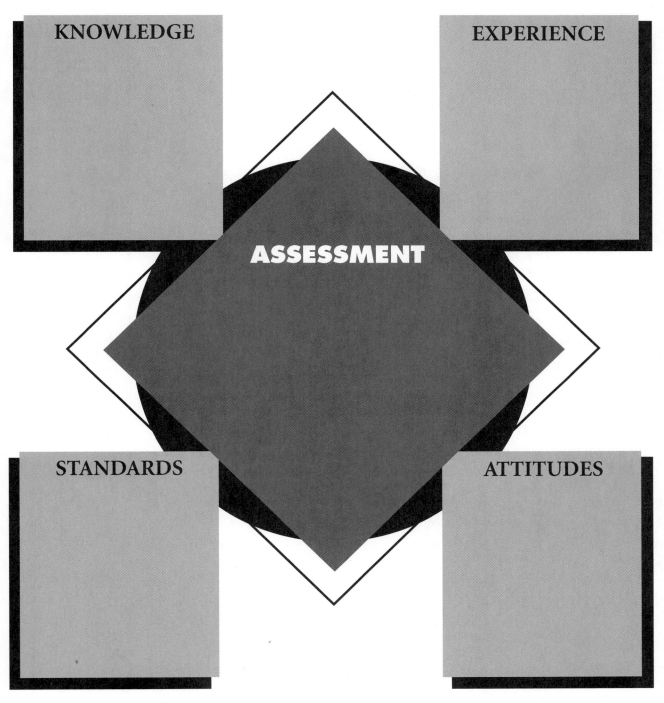

KNOWLEDGE

EXPERIENCE

ASSESSMENT

STANDARDS

ATTITUDES

Chapter 42 *Synthesis Model for Nursing Care Plan for* Acute Pain.

See answers on page 566.

Nutrition

Standards exist that clearly designate the needed care to promote optimal nutrition in all health care clients.

PRELIMINARY READING
Chapter 43, pp. 1323-1382

COMPREHENSIVE UNDERSTANDING

SCIENTIFIC KNOWLEDGE BASE

NUTRIENTS: THE BIOCHEMICAL UNITS OF NUTRITION

- The body requires fuel to provide energy for _____, _____, _____, and _____.

- Define the following terms:
  a. *Basal metabolic rate (BMR):* _____
  b. *Resting energy expenditure (REE):* _____
  c. *Nutrients:* _____
  d. *Nutrient density:* _____

- List the six categories of nutrients.
  a. _____
  b. _____
  c. _____
  d. _____
  e. _____
  f. _____

- Each gram of carbohydrate produces _____ kilocalories (kcal).

- Identify the three classifications of *carbohydrates.*
  a. _____
  b. _____
  c. _____

- Proteins provide a source of energy _____ kcal/g and are essential for _____.

- The simplest form of protein is _____ _____.

- Explain the two formsof protein.
  a. *Essential amino acids:* _____ _____
  b. *Nonessential amino acids:* _____ _____

- Define the following terms:
  a. *Complete protein:* _____ _____
  b. *Complementary proteins:* _____ _____
  c. *Nitrogen balance:* _____ _____

- *Lipids* (fats) are the most calorically dense nutrient, providing _____ kcal per gram.

- Describe the following composition of fats.
  a. *Triglycerides:* _____ _____
  b. *Fatty acids:* _____ _____

- *Lipogenesis* is _____ _____

- Define the following types of fats and give an example of each.
  a. *Saturated:* _____ _____
  b. *Unsaturated:* _____ _____
  c. *Monounsaturated:* _____
  d. *Polyunsaturated:* _____ _____

- Deficiencies occur when fat intake falls below _____ of daily nutrition.

- Briefly explain how Olestra (a fat replacer) works. _____ _____ _____ _____

- Water composes _____ of total body weight.

- _____ have the greatest percentage of total body weight as water, and people have the least.

- Fluid needs are met by _____ and by water produced during _____.

- *Vitamins* are _____ _____

- Identify the water-soluble vitamins. _____ _____

- Identify the fat-soluble vitamins. _____ _____

- *Minerals* are _____ _____

- Minerals are classified as _____ when the daily requirement is 100 mg or more; and _____ when less than 100 mg is needed daily.

ANATOMY AND PHYSIOLOGY OF DIGESTIVE SYSTEM

- Digestion of food consists of the mechanical breakdown and chemical reactions by which food is reduced to its simplest form.

- *Enzymes* are _____ _____

- The following activities of digestion are interdependent. Explain each one.
  a. Mechanical: _____ _____
  b. Chemical: _____ _____
  c. Hormonal: _____ _____

Chapter 43: Nutrition   289

- Match the food substance with the enzyme that aids its digestion.
  a. Substance
    1. Protein: _____

    _____

    2. Carbohydrate: _____

    _____

    3. Fat: _____

  a. Enzyme
    1. Ptyalin: _____

    2. Pepsin: _____

    3. Lipase: _____

    4. Polypeptidase: _____

    5. Amylase: _____

    6. Sucrase: _____

    7. Maltase: _____

    8. Lactase: _____

    9. Trypsin: _____

    _____

- The major portion of digestion occurs in the

  _____

  _____.

- Define the terms related to digestion.
  a. *Peristalsis:* _____

  _____

  b. *Dysphagia:* _____

  _____

  c. *Chyme:* _____

  _____

- The primary site of absorption is the _____

  _____.

- Absorption of water is the main function of the _____

  _____.

- In addition to water, electrolytes and minerals are absorbed, and bacteria in the colon synthesize _____ vitamins.

- *Metabolism* refers to _____

  _____.

- Describe the two types of metabolism.
  a. *Anabolism:* _____

  _____

  _____

  _____

  b. *Catabolism:* _____

  _____

  _____

  _____

- The body's major form of stored energy is _____ ,which is stored as _____.

- *Glycogen* is _____

  _____.

- Nutrient metabolism consists of three main processes. Explain each one.
  a. *Glycogenolysis:* _____

  _____

  b. *Glycogenesis:* _____

  _____

  c. *Gluconeogenesis:* _____

  _____

- Feces contain _____

  _____.

DIETARY GUIDELINES

- Explain the Dietary Reference Intakes (DRIs) format. _____

  _____

  _____

  _____

- The estimated average requirement (EAR) serves as a _____

  _____

  _____

  _____.

- The *tolerable upper intake level (UL)* is

  _____
  _____

- Using the space at the below, diagram and label the food guide pyramid developed by the U.S. Department of Agriculture (USDA).

- List the seven dietary guidelines for Americans issued by the USDA and the Department of Health and Human Services.

  a. _____
  _____
  b. _____
  _____
  c. _____
  _____
  d. _____
  _____
  e. _____
  _____
  f. _____
  _____
  g. _____
  _____

- Summarize the rationale for *daily values* on food labels: _____
  _____
  _____
  _____

- Summarize the differences between *Healthy People 2010* and *Healthy People 2000* goals:

  _____
  _____
  _____
  _____

NURSING KNOWLEDGE BASE

NUTRITION DURING HUMAN GROWTH AND DEVELOPMENT

Infants

- An energy intake of approximately _____ kcal/kg is needed in the first half of infancy, and an intake of _____ kcal/kg is needed in the second half.

- A full-term newborn is able to digest and absorb _____.

- Amylase is not present until _____ months of age.

- Infants need _____ ml/kg/day of fluid.

- List four nutrients that must be supplemented in the breast-fed infant.

  a. _____
  _____
  b. _____
  _____
  c. _____
  _____
  d. _____
  _____

- Explain why the following should not be used in infant formula.
  a. Cow's milk: _____
  _____
  b. Honey and corn syrup: _____
  _____

- List four indications of an infant's readiness to begin solid foods.

  a. _____
  _____

  b. _____
  _____

  c. _____
  _____

  d. _____
  _____

Toddlers and Preschoolers

- The toddler needs _____ calories but an increased amount of _____ in relation to body weight.

School-Age Children

- School-age children's diets should be assessed for _____
  _____.

- Explain some reasons for the increase in childhood obesity. _____
  _____

Adolescents

- Identify the common deficiencies in the following adolescent population.

  a. Girls: _____
  _____

  b. Boys: _____
  _____

  c. Those that eat fast-food: _____
  _____

  d. Those involved in intense exercise: _____
  _____
  _____

  e. Pregnant: _____
  _____

- Identify the diagnostic criteria for the following eating disorders:

  a. *Anorexia nervosa:* _____
  _____
  _____
  _____
  _____
  _____

  b. *Bulimia nervosa:* _____
  _____
  _____
  _____
  _____

Young and Middle Adults

- Obesity becomes a problem because of _____
  _____.

- Adult women who use oral contraceptives need extra _____
  _____.

- The energy requirements of pregnancy are related to _____
  _____.

- Explain the increased amounts of the following items that are required for pregnancy and lactation.

  a. Pregnancy

  1. Calories: _____
  _____

  2. Calcium: _____
  _____

  3. Iron: _____
  _____

  4. Vitamins: _____
  _____

  5. Fluids: _____
  _____

  b. Lactation

  1. Calories: _____
  _____

  2. Protein: _____
  _____

  3. Calcium: _____
  _____

  4. Vitamins: _____
  _____

  5. Fluids: _____
  _____

Older Adults

- List four factors that influence the nutritional status of the older adult. Using an asterisk, identify the one factor that is considered the most important.

  a. _____

  _____

  b. _____

  _____

  c. _____

  _____

  d. _____

  _____

ALTERNATIVE FOOD PATTERNS

- A common alternative dietary pattern is the vegetarian diet. Describe briefly. _____

  _____

  _____

  _____

  _____

  _____

NURSING PROCESS AND NUTRITION

- Close daily contact with clients and their families enables nurses to make observations about their physical status, food intake, weight gain or loss, and responses to therapy.

ASSESSMENT

- List the five components of a nutritional assessment.

  a. _____

  _____

  b. _____

  _____

  c. _____

  _____

  d. _____

  _____

  e. _____

  _____

- Define:

  a. *Anthropometry:* _____

  _____

  b. *Body mass index (BMI):* _____

  _____

  c. *Ideal body weight (IBW):* _____

  _____

  d. *Bioelectrical impedance analysis (BIA):* _____

  _____

- Identify the common laboratory tests used to study the nutritional status of a client:

  _____

  _____

  _____

  _____

- List the five factors on which a dietary history focuses.

  a. _____

  _____

  b. _____

  _____

  c. _____

  _____

  d. _____

  _____

  e _____

  _____

- List seven factors that influence dietary patterns.

  a. _____

  _____

  b. _____

  _____

  c. _____

  _____

  d. _____

  _____

  e. _____

  _____

  f. _____

  _____

  g. _____

  _____

- For each assessment area, list at least two signs of good and poor nutrition.
  a. General appearance
     1. _____
        _____
     2. _____
        _____
  b. General vitality
     1. _____
        _____
     2. _____
        _____
  c. Weight
     1. _____
        _____
     2. _____
        _____
  d. Hair
     1. _____
        _____
     2. _____
        _____
  e. Skin
     1. _____
        _____
     2. _____
        _____
  f. Mouth
     1. _____
        _____
     2. _____
        _____
  g. Eyes
     1. _____
        _____
     2. _____
        _____
  h. Gastrointestinal function
     1. _____
        _____
     2. _____
        _____
  i. Cardiovascular function
     1. _____
        _____
     2. _____
        _____

  j. Neurological function
     1. _____
        _____
     2. _____
        _____
  k. Musculoskeletal function
     1. _____
        _____
     2. _____
        _____

NURSING DIAGNOSIS

- List three potential or actual nursing diagnoses for altered nutritional status.
  a. _____
     _____
  b. _____
     _____
  c. _____
     _____

PLANNING

- Explain why the clients in the following situations are considered at risk for nutritional problems.
  a. Oral and throat surgery: _____
     _____
  b. GI surgery: _____
     _____
  c. Immobilization: _____
     _____

- List four goals for a client with nutritional problems.
  a. _____
     _____
  b. _____
     _____
  c. _____
     _____
  d. _____
     _____

IMPLEMENTATION

- List three situations that occur in the hospital setting that influence nutritional intake.

  a. _____

  b. _____
  _____

  c. _____
  _____

- List five ways that a nurse can stimulate the client's appetite.

  a. _____
  _____

  b. _____
  _____

  c. _____
  _____

  d. _____
  _____

  e. _____
  _____

Health Promotion

- Clients can prevent the development of many diseases by incorporating a knowledge of nutrition into their lifestyle.

- Summarize meal planning and identify the factors that should be considered. _____
  _____
  _____
  _____
  _____

Acute Care

- Clients who are NPO and only receive standard IV fluids for more than 7 days are at nutritional risk.

- Define *enteral nutrition (EN)*: _____
  _____

- Explain the beneficial effect of enteral feedings as compared to parenteral nutrition.
  _____
  _____
  _____
  _____
  _____
  _____
  _____
  _____
  _____

- Explain aspiration and the physiological changes that occur in the client. _____
  _____
  _____
  _____

- Identify the clients who are suitable for the following types of formulas.
  a. Protein: _____
  _____

  b. Elemental, or peptide based: _____
  _____

  c. Disease specific: _____
  _____

- Describe the following types of feeding tubes:
  a. Nasogastric: _____
  _____

  b. Gastrostomy: _____

  c. Peg _____
  _____

- Identify the tube type preferred for enteral tube feedings. _____
  _____
  _____
  _____

- The most reliable method for testing the placement of a small bore feeding tube is
  _____.

- Describe a method that the nurse may use to test the placement of a small-bore feeding tube. _____
  _____
  _____
  _____
  _____

- List the five major complications of enteral feedings.
  a. _____
     _____
  b. _____
     _____
  c. _____
     _____
  d. _____
     _____
  e. _____
     _____

- List the three factors on which safe administration of parenteral nutrition (PN) depends.
  a. _____
     _____
  b. _____
     _____
  c. _____
     _____

- *Lipid emulsions* are _____
  _____

- The adverse reactions to lipid emulsion include _____
  _____.

- Briefly describe the rationale for each action associated with the initiation and maintenance of total parenteral nutrition.
  a. Chest x-ray : _____
     _____
  b. Beginning an infusion: _____
     _____
  c. Infusion flow rate: _____
     _____

- List six potential complications of parenteral nutrition and identify the symptoms of each.
  a. _____
     _____
  b. _____
     _____
  c. _____
     _____
  d. _____
     _____
  e. _____
     _____
  f. _____
     _____

- Explain the goal of transition from PN to EN and/or oral feeding. _____
  _____
  _____

- *Medical nutrition therapy (MNT) is:* _____
  _____
  _____
  _____

Restorative and Continuing Care
- Restorative care includes both immediate post-surgical care and routine medical care and includes hospitalized and home care clients.

- Identify the nutritional interventions for the following common disease states:
  a. Peptic ulcers
     1. Inflammatory bowel disease: _____
        _____
     2. Malabsorption syndromes: _____
        _____
     3. Diverticulitis: _____
        _____
  b. Diabetes mellitus (DM)
     1. Type 1: _____
        _____
     2. Type 2: _____
        _____

c. Hypertension: _____

_____

d. COPD: _____

_____

e. Acute renal failure: _____

_____

f. Chronic renal failure: _____

_____

g. Cancer: _____

_____

h. Human immunodeficiency virus (HIV):

_____

_____

✎ EVALUATION

- Multidisciplinary collaboration remains essential in the provision of nutritional support.

Client Care

- The effectiveness of nutritional interventions delivered by the health care team is based on the expected outcomes.

- The client's ability to incorporate dietary changes into their lifestyle with the least amount of stress or disruption will ensure that outcome measures are successfully met.

Client Expectations

- Clients expect competent and accurate care. The plan of care must be altered if the outcomes aren't being met.

REVIEW QUESTIONS

The student should select the appropriate answer and cite the rationale for choosing that particular answer.

1. Which nutrient is the body's most preferred energy source?
   a. Protein
   b. Fat
   c. Carbohydrate
   d. Vitamin

   Answer: _____ Rationale: _____

   _____

   _____

2. Positive nitrogen balance would occur in which condition?
   a. Infection
   b. Starvation
   c. Burn injury
   d. Pregnancy

   Answer: _____ Rationale: _____

   _____

   _____

3. Mrs. Nelson is talking with the nurse about the dietary needs of her 23-month-old daughter, Laura. Which of the following responses by the nurse would be appropriate?
   a. "Use skim milk to cut down on the fat in Laura's diet."
   b. "Laura should be drinking at least 1 quart of milk per day."
   c. "Laura needs fewer calories in relation to her body weight now than she did as an infant."
   d. "Laura needs less protein in her diet now because she isn't growing as fast."

   Answer: _____ Rationale: _____

   _____

   _____

Chapter 43: Nutrition   297

4. All of the following clients are at risk for alteration in nutrition *except:*
   a. Client J, who is 86 years old, lives alone, and has poorly fitting dentures
   b. Client K, who has been NPO for 7 days following bowel surgery and is receiving 3000 ml of 10% dextrose per day
   c. Client L, whose weight is 10% above his ideal body weight
   d. Client M, who is a 17-year-old woman, weighs 90 lb, and frequently complains about her baby fat

Answer:_____   Rationale: _____
_____
_____

5. Which of the following is the most accurate method of bedside confirmation of placement of a small-bore nasogastric tube?
   a. Auscultate the epigastrium for gurgling or bubbling
   b. Test the pH of withdrawn gastric contents
   c. Assess the client's ability to speak
   d. Assess the length of the tube that is outside the client's nose

Answer:_____   Rationale: _____
_____
_____

6. A client who has been hospitalized after experiencing a heart attack will most likely receive a diet consisting of:
   a. Low fat, low sodium, and high carbohydrates
   b. Low fat, high protein, and high carbohydrates
   c. Low fat, low sodium, and low carbohydrates
   d. Liquids for several days, progressing to a soft and then a regular diet

Answer:_____   Rationale: _____
_____
_____

SYNTHESIS MODEL FOR NURSING CARE PLAN FOR ALTERED NUTRITION: LESS THAN BODY REQUIREMENTS

Imagine that you are Marie, the nurse in the Care Plan on page 1354 of your text. Complete the *Planning phase* of the synthesis model by writing your answers in the appropriate boxes of the model shown. Think about the following:

• In developing Mrs. Cooper's plan of care, what **knowledge** did Marie apply?

• In what ways might Marie's previous **experience** assist in developing Mrs. Cooper's plan of care?

• When developing a plan of care for Mrs. Cooper what intellectual and professional **standards** were applied?

• What critical thinking **attitudes** might have been applied in developing Mrs. Cooper's plan of care?

• How will Marie accomplish these goals?

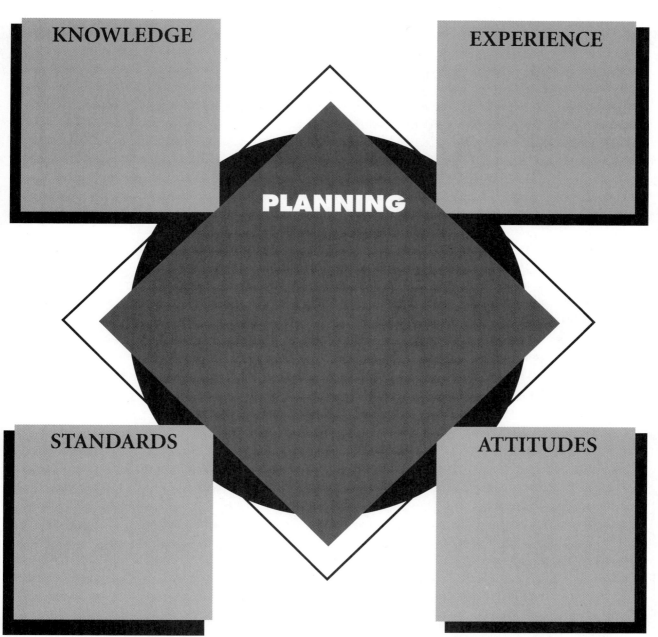

KNOWLEDGE

EXPERIENCE

PLANNING

STANDARDS

ATTITUDES

Chapter 43 *Synthesis model for Nursing Care Plan for* Altered Nutrition: Less Than Body Requirements.

See answers on page 567.

Urinary Elimination

 If the urinary system fails to function properly, virtually all organ systems will be eventually affected.

PRELIMINARY READING
Chapter 44, pp. 1383-1435

COMPREHENSIVE UNDERSTANDING

SCIENTIFIC KNOWLEDGE BASE

• Summarize the function of each of the following organs in the urinary system:

a. Kidneys: _____

_____

b. Ureters: _____

_____

c. Bladder: _____

_____

d. Urethra: _____

_____

• Define the following terms related to urine elimination.

a. *Nephron:* _____

b. *Proteinuria:* _____

c. *Erythropoietin:* _____

d. *Renin:* _____

e. *Micturation:* _____

f. *Meatus:* _____

ACT OF URINATION

• Number the steps describing the normal act of micturition in sequential order.

_____ Parasympathetic impulses from the micturition center cause the detrusor muscle to begin contracting.

_____ The external bladder sphincter relaxes.

_____ Impulses travel to the cerebral cortex, making the person conscious of the need to void.

_____ The detrusor muscle contracts.

_____ The internal urethral sphincter relaxes, allowing urine to enter the urethra.

_____ Urine passes through the urethral meatus.

_____ Urine volume stretches the bladder walls, sending impulses to the spinal cord.

- Explain the following two alterations with elimination.
  a. *Reflex bladder:* _____

  b. *Urinary retention:* _____

- Problems related to the act of urination may be the result of cognitive, functional, or physical means and may result in incontinence, retention, or infection.

- Disease processes that primarily affect renal function (changes in urine volume or quality) are generally categorized as the following. Briefly explain.
  a. Prerenal: _____

  b. Renal: _____

  c. Postrenal: _____

- Define *oliguria:* _____

- Define *anuria:* _____

- List the characteristic signs of the *uremic syndrome.* _____

- Briefly describe the two methods of dialysis.
  a. Peritoneal: _____

  b. Hemodialysis: _____

- Identify some indications for dialysis.
  _____

Growth and Development
- Briefly explain the normal micturition patterns that occur in the following developmental stages.
  a. Infants: _____

  b. Children: _____

  c. Adults: _____

  d. Older adults: _____

- Define the following terms related to urination.
  a. *Nocturia:* _____

  b. *Urinary frequency:* _____

  c. *Residual urine:* _____

- Briefly explain the following factors that influence urination.
  a. Sociocultural factors: _____

  b. Psychological factors: _____

  c. Muscle tone: _____

Chapter 44: Urinary Elimination   301

- Explain how the following affect the balance of urine excreted.
  a. Alcohol: _____
  _____
  _____
  _____

  b. Caffeine drinks: _____
  _____
  _____
  _____

  c. Fruits and vegetables: _____
  _____
  _____
  _____

  d. Febrile conditions: _____
  _____
  _____
  _____

- Briefly explain how the stress of surgery affects urine output. _____
  _____
  _____
  _____
  _____

- Briefly explain how anesthetics and narcotic analgesics affect urine output. _____
  _____
  _____
  _____
  _____

- A *urinary diversion* is: _____
  _____

- List five medications that affect urination.
  a. _____
  _____
  b. _____
  _____
  c. _____
  _____
  d. _____
  _____
  e. _____
  _____

- Explain what a cystoscopy is and how it may affect urination. _____
  _____
  _____
  _____

- Clients with urinary problems have disturbances in the act of micturition that involve a failure to store urine or a failure to empty urine. List the three most common.
  a. _____
  _____
  b. _____
  _____
  c. _____
  _____

- Define *urinary retention:* _____
  _____

- Define *retention with overflow:* _____
  _____

- List six signs or symptoms of urinary tract infections (UTIs).
  a. _____
  _____
  b. _____
  _____
  c. _____
  _____
  d. _____
  _____
  e. _____
  _____
  f. _____
  _____

- Identify the most common cause of UTIs.
  _____
  _____
  _____
  _____

- Identify the three common causes of UTIs in women.
  a. _____
  _____
  b. _____
  _____
  c. _____
  _____

- Define the following terms related to UTIs.
  a. *Bacteriuria:* _____
  _____
  b. *Dysuria:* _____
  _____
  c. *Hematuria:* _____
  _____
  d. *Pyelonephritis:* _____
  _____

- Define *urinary incontinence:* _____
  _____

- Briefly describe the five types of urinary incontinence.
  a. Functional: _____
  _____
  b. Overflow: _____
  _____
  c. Reflex: _____
  _____
  d. Stress: _____
  _____
  e. Urge: _____
  _____

- Identify some indications for *urinary diversions.* _____
  _____
  _____
  _____

- Briefly describe the following *urinary diversions.*
  a. Ileal loop or conduit: _____
  _____
  _____
  _____

  b. *Ureterostomy:* _____
  _____
  _____
  _____

  c. *Nephrostomy:* _____
  _____
  _____
  _____

NURSING KNOWLEDGE BASE
- The nurse needs to know concepts other than anatomy and physiology, such as infection control, hygiene measures, growth and development, and psychosocial influences.

INFECTION CONTROL AND HYGIENE
- Although the urinary tract is considered sterile, it is a common site for infections. Many UTIs are caused by _____
  _____.

- Hospital acquired UTIs are related to _____, _____, or _____.

DEVELOPMENTAL CONSIDERATIONS
- Briefly summarize the developmental changes that may influence urination.
  _____
  _____
  _____
  _____
  _____
  _____

PSYCHOSOCIAL CONSIDERATIONS
- Identify the psychosocial factors that may influence urination.
  _____
  _____
  _____
  _____

NURSING PROCESS AND ALTERATIONS IN URINARY FUNCTION

🙣 ASSESSMENT

Nursing History
- List the three major factors to be explored during a nursing history in regard to urinary elimination.

  a. _____
  _____

  b. _____
  _____

  c. _____
  _____

- Describe the following symptoms of urinary alterations.

  a. Urgency: _____
  _____

  b. Dysuria: _____

  c. Frequency _____

  d. Hesitancy: _____
  _____

  e. Polyuria: _____

  f. Oliguria: _____
  _____

  g. Nocturia: _____
  _____

  h. Dribbling: _____
  _____

  i. Incontinence: _____
  _____

  j. Hematuria: _____

  k. Retention: _____
  _____

  l. Residual urine: _____
  _____

- List and briefly explain the organs that the nurse would assess to determine the presence and severity of urinary problems.

  a. _____
  _____

  b. _____
  _____

  c. _____
  _____

  d. _____
  _____

- Assessment of urine involves _____ and _____.

- Describe the following characteristics of urine.

  a. Color: _____
  _____
  _____
  _____

  b. Clarity: _____
  _____
  _____

  c. Odor: _____
  _____
  _____

- Describe the following types of urine specimens collected for testing.

  a. Random: _____
  _____
  _____

  b. Clean-voided or midstream: _____
  _____
  _____

  c. Sterile: _____
  _____
  _____

  d. Timed urine: _____
  _____
  _____
  _____

- Common urine tests include the following. Briefly explain each.
  a. Urinalysis: _____
  _____
  _____
  _____

  b. Specific gravity: _____
  _____
  _____
  _____

  c. Urine culture: _____
  _____
  _____
  _____

- Briefly explain the following types of diagnostic examinations and give the nursing implications for each.
  a. Abdominal roentgenogram: _____
  _____
  _____
  _____
  _____

  b. Intravenous pyelogram (IVP): _____
  _____
  _____
  _____
  _____
  _____

- Identify the specific nursing implications for a client receiving an IVP.
  a. _____
  _____
  b. _____
  _____
  c. _____
  _____

- Identify the specific nursing implications for a client after an IVP test.
  a. _____
  _____
  b. _____
  _____

  c. _____
  _____
  d. _____
  _____

- List the nursing implications for a client before a renal scan.
  a. _____
  _____
  b. _____
  _____
  c. _____
  _____
  d. _____
  _____
  e. _____
  _____

- Name two nursing implications for a client during a renal scan.
  a. _____
  _____
  b. _____
  _____

- Briefly explain the following diagnostic tests, and give the nursing implications for each.
  a. Computerized axial tomography (CT):
  _____
  _____
  _____
  _____

  b. Renal ultrasound: _____
  _____
  _____
  _____

- List the three types of invasive procedures.
  a. _____
  _____
  b. _____
  _____
  c. _____
  _____

- List the nursing implications for a cystoscopy.
  a. *Before the test:*
    1. _____
       _____
    2. _____
       _____
    3. _____
       _____
    4. _____
       _____
    5. _____
       _____
    6. _____
       _____
    7. _____
       _____
    8. _____
       _____

  b. *During the test:*
    1. _____
       _____
    2. _____
       _____
    3. _____
       _____
    4. _____
       _____

  c. *After the test:*
    1. _____
       _____
    2. _____
       _____
    3 _____
       _____
    4. _____
       _____
    5. _____
       _____
    6. _____
       _____

- List the nursing implications related to an angiography (arteriogram).
  a. *Before the test:*
    1. _____
       _____
    2. _____
       _____
    3. _____
       _____
    4. _____
       _____
    5. _____
       _____

  b. *After the test:*
    1. _____
       _____
    2. _____
       _____
    3. _____
       _____
    4. _____
       _____
    5. _____
       _____
    6. _____
       _____

- Explain the responsibilities of the nurse who is caring for a client who had a cystometrogram (CMG). _____
  _____
  _____
  _____

NURSING DIAGNOSIS

- List six potential or actual nursing diagnoses related to urinary elimination.
  a. _____
     _____
  b. _____
     _____
  c. _____
     _____
  d. _____
     _____
  e. _____
     _____
  f. _____
     _____

PLANNING

- List the six goals appropriate for a client with a urinary elimination problem.

  a. _____
  _____

  b. _____
  _____

  c. _____
  _____

  d. _____
  _____

  e. _____
  _____

  f. _____
  _____

IMPLEMENTATION

Health promotion

- List five teaching strategies aimed at eradicating or minimizing urinary elimination problems.

  a. _____
  _____

  b. _____
  _____

  c. _____
  _____

  d. _____
  _____

  e. _____
  _____

- List five techniques that may be used to stimulate the micturition reflex.

  a. _____
  _____

  b. _____
  _____

  c. _____
  _____

  d. _____
  _____

  e. _____
  _____

- Identify at least two types of treatment options to promote micturition in the following types of urinary incontinence.

  a. Functional incontinence: _____
  _____
  _____

  b. Overflow incontinence: _____
  _____
  _____

  c. Reflex incontinence: _____
  _____
  _____

  d. Stress incontinence: _____
  _____
  _____

  e. Urge incontinence: _____
  _____
  _____

- Urine is normally acidic and tends to inhibit the growth of microorganisms. List four types of foods that increase urine acidity.

  a. _____
  _____

  b. _____
  _____

  c. _____
  _____

  d. _____
  _____

Acute Care

- Briefly explain how the nurse could help the hospitalized client maintain normal elimination habits. _____
  _____
  _____
  _____

- List and explain three types of medications that can be used to treat incontinence or retention.

  a. _____

  _____

  b. _____

  _____

  c. _____

  _____

- Briefly describe the following types of catheters.

  a. Straight single-use: _____

  _____

  _____

  _____

  b. Indwelling: _____

  _____

  _____

  _____

  c. Coude': _____

  _____

  _____

  _____

- Give an example of the following indications for catheterization.

  a. Intermittent: _____

  _____

  b. Short-term indwelling: _____

  _____

  c. Long-term indwelling: _____

  _____

- Explain the nursing measures taken to prevent infection and maintain an unobstructed flow of urine in catheterized clients.

  a. Fluid intake: _____

  _____

  _____

  _____

  b. Perineal hygiene: _____

  _____

  c. Catheter care: _____

  _____

- Identify the sites of infection in the catheterized client. _____

  _____

  _____

  _____

- Briefly describe catheter irrigations and instillations. _____

  _____

  _____

  _____

- Name two important principles to follow when removing an indwelling catheter.

  a. _____

  _____

  b. _____

  _____

- Briefly explain the two alternatives for urinary drainage and give the nursing implications for each.

  a. Suprapubic catheter: _____

  _____

  _____

  _____

  _____

  b. Condom catheter: _____

  _____

  _____

  _____

  _____

- Name two precautions that should be taken to ensure client safety and comfort when using a condom catheter.

  a. _____

  _____

  b. _____

  _____

Restorative Care

- Define *Pelvic Floor Exercises (PFEs/Kegel exercises):* _____
_____
_____
_____

- Identify the goal of bladder retraining.
_____
_____
_____
_____

- List eleven measures the nurse can teach the incontinent client to gain control over urination.
  a. _____
  _____
  b. _____
  _____
  c. _____
  d. _____
  _____
  e. _____
  _____
  f. _____
  _____
  g. _____
  _____
  h. _____
  _____
  i. _____
  _____
  j. _____
  _____
  k. _____
  _____

- A client with functional incontinence may benefit from habit training, which helps clients improve voluntary control over urination.

- List the nursing measures used to maintain skin integrity when urine comes in contact with the skin.
  a. _____
  _____
  b. _____
  _____
  c. _____
  _____
  d. _____
  _____

- List two comfort measures for a client with the following sources of discomfort.
  a. Incontinence
    1. _____
    _____
    2. _____
    _____
  b. Dysuria
    1. _____
    _____
    2. _____
    _____
  c. Painful distention
    1. _____
    _____
    2. _____
    _____

EVALUATION

Client Care

- Client care evaluates the actual care delivered by the health care team based on the expected outcomes.

- The nurse evaluates for change in the _____, _____, and _____.

Client Expectations

- Client expectations evaluate care from the client's perspective.

- The nurse can also assist the client in redefining unrealistic goals when an impairment is not likely to be altered as completely as the client might like.

REVIEW QUESTIONS

The student should select the appropriate answer and cite the rationale for choosing that particular answer.

1. All of the following factors will influence the production of urine *except:*
   a. Anxiety
   b. Acute renal disease
   c. Febrile conditions
   d. Diuretic medications

   Answer:_____   Rationale: _____
   _____
   _____

2. Mrs. Rantz complains of leaking urine when she coughs or laughs. This is known as:
   a. Functional incontinence
   b. Stress incontinence
   c. Urge incontinence
   d. Reflex incontinence

   Answer:_____   Rationale: _____
   _____
   _____

3. Ms. Hathaway has a urinary tract infection. Which of the following symptoms would you expect her to exhibit?
   a. Proteinuria
   b. Dysuria
   c. Oliguria
   d. Polyuria

   Answer:_____   Rationale: _____
   _____
   _____

4. The nurse is working in the radiology department with a client who is having an intravenous pyelogram. Which of the following complaints by the client is an abnormal response?
   a. Shortness of breath and audible wheezing
   b. Feeling dizzy and warm with obvious facial flushing
   c. Thirst and feeling "worn out"
   d. Frequent, loose stools

   Answer:_____   Rationale: _____
   _____
   _____

5. The urinalysis of Ms. Hathaway reveals a high bacteria count. Ampicillin is prescribed for her urinary tract infection. The teaching plan for a UTI should include all of the following *except:*
   a. Drink at least 2000 ml of fluid daily.
   b. Always wipe perineum from front to back.
   c. Explain the possible side effects of medication.
   d. Drink plenty of orange and grapefruit juices.

   Answer:_____   Rationale: _____
   _____
   _____

SYNTHESIS MODEL FOR NURSING CARE PLAN FOR FUNCTIONAL INCONTINENCE

Imagine that you are Judi, the student nurse in the Care Plan on page 1410 of your text. Complete the *Assessment phase* of the synthesis model by writing your answers in the appropriate boxes of the model shown. Think about the following:

• What **knowledge** base was applied to the care of Judi's grandmother?

• In what way might Judi's previous **experience** assist in this case?

• What intellectual or professional **standards** were applied to Judi's grandmother?

• What critical thinking **attitudes** did you utilize in assessing Judi's grandmother?

• As you review the **assessment** what key areas did Judi cover?

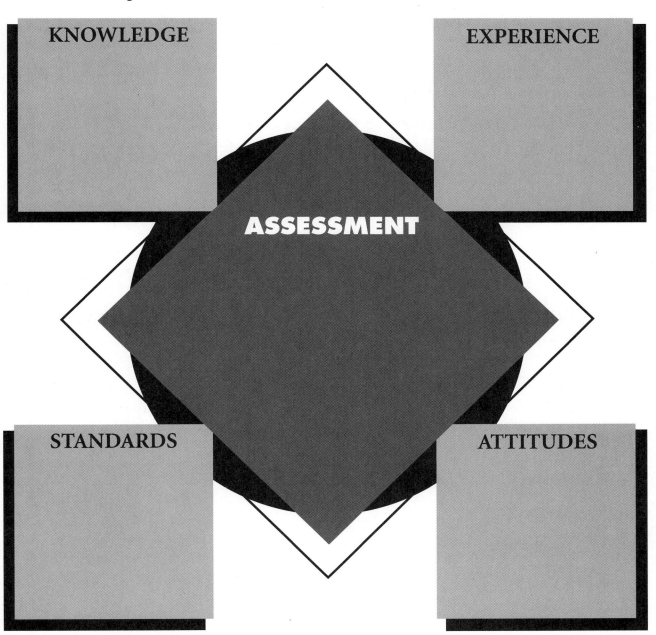

Chapter 44 *Synthesis Model for Nursing Care Plan for* Functional Incontinence.

See answers on page 568.

Bowel Elimination

To manage clients' elimination problems, the nurse must understand normal elimination and the factors that promote, impede, or cause alterations in elimination.

PRELIMINARY READING
Chapter 45, pp. 1436-1484

COMPREHENSIVE UNDERSTANDING

SCIENTIFIC KNOWLEDGE BASE

- The volume of fluids absorbed by the GI tract is high, making fluid balance a key function of the GI system.

- Summarize the functions of the following.
  a. Mouth: _____
  _____
  b. Esophagus: _____
  _____
  c. Stomach: _____
  _____
  d. Small intestine: _____
  _____
  e. Large intestine: _____
  _____

- Define the following terms and identify the portion of the GI tract to which they relate.
  a. *Masticate:* _____
  b. *Bolus:* _____
  c. *Refluxing:* _____
  d. *Peristalsis:* _____
  e. *Chyme:* _____
  f. *Haustral contractions:* _____
  g. *Flatus:* _____
  h. *Feces:* _____
  i. *Valsalva maneuver:* _____

- List and briefly describe the four functions of the colon.

  a. _____

  _____

  b. _____

  _____

  c. _____

  _____

  d. _____

  _____

- Indicate the correct sequence of mechanisms involved in normal defecation.

  _____ Increased intraabdominal pressure or the Valsalva maneuver occurs.

  _____ The external sphincter relaxes.

  _____ The internal sphincter relaxes and awareness of the need to defecate occurs.

  _____ The levator ani muscles relax.

  _____ Sensory nerves are stimulated via rectal distention.

NURSING KNOWLEDGE BASE

FACTORS AFFECTING BOWEL ELIMINATION

- Briefly describe the normal elimination pattern of an infant. _____

  _____

  _____

  _____

  _____

  _____

- List six changes that occur in the GI system of the older adult that impair normal digestion and elimination.

  a. _____

  _____

  b. _____

  _____

  c. _____

  _____

  d. _____

  _____

  e. _____

  _____

  f. _____

  _____

- Identify the mechanisms that cause high-fiber diets to promote elimination. _____

  _____

  _____

  _____

  _____

- List five types of foods that are considered high in fiber (bulk).

  a. _____

  _____

  b. _____

  _____

  c. _____

  _____

  d. _____

  _____

  e. _____

  _____

- Define *lactose intolerance:* _____

  _____

- Summarize how an inadequate intake of fluids can affect the character of feces. _____

  _____

  _____

  _____

  _____

  _____

- Physical activity _____ peristalsis; immobilization _____ peristalsis.

- Weakened abdominal and pelvic floor muscles impair the ability to _____ and to _____.

- List three diseases of the GI tract that may be associated with stress.

  a. _____

  _____

  b. _____

  _____

  c. _____

  _____

- Summarize how the stress response affects elimination. _____
_____
_____
_____

- List four personal elimination habits that influence bowel function.
  a. _____
  _____
  b. _____
  _____
  c. _____
  _____
  d. _____
  _____

- Describe how the position of squatting facilitates defecation. _____
_____
_____
_____
_____
_____

- List conditions that may result in painful defecation.
  a. _____
  _____
  b. _____
  _____
  c. _____
  _____
  d. _____
  _____

- Identify the common problems related to defecation that occur during pregnancy and explain why they occur. _____
_____
_____
_____

- Summarize the effects of anesthetic agents and peristalsis on defecation. _____
_____
_____
_____

- Describe the effect of each medication on elimination.
  a. Mineral oil: _____
  _____
  b. Dicyclomine HCl (Bentyl): _____
  c. Narcotics: _____
  _____
  d. Anticholinergics: _____
  _____
  e. Antibiotics: _____
  _____

- List three types of diagnostic tests for visualization of GI structures.
  a. _____
  _____
  b. _____
  _____
  c. _____
  _____

COMMON BOWEL ELIMINATION PROBLEMS

- List four factors that place a client at risk for elimination problems.
  a. _____
  _____
  b. _____
  _____
  c. _____
  _____
  d. _____
  _____

- Define *constipation:* _____
_____

- List and briefly describe four causes of constipation.
  a. _____
  _____
  b. _____
  _____
  c. _____
  _____
  d. _____
  _____

- List three groups of clients in whom constipation could pose a significant health hazard.

  a. _____

  b. _____

  c. _____

- Describe how the Valsalva maneuver can be avoided. _____

- Define *fecal impaction*: _____

- List four signs and symptoms of fecal impaction.

  a. _____

  b. _____

  c. _____

  d. _____

- Define *diarrhea:* _____

- Name the two major complications associated with diarrhea.

  a _____

  b _____

- List five conditions and the physiological effects that cause diarrhea.

  a. _____

  b. _____

  c. _____

  d. _____

  e. _____

- List six nursing responsibilities in the management of diarrhea.

  a. _____

  b. _____

  c. _____

  d. _____

  e _____

  f. _____

- Define *fecal incontinence:* _____

- *Flatulence* is _____.
  It is a common cause of _____,
  _____, and _____.

- Define *hemorrhoids:* _____

- List four conditions that cause hemorrhoids.

  a. _____

  b. _____

  c. _____

  d. _____

BOWEL DIVERSIONS

- Define the following:
  a. *Stoma:* _____

  _____

  b. *Ostomies:* _____

  _____

  c. *Ileostomy:* _____

  _____

  d. *Colostomy:* _____

  _____

  e. *Incontinent ostomy:* _____

  _____

  f. *Continent ostomy:* _____

  _____

- The location of the ostomy determines the consistency of the stool.

- Describe the normal consistency and appearance of feces the nurse would expect from:
  a. An ileostomy: _____

  _____

  b. A sigmoid colostomy: _____

  _____

  c. A transverse colostomy: _____

  _____

  d. An ascending colostomy: _____

  _____

- List and briefly describe three types of colostomy construction.
  a. _____

  _____

  b. _____

  _____

  c. _____

  _____

- Briefly describe the following surgical procedures that provide continence for selected colectomy clients.
  a. Ileoanal reservoir: _____

  _____

  _____

  b. Kock continent ileostomy: _____

  _____

  _____

  _____

- Identify a major physiological concern of osstomy clients. _____

  _____

  _____

  _____

NURSING PROCESS AND BOWEL ELIMINATION

ASSESSMENT

- List fourteen factors to include in a nursing history for clients with altered elimination status.
  a. _____

  _____

  b. _____

  _____

  c. _____

  _____

  d. _____

  _____

  e. _____

  _____

  f. _____

  _____

  g. _____

  _____

  h. _____

  _____

  i. _____

  _____

  j. _____

  _____

  k. _____

  _____

  l. _____

  _____

  m. _____

  _____

  n. _____

  _____

- Summarize the following steps for assessing the abdomen.
  a. Inspection: _____
  _____
  _____

  b. Auscultation: _____
  _____
  _____

  c. Palpation: _____
  _____
  _____
  _____

  d. Percussion: _____
  _____
  _____
  _____

- Summarize the assessment of the rectum.
  _____
  _____
  _____
  _____

- Briefly describe the appropriate technique for collecting a fecal specimen.
  _____
  _____
  _____
  _____
  _____
  _____

- Define *guaiac test:* _____
  _____

- Describe the normal fecal characteristics.
  a. Color: _____

  b. Odor: _____
  _____

- c. Consistency: _____
  _____

  d. Frequency: _____
  _____

  e. Amount: _____
  _____

  f. Shape: _____
  _____

  g. Constituents: _____
  _____

- Indicate the possible cause for each of the following fecal characteristics.
  a. White or clay color: _____
  _____

  b. Black or tarry: _____
  _____

  c. Melena: _____
  _____

  d. Liquid consistency: _____
  _____

  e. Narrow, pencil shaped: _____
  _____

- Define *endoscopy* or *gastroscopy:* _____
  _____

- List the nursing implications for a client prior to having an UGI endoscopy or gastroscopy.
  a. _____
  _____

  b. _____
  _____

  c. _____
  _____

  d. _____
  _____

  e. _____
  _____

  f. _____
  _____

- List the nursing implications related to a client undergoing a sigmoidoscopy or proctoscopy.

   a. _____

   _____

   b. _____

   _____

   c. _____

   _____

   d. _____

   _____

   e. _____

   _____

   f. _____

   _____

   g. _____

   _____

   h. _____

   _____

   i. _____

   _____

- List the nursing implications following the test.

   a _____

   _____

   b. _____

   _____

   c. _____

   _____

- Define *UGI:* _____

   _____

- List the nursing implications appropriate for a client prior to a UGI.

   a. _____

   _____

   b. _____

   _____

   c. _____

   _____

   d. _____

   _____

- Define *small bowel follow-through:*

   _____

   _____

NURSING DIAGNOSIS

- List six potential or actual nursing diagnoses for a client with alteration in bowel elimination.

   a. _____

   _____

   b. _____

   _____

   c. _____

   _____

   d. _____

   _____

   e. _____

   _____

   f. _____

   _____

PLANNING

- List seven goals appropriate for clients with elimination problems.

   a. _____

   _____

   b. _____

   _____

   c. _____

   _____

   d. _____

   _____

   e. _____

   _____

   f. _____

   _____

   g. _____

   _____

IMPLEMENTATION

Health Promotion

- Explain how the following can assist the client to evacuate their bowels.

   a. Squatting position: _____

   b. Positioning on the bedpan: _____

   _____

- Explain the proper technique for positioning a client on a bedpan. _____
  _____
  _____
  _____

- Identify the primary action of the following:
  a. Cathartics: _____
  _____
  b. Laxatives: _____
  _____
  c. Antidiarrheals: _____
  _____

- List four types of *laxatives* and *cathartics* and give an example of each.
  a. _____
  _____
  b. _____
  _____
  c. _____
  _____
  d. _____
  _____

Acute Care
- The primary reason for an *enema* is
  _____
  _____.

- Briefly describe the following types of enemas.
  a. Tap water: _____
  _____
  b. Normal saline: _____
  _____
  c. Soapsuds solution: _____
  _____
  d. Low-volume hypertonic saline: _____
  _____
  e. Oil-retention: _____
  _____
  f. Carminative: _____
  _____
  g. Harris flush: _____
  _____
  h. Medicated: _____
  _____

- Explain the physician's order, "Give enemas till clear." _____
  _____
  _____
  _____

- List three complications of digital removal of stool.
  a. _____
  _____
  b. _____
  _____
  c. _____
  _____

CARE OF OSTOMIES
- List five factors to consider when selecting a pouching system for an ostomate.
  a. _____
  _____
  b. _____
  _____
  c. _____
  _____
  d. _____
  _____
  e. _____
  _____

- List six contraindications to colostomy irrigation.
  a. _____
  _____
  b. _____
  _____
  c. _____
  _____
  d. _____
  _____
  e. _____
  _____
  f. _____
  _____

Chapter 45: Bowel Elimination   319

- List four reasons to insert a nasogastric tube for decompression.

  a. _____

  _____

  b. _____

  _____

  c. _____

  _____

  d. _____

  _____

- Explain how the salem sump tube works.

  _____

  _____

  _____

  _____

- Explain how the nurse would provide comfort to a client with a NG tube. _____

  _____

  _____

  _____

- Explain how an NG tube can cause distention and how it can be prevented. _____

  _____

  _____

Restorative and Continuing Care

- Summarize the goals of a bowel training program. _____

  _____

  _____

  _____

  _____

  _____

  _____

- Summarize the diet restrictions for ostomy clients. _____

  _____

  _____

  _____

  _____

  _____

  _____

- Describe two exercises that help prevent of constipation in the bedridden client.

  a. _____

  _____

  b. _____

  _____

- Describe two nursing interventions that promote comfort for clients who experience the following:

  a. *Hemorrhoids:*

  1. _____

  _____

  2. _____

  _____

  b. *Flatulence:*

  1. _____

  _____

  2. _____

  _____

  c. Skin breakdown:

  1. _____

  _____

  2. _____

  _____

- List and describe six interventions that may assist in restoring self-concept in a client with bowel elimination problems.

  a. _____

  _____

  b. _____

  _____

  c. _____

  _____

  d. _____

  _____

  e. _____

  _____

  f. _____

  _____

EVALUATION

Client Care

- Client care evaluates the actual care delivered by the health team based on expected outcomes.

- The client is the only one who is able to determine if the bowel elimination problems have been relieved and which therapies were the most effective.

Client Expectations
- Client expectations evaluate care from the client's perspective.

REVIEW QUESTIONS

The student should select the appropriate answer and cite the rationale for choosing that particular answer.

1. Most nutrients and electrolytes are absorbed in the:
   a. Esophagus
   b. Small intestine
   c. Colon
   d. Stomach

   Answer:_____   Rationale: _____
   _____
   _____

2. Which of the following should be included in the teaching plan for the client who is scheduled for a gastroscopy?
   a. Avoid eating and drinking for 2 to 4 hours after the test
   b. A cleansing enema will be given the evening before the procedure
   c. General anesthetic is usually used for the procedure
   d. Moderate abdominal pain is common after the procedure

   Answer:_____   Rationale: _____
   _____
   _____

3. Mrs. Anthony is concerned about her breast-fed infant's stool, stating that it is yellow instead of brown. The nurse explains to Mrs. Anthony that:
   a. A change to formula may be necessary
   b. Her infant is dehydrated and she should increase his fluid intake
   c. The stool is normal for an infant
   d. It will be necessary to send a stool specimen to the lab

   Answer:_____   Rationale: _____
   _____
   _____

4. After positioning a client on the bedpan, the nurse should:
   a. Leave the head of the bed flat
   b. Raise the head of the bed 30 degrees
   c. Raise the head of the bed to a 90-degree angle
   d. Raise the bed to the highest working level

   Answer:_____   Rationale: _____
   _____
   _____

5. The physician has ordered a cleansing enema for 7-year-old Michael. The nurse realizes the maximum volume to be given would be:
   a. 100 to 150 ml
   b. 150 to 250 ml
   c. 300 to 500 ml
   d. 600 to 700 ml

   Answer:_____   Rationale: _____
   _____
   _____

SYNTHESIS MODEL FOR NURSING CARE PLAN FOR CONSTIPATION

Imagine that you are Javier, the nurse in the Care Plan on page 1457 of your text. Complete the *Planning phase* of the synthesis model by writing your answers in the appropriate boxes of the model shown. Think about the following:

• In developing Larry's plan of care, what **knowledge** did Javier apply?

• In what way might Javier's previous **experience** assist in developing a plan of care for Larry?

• When developing a plan of care what intellectual and professional **standards** were applied?

• What critical thinking **attitudes** might have been applied in developing a plan for Larry?

• How will Javier accomplish the goals?

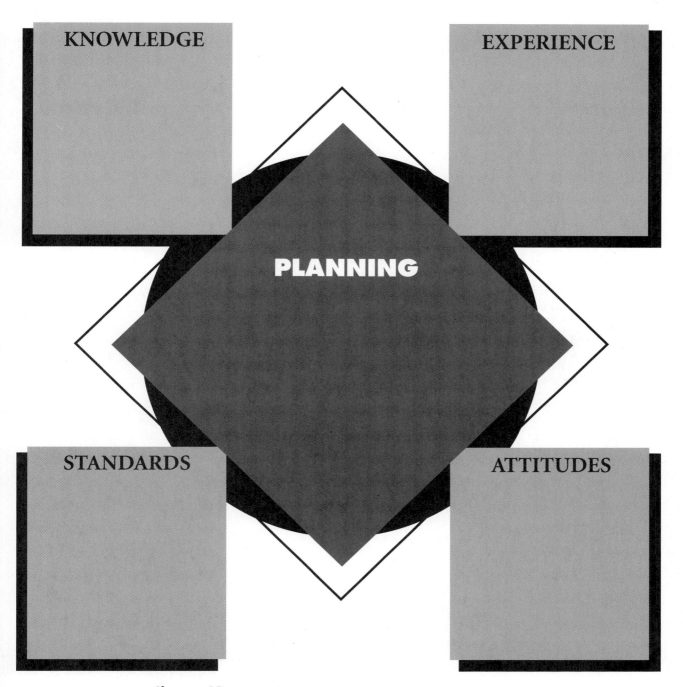

KNOWLEDGE

EXPERIENCE

PLANNING

STANDARDS

ATTITUDES

Chapter 45 *Synthesis Model for Nursing Care Plan for* Constipation.

See answers on page 569.

Mobility and Immobility

To maintain optimal physical mobility, the nervous, muscular, and skeletal systems of the body must be intact and functioning.

PRELIMINARY READING
Chapter 46, pp. 1485-1543

COMPREHENSIVE UNDERSTANDING
• *Mobility* refers to _____.

SCIENTIFIC KNOWLEDGE BASE

PHYSIOLOGY AND PRINCIPLES OF BODY MECHANICS
• Define the following:
 a. *Body mechanics:* _____
 b. *Body alignment:* _____
 c. *Body balance:* _____

• Balance is required for _____, _____, and
 _____.

• The ability to balance can be compromised by _____, _____,
 _____, and _____.

Gravity and Friction
• Define *friction*: _____

• List two techniques that minimize friction.
 a. _____
 b. _____

REGULATION OF MOVEMENT
• List three systems responsible for coordinating body movements.
 a. _____
 b. _____
 c. _____

Skeletal System

- List four functions of the skeletal system.

  a. _____
  _____

  b. _____
  _____

  c. _____
  _____

  d. _____
  _____

- Describe the following:

  a. *Long bones:* _____
  _____

  b. *Short bones:* _____
  _____

  c. *Pathological fractures:* _____
  _____

  d. *Flat bones:* _____
  _____

  e. *Irregular bones:* _____
  _____

- *Leverage* is _____
  _____

- The characteristics of bone include
  _____, _____,
  and _____.

- Describe the following types of joints and give an example of each.

  a. *Synostotic joint:* _____
  _____

  b. *Cartilaginous joint:* _____
  _____

  c. *Fibrous joint:* _____
  _____

  d. *Synovial joint:* _____
  _____

- *Ligaments* are _____
  _____

- *Tendons* are _____
  _____

- *Cartilage* is _____
  _____

Skeletal Muscle

- Briefly describe how skeletal muscles affect movement. _____
  _____
  _____
  _____

- Briefly describe the two types of muscle contractions.

  a. *Isotonic:* _____
  _____

  b. *Isometric:* _____
  _____

- Define *posture* and name the associated muscles. _____
  _____
  _____
  _____

- Briefly explain how posture and movement are coordinated and regulated. _____
  _____
  _____
  _____

Nervous System

- Briefly describe how movement and posture are regulated by the nervous system.
  _____
  _____
  _____
  _____

- Define *neurotransmitter:* _____
  _____

PATHOLOGICAL INFLUENCES ON MOBILITY

- Briefly explain how the following pathological conditions affect mobility.
  a. Postural abnormalities: _____
  _____
  _____
  _____

  b. Impaired muscle development: _____
  _____
  _____
  _____

  c. Damage to the central nervous system:
  _____
  _____
  _____

  d. Direct trauma to the musculoskeletal system: _____
  _____
  _____
  _____

NURSING KNOWLEDGE BASE

MOBILITY-IMMOBILITY

- Define *bed rest:* _____
  _____

- *Impaired physical mobility* is defined as
  _____
  _____

Systemic Effects

- When there is an alteration in mobility, each body system is at risk. Identify at least two hazards of immobility for each area.
  a. Metabolic changes:
     a. _____
     _____
     b. _____
     _____

  b. Respiratory changes:
     a. _____
     _____
     b. _____
     _____

  c. Cardiovascular changes:
     a. _____
     _____
     b. _____
     _____

  d. Musculoskeletal changes:
     a. _____
     _____
     b. _____
     _____

  e. Urinary elimination changes:
     a. _____
     _____
     b. _____
     _____

  f. Integumentary changes:
     a. _____
     _____
     b. _____
     _____

- Identify the most common psychological changes that occur with immobilization.
  _____
  _____
  _____
  _____

Developmental Changes

- Identify the descriptive characteristics of body alignment and mobility related to the following developmental stages:
  a. Infants: _____
  _____
  _____
  _____

  b. Toddlers: _____
  _____
  _____
  _____

  c. Preschool children: _____
  _____
  _____
  _____

  d. Adolescents: _____
  _____
  _____
  _____

e. Adults: _____

_____

_____

f. Older adults: _____

_____

_____

_____

NURSING PROCESS FOR IMPAIRED BODY ALIGNMENT AND MOBILITY

ASSESSMENT

- Briefly describe the four major areas for assessment of client mobility.

  a. *Range of motion:* _____

  _____

  b. *Gait:* _____

  _____

  c. *Exercise and activity tolerance:* _____

  _____

  d. *Body alignment:* _____

  _____

Immobility

- Briefly describe the physiological hazards of immobility in relation to the following systems:

  a. Metabolic: _____

  _____

  _____

  b. Respiratory: _____

  _____

  _____

  c. Cardiovascular: _____

  _____

  _____

  d. Musculoskeletal: _____

  _____

  _____

  e. Integumentary: _____

  _____

  _____

  f. Gastrointestinal: _____

  _____

  _____

- List four areas of assessment for the older adult.

  a. _____

  _____

  b. _____

  _____

  c. _____

  _____

  d. _____

  _____

NURSING DIAGNOSIS

- List six actual or potential nursing diagnoses related to an immobilized or partially immobilized client.

  a _____

  _____

  b. _____

  _____

  c. _____

  _____

  d. _____

  _____

  e. _____

  _____

  f. _____

  _____

PLANNING

- The nurse plans therapies according to severity of risks to the client, and the plan is individualized according to the client's

  _____, _____,

  and _____.

IMPLEMENTATION

Health Promotion

- List the criteria the nurse needs to assess before lifting a client or object. _____

  _____

  _____

  _____

  _____

  _____

Chapter 46: Mobility and Immobility   327

Exercise
- Briefly explain the benefits of exercise.

  _____

  _____

  _____

  _____

Acute Care
- Identify two nursing interventions to meet each of the following goals for the immobilized client.

  a. Maintain optimal nutritional (metabolic) state:

  1. _____

  _____

  2. _____

  _____

  b. Promote lung expansion of chest and lungs:

  1. _____

  _____

  2. _____

  _____

  c. Prevent stasis of pulmonary secretions:

  1. _____

  _____

  2. _____

  _____

  d. Maintain patent airway:

  1. _____

  _____

  2. _____

  _____

  e. Reduce orthostatic hypotension:

  1. _____

  _____

  2. _____

  _____

  f. Reduce cardiac workload:

  1. _____

  _____

  2. _____

  _____

  g. Prevent thrombus formation:

  1. _____

  _____

  2. _____

  _____

  h. Maintain muscle strength and joint mobility:

  1. _____

  _____

  2. _____

  _____

  i. Prevent pressure ulcers:

  1. _____

  _____

  2. _____

  _____

  j. Maintain normal elimination patterns:

  1. _____

  _____

  2. _____

  _____

  k. Maintain usual psychosocial state:

  1. _____

  _____

  2. _____

  _____

- Identify two nursing interventions for the following immobilized clients.

  a. Young child

  1. _____

  _____

  2. _____

  _____

  b. Older adult

  1. _____

  _____

  2. _____

  _____

- Indicate the correct use for each positioning device listed.

Device	Uses
Pillow	
Footboard	
Trochanter roll	
Sandbag	
Hand-wrist splints	
Trapeze bar	
Restraints	
Side rails	
Bed board	

- List four areas the nurse needs to consider to determine if assistance is required when moving a client in bed.

  a. _____

  _____

  b. _____

  _____

  c. _____

  _____

  d. _____

  _____

- List some general guidelines to apply in any transfer procedure. _____

  _____

  _____

  _____

  _____

  _____

  _____

  _____

Restorative Care

- The goal of restorative care is to _____

  _____.

- Instrumental activities of daily living (IADLs) are _____

  _____.

- List the common trouble areas for the clients in the following positions.

Positions Give a brief description of the position.	Trouble Areas
Fowler's	a.
	b.
	c.
	d.
	e.
	f.
	g.
Supine	a.
	b.
	c.
	d.
	e.
	f.
	g.
	h.
Prone	a.
	b.
	c.
	d.
Side-lying	a.
	b.
	c.
	d.
	e.
Sims'	a.
	b.
	c.
	d.

Joint Mobility

- Indicate the type of joint and range of motion exercises for the body parts listed in the table below:

Body Part	Type of Joint	Type of Movement
Neck		
Shoulder		
Elbow		
Forearm		
Wrist		
Fingers and thumb		
Hip		
Knee		
Ankle and foot		
Toes		

Walking

- Identify the steps the nurse should take to prepare to assist a client to walk. _____
  _____
  _____
  _____
  _____

- Describe how the nurse would assist clients with the following:
  a. *Hemiplegia:* _____
  _____

  b. *Hemiparesis:* _____
  _____

☙ EVALUATION

Client Care

- Client care evaluates the actual care delivered by the health care team based on expected outcomes.

- The optimal outcomes are the client's ability to maintain or improve body alignment and joint mobility.

Client Expectations

- Client expectations evaluate care from the client's perspective.

REVIEW QUESTIONS

The student should select the appropriate answer and cite the rationale for choosing that particular answer.

1. The nurse would expect all of the following physiological effects of exercise on the body systems *except:*
   a. Decreased cardiac output
   b. Increased respiratory rate and depth
   c. Increased muscle tone, size, and strength
   d. Change in metabolic rate

Answer:_____   Rationale: _____
_____
_____

2. Which of the following is a potential hazard that the nurse should assess when the client is in the prone position?
   a. Unprotected pressure points at the sacrum and heels
   b. Internal rotation of the shoulder
   c. Increased cervical flexion
   d. Plantar flexion

   Answer:_____   Rationale: _____
   _____
   _____

3. Which of the following is a physiological effect of prolonged bed rest?
   a. A decrease in urinary excretion of nitrogen
   b. An increase in cardiac output
   c. A decrease in lean body mass
   d. A decrease in lung expansion

   Answer:_____   Rationale: _____
   _____
   _____

4. All of the following measures are used to assess for deep vein thrombosis *except:*
   a. Measuring the circumference of each leg daily, placing the tape measure at the midpoint of the knee
   b. Observing the dorsal aspect of lower extremities for redness, warmth, and tenderness
   c. Asking the client about the presence of calf pain
   d. Checking for a positive Homans' sign

   Answer:_____   Rationale: _____
   _____
   _____

5. Which of the following is an appropriate intervention to maintain the respiratory system of the immobilized client?
   a. Turn the client every 4 hours
   b. Maintain a maximum fluid intake of 1500 ml per day
   c. Apply an abdominal binder continuously while in bed
   d. Encourage the use of an incentive spirometer

   Answer:_____   Rationale: _____
   _____
   _____

SYNTHESIS MODEL FOR NURSING CARE PLAN FOR IMPAIRED MOBILITY

Imagine that you are the student nurse, in the Care Plan on page 1512 of your text. Complete the *evaluation phase* of the synthesis model by writing your answers in the appropriate boxes of the model shown. Think about the following:

- What **knowledge** did you apply in evaluating Miss Adams' care?

- In what way might your previous **experience** influence your evaluation of Miss Adams?

- During evaluation, what intellectual and professional **standards** were applied to Miss Adams' care?

- In what ways does critical thinking **attitudes** play a role in how you approach evaluation of Miss Adam's care?

- How might you adjust Miss Adam's care?

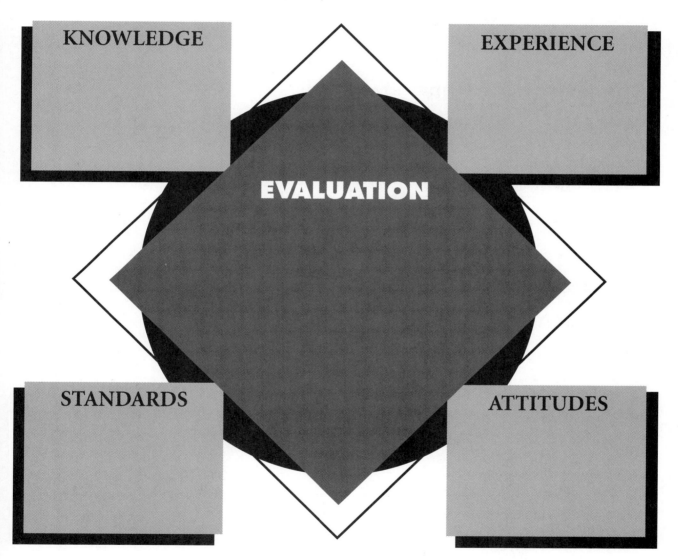

KNOWLEDGE

EXPERIENCE

EVALUATION

STANDARDS

ATTITUDES

Chapter 46 *Synthesis Model for Nursing Care Plan for Impaired Mobility.*

See answers on page 570.

Skin Integrity and Wound Care

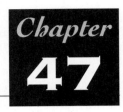

Chapter 47

 Injury to the integument poses risks to safety and triggers a complex healing response.

PRELIMINARY READING
Chapter 47, pp. 1544-1629

COMPREHENSIVE UNDERSTANDING

SCIENTIFIC KNOWLEDGE BASE

NORMAL INTEGUMENT

- There are two principal layers of the integument.
  a. _____
  b. _____

- Describe the function of each of the following.
  a. *Epidermis:* _____
  b. *Dermis:* _____

- List the normal changes that occur in older adults. _____
  _____
  _____
  _____

PRESSURE ULCERS

- Define *pressure ulcer:* _____

- Define the following terms:
  a. *Tissue ischemia:* _____
  b. *Blanching:* _____
  c. *Capillary closing pressure:* _____
  d. *Normal reactive hyperemia:* _____
  e. *Abnormal reactive hyperemia:* _____

- Briefly explain how the following factors contribute to an increased risk for pressure ulcers.
  a. Impaired sensory input: _____
  _____
  _____
  _____

  b. Impaired motor function: _____
  _____
  _____
  _____

  c. Alterations in level of consciousness:
  _____
  _____
  _____
  _____

  d. Orthopedic devices: _____
  _____
  _____
  _____

- Identify the three elements of pressure ulcer development.
  a. _____
  b. _____
  _____
  c. _____
  _____

- Identify the most common sites of pressure ulcers development and explain why.
  _____
  _____
  _____
  _____
  _____
  _____

CLASSIFICATION OF PRESSURE ULCER STAGING OR COLOR

- Staging systems for pressure ulcers are based on the depth of tissue destroyed. Briefly describe each stage.
  I: _____
  _____

II: _____
_____

III: _____
_____

IV: _____
_____

- Describe the following wound classifications by color.
  a. Black wounds: _____
  _____
  b. Yellow wounds: _____
  _____
  c. Red wounds: _____
  _____

- Describe the physiological process involved with wound healing.
  a. *Primary intention:* _____
  _____
  _____
  _____

  b. *Secondary intention:* _____
  _____
  _____
  _____

- Healing by primary intention occurs in three stages. Explain each one.
  a. Inflammatory phase (reaction):
  _____
  _____
  _____

  b. Proliferative phase (regeneration):
  _____
  _____
  _____
  _____

  c. Maturation (remodeling): _____
  _____
  _____
  _____

- Explain the following terms related to healing by secondary intention.
  a. *Granulation tissue:* _____
  _____
  _____
  _____

  b. *Epithelization:* _____
  _____
  _____
  _____

  c. *Wound contraction:* _____
  _____
  _____
  _____

- Briefly explain the following complications of wound healing.
  a. *Hemorrhage:* _____
  _____
  _____
  _____
  _____

  b. *Infection:* _____
  _____
  _____
  _____
  _____
  _____

  c. *Dehiscence:* _____
  _____
  _____
  _____
  _____
  _____

  d. *Evisceration:* _____
  _____
  _____
  _____
  _____
  _____

  e. *Fistulas:* _____
  _____
  _____
  _____
  _____
  _____

  f. Delayed wound healing: _____
  _____
  _____
  _____
  _____

- Identify and define the types of wound drainage.
  a. _____
  _____

  b. _____
  _____

  c. _____
  _____

  d. _____
  _____

NURSING KNOWLEDGE BASE

PREDICTION AND PREVENTION OF PRESSURE ULCERS

- Explain the following risk assessment scales.
  a. Norton scale: _____
  _____
  _____

  b. Gosnell scale: _____
  _____
  _____

  c. Braden scale: _____
  _____
  _____

- Identify the prevalence of pressure ulcers in the following settings.
  a. Acute care: _____

  _____

  _____

  _____

  b. Restorative care: _____

  _____

  _____

  _____

  c. Home care: _____

  _____

  _____

  _____

FACTORS INFLUENCING PRESSURE ULCER FORMATION AND WOUND HEALING

- Describe why each of the following factors increase the client's risk for pressure ulcer development.
  a. *Shearing force:* _____

  _____

  _____

  _____

  _____

  b. Friction: _____

  _____

  _____

  _____

  _____

  c. Moisture: _____

  _____

  _____

  _____

  _____

  d. Nutrition: _____

  _____

  _____

  _____

  _____

  _____

  e. *Anemia* _____

  _____

  _____

  _____

  _____

  f. *Cachexia:* _____

  _____

  _____

  _____

  g. Obesity: _____

  _____

  _____

  _____

  _____

  _____

  h. Infection: _____

  _____

  _____

  _____

  _____

  i. Impaired peripheral circulation: _____

  _____

  _____

  _____

  _____

  j. Age: _____

  _____

  _____

  _____

PSYCHOSOCIAL IMPACT OF WOUNDS

- Identify the factors that may affect the client's perception of the wound.

  _____

  _____

  _____

  _____

  _____

CRITICAL THINKING
SYNTHESIS
NURSING PROCESS

ASSESSMENT

• Because of the multiple etiological factors, pressure ulcers assessment includes several dimensions.

• A benefit of the predictive instruments is

_____

_____

_____

_____ .

• Identify nursing assessment data for the following dimensions.

a. Skin: _____

_____

_____

_____

b. Mobility: _____

_____

_____

_____

c. Nutritional status: _____

_____

_____

_____

d. Pain: _____

_____

_____

_____

• Briefly explain how the assessment differs under the following conditions.

a. In the emergency setting: _____

_____

_____

b. In the stable setting: _____

_____

_____

• Explain how the nurse assesses the following:

a. Wound appearance: _____

_____

_____

_____

b. Drains: _____

_____

_____

_____

c. Wound closures: _____

_____

_____

_____

d. Palpation of the wound: _____

_____

_____

_____

NURSING DIAGNOSIS

• List three nursing diagnoses related to impaired skin integrity.

a. _____

_____

b. _____

_____

c. _____

_____

PLANNING

• List six possible goals for the client at risk for pressure ulcers.

a. _____

_____

b. _____

_____

c. _____

_____

d. _____

_____

e. _____

_____

f. _____

_____

Health Promotion

- Briefly explain the following nursing interventions for the prevention of pressure ulcers.

  a. Hygiene and skin care: _____

  _____

  _____

  _____

  b. Positioning: _____

  _____

  _____

  _____

  c. Support surfaces: _____

  _____

  _____

  _____

Acute Care

- Aspects of pressure ulcer treatment include local care of the wound and supportive measures. Briefly explain the principles of wound care in relation to debridement.

  _____

  _____

  _____

  _____

- Describe the three methods of debridement.

  a. _____

  _____

  b. _____

  _____

  c. _____

  _____

- Define *moist wound-healing* and list the appropriate steps to take to accomplish it.

  _____

  _____

  _____

  _____

  _____

  _____

- Identify other methods achieving local wound healing. _____

  _____

  _____

  _____

- Describe two nursing interventions that relate to nutritional status in the treatment of pressure ulcers.

  a. _____

  _____

  b. _____

  _____

- First aid for wounds includes the following. Briefly explain each one.

  a. Hemostasis: _____

  _____

  _____

  _____

  b. Cleansing: _____

  _____

  _____

  _____

  c. Protecting: _____

  _____

  _____

  _____

- List the purposes for dressings.

  a. _____

  _____

  b. _____

  _____

  c. _____

  _____

  d. _____

  _____

  e. _____

  _____

  f. _____

  _____

  g. _____

  _____

Chapter 47: Skin Integrity and Wound Care   339

- List the clinical guidelines to use when selecting the appropriate dressing.

  a. _____
  _____

  b. _____
  _____

  c. _____
  _____

  d. _____
  _____

  e. _____
  _____

  f. _____
  _____

  g. _____
  _____

- Briefly describe the following types of dressings and their uses.

  a. Gauze: _____
  _____
  _____
  _____

  b. Wet -to-dry: _____
  _____
  _____
  _____

  c. Film: _____
  _____
  _____
  _____

  d. Hydrocolloid (HCD): _____
  _____
  _____
  _____

  e. Hydrogel: _____
  _____
  _____
  _____

  f. Alginate: _____
  _____
  _____
  _____

- To prepare for a dressing change, the nurse must know _____,
  _____, and
  _____.

- The physician's order for changing a dressing should indicate the _____,
  _____, and
  _____ to the wound.

- In relation to sterile versus clean dressing, the AHCPR 1994 clinical practice guidelines recommend that _____
  be used on pressure ulcers.

- The first step in packing a wound is to assess the _____,
  _____, and
  _____ of the wound.

- Summarize the principles of packing a wound. _____
  _____
  _____
  _____
  _____
  _____

- To secure the dressing the nurse considers the _____,
  _____,
  _____,
  _____, and
  _____.

- Identify three principles that are important when cleaning an incision.

  a. _____
  _____

  b. _____
  _____

  c. _____
  _____

- Irrigation of a wound requires _____
  _____ technique.

- Irrigations are used for _____
  _____.

- Summarize the nursing responsibilities for suture care. _____
_____
_____
_____
_____

- The most important principle in suture removal is to _____
_____.

- Explain the purpose for drainage evacuation.
_____
_____
_____
_____

- Explain the benefits of binders and bandages.
  a. _____
  _____
  b. _____
  _____
  c. _____
  _____
  d. _____
  _____
  e. _____
  _____
  f. _____
  _____

- List the nursing responsibilities when applying a bandage or binder.
  a. _____
  _____
  b. _____
  _____
  c. _____
  _____
  d. _____
  _____

- Describe the following types of binders.
  a. Abdominal: _____
  _____
  b. T: _____
  _____

- Sling supports are used for _____
_____

- Summarize the body's responses to heat and cold. _____
_____
_____
_____
_____
_____

- Describe the physiologic responses to the following:
  a. Heat applications: _____

  b. Cold applications: _____
  _____

- List the factors that influence heat and cold tolerance.
  a. _____
  _____
  b. _____
  _____
  c. _____
  _____
  d. _____
  _____
  e. _____
  _____
  f. _____
  _____

- Prior to applying heat or cold therapies the nurse assesses for temperature tolerance by
_____
_____
_____
_____
_____

- Cold therapy is contraindicated for
_____
_____.

- Heat and cold applications can be administered in _____ or
_____ forms.

Chapter 47: Skin Integrity and Wound Care   341

- Dry and moist applications each have advantages and disadvantages. Give some examples of each.
  a. Moist: _____
  _____
  _____
  _____

  b. Dry: _____
  _____
  _____
  _____

- Explain the following types of heat and cold applications, and give the nursing implications for each.
  a. Warm soaks: _____
  _____
  _____
  _____

  b. Sitz baths: _____
  _____
  _____
  _____

  c. Aquathermia pads: _____
  _____
  _____
  _____

  d. Warm air blower: _____
  _____
  _____
  _____

  e. Commercial hot packs: _____
  _____
  _____
  _____

  f. Cold, moist, and dry compresses: _____
  _____
  _____
  _____

✎ EVALUATION

Client Care
- Client care evaluates the actual care delivered by the health care team based on the expected outcomes.

- The optimal outcomes are to _____,
  _____, and
  _____.

Client Expectations
- Client expectations evaluate care from the client's perspective.

- Clients with chronic wounds are often cared for in the home and have certain expectations about their level of _____,
  _____, _____,
  and _____.

REVIEW QUESTIONS

The student should select the appropriate answer and cite the rationale for choosing that particular answer.

1. Ischemia is defined as:
   a. Increased tissue buildup during the healing process
   b. A deficiency of blood supply to a part
   c. Decreased fluid to the tissues
   d. Increased irritability of nerves

   Answer: _____   Rationale: _____
   _____
   _____

2. Mr. Post is in a Fowler's position to improve his oxygenation status. The nurse notes that he frequently slides down in the bed and needs to be repositioned. Mr. Post is at risk for developing a pressure ulcer on his coccyx because of:
   a. Friction
   b. Shearing force
   c. Maceration
   d. Impaired peripheral circulation

   Answer: _____   Rationale: _____
   _____
   _____

3. Which of the following is *not* a subscale on the Braden scale for predicting pressure ulcer risk?
   a. Age
   b. Sensory perception
   c. Moisture
   d. Activity

   Answer:_____ Rationale: _____
   _____
   _____

4. Which of these clients has a nutritional risk for pressure ulcer development?
   a. Client A has an albumin level of 3.5.
   b. Client B has a hemoglobin level within normal limits.
   c. Client C has a protein intake of 0.5 gm per kilogram per day.
   d. Client D has a body weight that is 5% greater than his ideal weight.

   Answer:_____ Rationale: _____
   _____
   _____

5. Mrs. Greer is an immobilized client. Which of the following is *not* a factor that will increase her risk of pressure development?
   a. She has unrelieved pressure to her hip of greater than 32 mm Hg.
   b. She displays reactive hyperemia on her coccyx that lasts for 30 minutes after being turned to her side.
   c. She has low intensity pressure over a long period to her heels as a result of elastic stockings.
   d. She is positioned so that she has an unequal distribution of body weight.

   Answer:_____ Rationale: _____
   _____
   _____

6. Mr. Perkins has a stage II ulcer of his right heel. What would be the most appropriate treatment for this ulcer?
   a. Apply a thick layer of enzymatic ointment to the ulcer and the surrounding skin.
   b. Apply a calcium alginate dressing and change when strike through is noted.
   c. Apply a heat lamp to the area for 20 minutes twice daily.
   d. Apply a hydrocolloid dressing and change it as necessary.

   Answer:_____ Rationale: _____
   _____
   _____

SYNTHESIS MODEL FOR NURSING CARE PLAN FOR IMPAIRED SKIN INTEGRITY

Imagine that you are the student nurse in the Care Plan on page 1577 of your text. Complete the *Assessment phase* of the synthesis model by writing your answers in the appropriate boxes of the model shown. Think about the following:

- What **knowledge** base was applied to Mrs. Stein?

- In what way might your previous **experience** assist you in this case?

- What intellectual or professional standards were applied to Mrs. Stein?

- What critical thinking **attitudes** did you use in assessing Mrs. Stein?

- As you review your **assessment** what key areas did you cover?

are 343

grity and Wound Care

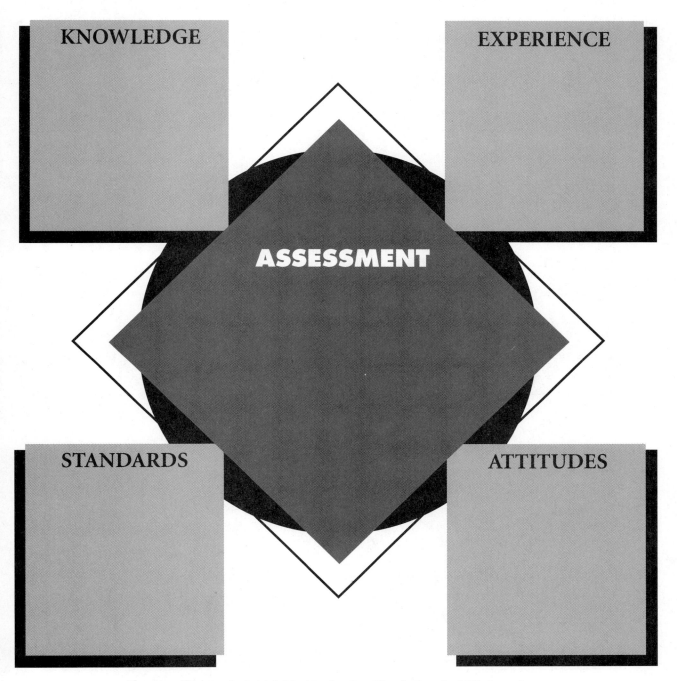

KNOWLEDGE

EXPERIENCE

ASSESSMENT

STANDARDS

ATTITUDES

Chapter 47 *Synthesis Model for Nursing Care Plan for* Impaired Skin Integrity.

See answers on page 571.

Sensory Alterations

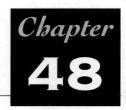

Many sources inside and outside of the body provides us with stimulation. We use the senses of sight (visual), hearing (auditory), touch (tactile), smell (olfactory), and taste (gustatory) to process the information.

PRELIMINARY READING

Chapter 48, pp. 1630-1658

COMPREHENSIVE UNDERSTANDING

SCIENTIFIC KNOWLEDGE BASE

NORMAL SENSATION

- List and briefly explain the three functional components necessary for any sensory experience.
  - a. _____
  - b. _____
  - c. _____

SENSORY ALTERATIONS

- The types of sensory alterations commonly seen by the nurse are _____, _____, and _____.

- When a client suffers from more than one sensory alteration, the ability to function and relate effectively within the environment is seriously impaired.

- List eight factors that influence sensory function and give an example of each.
  - a. _____
  - b. _____
  - c. _____
  - d. _____
  - e. _____
  - f. _____
  - g. _____
  - h. _____

- Define *sensory deficit:* _____

- List the three major types of sensory deprivation and give an example of each.
  a. _____
     _____
  b. _____
  c. _____
     _____

- Define *sensory overload:* _____
  _____

- Identify the behavioral changes that are associated with sensory overload. _____
  _____
  _____
  _____
  _____

NURSING KNOWLEDGE BASE

FACTORS AFFECTING SENSORY FUNCTION

- Explain how and why the following factors affect sensory function.
  a. Persons at risk: _____
     _____
     _____
     _____

  b. Meaningful stimuli: _____
     _____
     _____
     _____

  c. Amount of stimuli: _____
     _____
     _____
     _____

  d. Family factors: _____
     _____
     _____
     _____

  e. Environmental factors: _____
     _____
     _____
     _____

  f. Hazards: _____
     _____
     _____
     _____

  g. Cultural factors: _____
     _____
     _____
     _____

CRITICAL THINKING SYNTHESIS NURSING PROCESS

ASSESSMENT

- The nurse collects a history that assesses the client's current sensory status and the degree to which a sensory deficit affects the client's
  _____, _____, _____,
  _____, and _____.

- When assessing the client's mental status the nurse needs to evaluate each of the following Give an example of each.
  a. Physical appearance and behavior:_____
     _____
     _____
     _____

  b. Cognitive ability: _____
     _____
     _____
     _____

  c. Emotional stability: _____
     _____
     _____
     _____

- Complete the grid by describing at least one assessment technique for the identified sensory function and the behaviors for an adult and child that would indicate a sensory deficit.

Sense	Assessment Technique	Child Behavior	Adult Behavior
Vision			
Hearing			
Touch			
Smell			
Taste			
Position sense			

- When assessing the client's functional abilities, the nurse assesses _____, _____, _____, and _____ activities.

- Identify three questions that the nurse may ask the client to describe a sensory deficit.

  a. _____
     _____
  b. _____
     _____
  c. _____
     _____

- Identify some questions the nurse may ask the client to elicit knowledge about the onset and duration of sensory alteration. _____
  _____
  _____
  _____
  _____
  _____

- The nurse also assesses a client's compliance with routine health screening. Identify three questions related to this.

  a. _____
     _____
  b. _____
     _____
  c. _____
     _____

- Clients with existing sensory deficits often develop alternative ways of communicating. Give two examples.

  a. _____
  _____

  b. _____
  _____

- Define the following types of aphasia.
  a. *Expressive:* _____
  _____

  b. *Receptive:* _____
  _____

NURSING DIAGNOSIS

- List six actual or potential nursing diagnoses for a client with sensory alterations.

  a. _____
  _____

  b. _____
  _____

  c. _____
  _____

  d. _____
  _____

  e. _____
  _____

  f. _____
  _____

PLANNING

- List eight goals appropriate for clients with sensory alterations.

  a. _____
  _____

  b. _____
  _____

  c. _____
  _____

  d. _____
  _____

  e. _____
  _____

  f. _____
  _____

  g. _____
  _____

  h. _____
  _____

IMPLEMENTATION

- The most effective interventions enable the client with sensory alterations to function safely with existing deficits.

Health promotion
- List the three recommended screening interventions.

  a. _____
  _____

  b. _____
  _____

  c. _____
  _____

- The most common visual problem is _____
  _____.

- Explain how hearing loss occurs from loud noises. _____
  _____
  _____
  _____
  _____

- Identify the common trauma injuries that result in hearing or vision loss in both adults and children.
  a. Adults _____
  _____
  _____
  _____

  b. Children _____
  _____
  _____
  _____

- Explain the measures to take to maintain sensory function at the highest level with the use of assistive devices. _____
  _____
  _____
  _____
  _____
  _____

- Complete the grid by filling in the normal physiological changes that occur and cite how the nurse can minimize the loss.

Senses	Physiological Change	Interventions
Vision		
Hearing		
Taste and Smell		
Touch		
Trachea		

- List three methods of establishing a safe environment with regard to the following adaptations:

  a. Visual loss:

  1. _____

  _____

  2. _____

  _____

  3. _____

  _____

  b. Reduced hearing:

  1. _____

  _____

  2. _____

  _____

  3. _____

  _____

  c. Reduced olfaction:

  1. _____

  _____

  2. _____

  _____

  3. _____

  _____

  d. Reduced tactile sensation:

  1. _____

  _____

  2. _____

  _____

  3. _____

  _____

- Describe six communication methods that are appropriate for clients with a hearing impairment.

  a. _____

  _____

  b. _____

  _____

  c. _____

  d. _____

  e. _____

  _____

  f. _____

  _____

Acute Care

- When clients enter acute care settings for therapeutic management of sensory deficits or as a result of traumatic injury, the following approaches are used to maximize sensory function. Briefly explain each.

  a. Orientation to the environment: _____

  _____

  _____

  _____

  _____

  _____

  b. Communication: _____

  _____

  _____

  _____

  _____

  _____

  c. Controlling sensory stimuli: _____

  _____

  _____

  _____

  _____

  _____

  d. Safety measures: _____

  _____

  _____

  _____

  _____

  _____

Restorative and Continuing Care

- After a client experiences a sensory loss, it becomes important to understand the implications of the loss and to make the adjustments needed to continue a normal lifestyle. Briefly explain.

  a. Understanding sensory loss: _____

  _____

  _____

  _____

  _____

  b. Socialization: _____

  _____

  _____

  _____

  _____

  _____

  c. Promoting self-care: _____

  _____

  _____

  _____

  _____

  _____

EVALUATION

Client Care

- Client care evaluates the actual care delivered by the health care team based on expected outcomes.

- The client is the only one who will know if their sensory abilities are improved and which specific interventions or therapies are most successful in facilitating a change in their performance.

Client Expectations

- Client expectations evaluate care from the client's perspective.

REVIEW QUESTIONS

The student should select the appropriate answer and cite the rationale for choosing that particular answer.

1. All of the following are true of age-related factors that influence sensory function *except:*
   a. Refractive errors are the most common types of visual disorders in children.
   b. Visual changes in adulthood include presbyopia.
   c. Older adults hear high-pitched sounds the best.
   d. Neonates are unable to discriminate sensory stimuli.

   Answer:_____ Rationale: _____
   _____
   _____

2. Mr. Green, a 62-year-old farmer, has been hospitalized for 2 weeks for thrombophlebitis. He has no visitors, and the nurse notices that he appears bored, restless, and anxious. The type of alteration occurring because of sensory deprivation is:
   a. Affective
   b. Cognitive
   c. Perceptual
   d. Receptual

   Answer:_____ Rationale: _____
   _____
   _____

3. Which of the following would *not* provide meaningful stimuli for a client?
   a. A clock or calendar with large numbers
   b. A television that is kept on all day at a low volume
   c. Family pictures and personal possessions
   d. Interesting magazines and books

   Answer:_____ Rationale: _____
   _____
   _____

4. Clients with existing sensory loss must be protected from injury. What determines the safety precautions taken?
   a. The existing dangers in the environment
   b. The financial availability to make needed safety changes
   c. The nature of the client's actual or potential sensory loss
   d. The availability of a support system to enable the client to exist in his or her present environment

   Answer:_____ Rationale: _____
   _____
   _____

5. A client who is unable to name common objects or express simple ideas in words or writing suffers from:
   a. Expressive aphasia
   b. Receptive aphasia
   c. Global aphasia
   d. Mental retardation

   Answer:_____ Rationale: _____
   _____
   _____

SYNTHESIS MODEL FOR NURSING CARE PLAN FOR SENSORY PERCEPTUAL ALTERATIONS

Imagine that you are the community health nurse in the Care Plan on page 1645 of your text. Complete the *Planning phase* of the synthesis model by writing your answers in the appropriate boxes of the model shown. Think about the following:

- In developing Judy's plan of care, what **knowledge** did you apply?

- In what way might your previous **experience** assist in developing a plan of care for Judy?

- When developing a plan of care what intellectual and professional «Xtags error: No such font: tag f»standards were applied?

- What critical thinking **attitudes** might have been applied developing Judy's plan?

- How will you accomplish the goals?

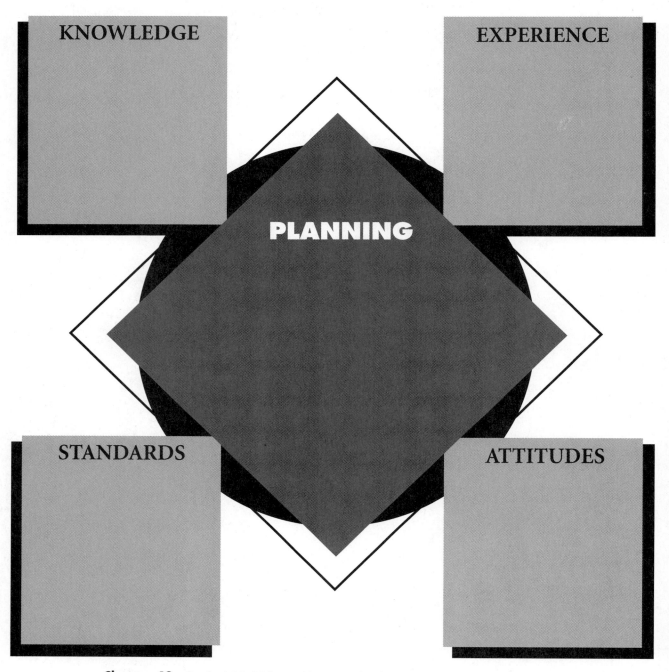

KNOWLEDGE

EXPERIENCE

PLANNING

STANDARDS

ATTITUDES

Chapter 48 *Synthesis Model for Nursing Care Plan for Sensory Perceptual Alterations.*

See answers on page 572.

Surgical Client

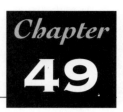

Perioperative nursing care includes nursing care given before (preoperative), during (intraoperative), and after surgery (postoperative).

PRELIMINARY READING

Chapter 49, pp. 1659-1715

COMPREHENSIVE UNDERSTANDING

HISTORY OF SURGICAL NURSING

• Summarize the historical changes that have occurred in surgical nursing. _____
_____
_____

AMBULATORY SURGERY

• List the benefits of ambulatory surgery.
    a. _____
    b. _____
    c. _____
    d. _____

SCIENTIFIC KNOWLEDGE BASE

CLASSIFICATION OF SURGERY

• Define the following surgical procedure classifications:
    a. *Palliative:* _____
    b. *Ablative:* _____
    c. *Emergency:* _____
    d. *Minor:* _____
    e. *Urgent:* _____
    f. *Major:* _____
    g. *Reconstructive:* _____
    h. *Constructive:* _____
    i. *Elective:* _____
    j. *Transplant:* _____
    k. *Diagnostic:* _____

Chapter 49: Surgical Client   355

- Briefly explain the following factors that increase the client's risk in surgery:
  a. Age: _____
  _____
  _____
  _____
  _____

  b. Nutrition: _____
  _____
  _____
  _____
  _____

  c. Obesity: _____
  _____
  _____
  _____
  _____

  d. Radiotherapy: _____
  _____
  _____
  _____
  _____

  e. Fluid and electrolyte balance: _____
  _____
  _____
  _____
  _____
  _____

  f. Pregnancy: _____
  _____
  _____
  _____
  _____

NURSING KNOWLEDGE BASE

- In the preoperative or preanesthetic phase, the nurse's role centers on:
  a. _____
  _____
  b. _____
  _____
  c. _____
  _____

- In the postoperative or postanesthesia phase, the nurse's responsibilities include:
  a. _____
  _____
  b. _____
  _____
  c. _____
  _____

CRITICAL THINKING SYNTHESIS THE NURSING PROCESS IN THE PREOPERATIVE SURGICAL PHASE

- List and describe six nursing responsibilities during the preoperative phase.
  a. _____
  _____
  b. _____
  _____
  c. _____
  _____
  d. _____
  _____
  e. _____
  _____
  f. _____
  _____

ASSESSMENT

- Assessment of the surgical client involves collecting a nursing history, performing a physical examination, reviewing the client's and family members' emotional health, and analyzing risk factors and diagnostic data.

- Identify the data the nurse would collect from the client's medical history.

- Describe how each of the following conditions increases the risk associated with surgery.
  a. Bleeding disorders: _____

  b. Diabetes mellitus: _____

  c. Heart disease: _____

  d. Respiratory infections: _____

  e. Liver disease: _____

  f. Fever: _____

  g. Chronic respiratory disease: _____

  h. Immunological disorders: _____

  i. Chronic pain: _____

- A client's past experience with surgery can influence physical and psychological responses to a procedure. List four factors to assess.
  a. _____

  b. _____

  c. _____

  d. _____

- Briefly explain how the nurse can prepare clients and their family members for the surgical experience. _____

- Describe how each of the following drugs has special implications for the surgical client.
  a. Antibiotics: _____

  b. Antidysrhythmics: _____

  c. Anticoagulants: _____

  d. Anticonvulsants: _____

  e. Antihypertensives: _____

  f. Corticosteroids: _____

  g. Insulin: _____

  h. Diuretics: _____

  i. Nonsteroidal antiinflammatory (NSAIDS): _____

- Briefly describe how the following factors may place the client at risk for a surgical procedure.
  a. Allergies: _____

  b. Smoking habits: _____

  c. Alcohol ingestion and substance abuse: _____

  d. Family support: _____

  e. Occupation: _____

Chapter 49: Surgical Client   357

- Briefly explain each of the following factors that need to be assessed in order to understand the impact of surgery on a client's and family's emotional health.

  a. Feelings: _____
  _____
  _____
  _____

  b. Self-concept: _____
  _____
  _____
  _____

  c. Body image: _____
  _____
  _____
  _____

  d. Coping resources: _____
  _____
  _____
  _____

- Cultural differences influence the surgical experience. Give an example of each.

  a. Native Americans: _____
  _____
  _____
  _____

  b. Arab Americans: _____
  _____
  _____
  _____

  c. African Americans: _____
  _____
  _____
  _____

  d. Vietnamese Americans: _____
  _____
  _____
  _____

- Briefly describe the findings on which the nurse would focus related to the physical examination of the following body systems:

  a. General survey: _____
  _____
  _____
  _____
  _____

  b. Head and neck: _____
  _____
  _____
  _____
  _____

  c. Integument: _____
  _____
  _____
  _____
  _____

  d. Thorax and lungs: _____
  _____
  _____
  _____
  _____

  e. Heart and vascular system: _____
  _____
  _____
  _____

  f. Abdomen: _____
  _____
  _____
  _____

  g. Neurological status: _____
  _____
  _____
  _____
  _____

- Describe the following routine screening tests for surgical clients.
  a. CBC: _____
  _____
  _____
  _____

  b. Serum electrolytes: _____
  _____
  _____
  _____

  c. Coagulation studies _____
  _____
  _____
  _____

  d. Serum creatinine: _____
  _____
  _____
  _____

  e. Urinalysis: _____
  _____
  _____
  _____

NURSING DIAGNOSIS

- List ten potential or actual nursing diagnoses appropriate for the preoperative client.
  a. _____
  _____
  b. _____
  _____
  c. _____
  _____
  d. _____
  _____
  e. _____
  _____
  f. _____
  _____
  g. _____
  _____
  h. _____
  _____
  i. _____
  _____
  j. _____
  _____

PLANNING

- List eight goals of care for the perioperative client.
  a. _____
  _____
  b. _____
  _____
  c. _____
  _____
  d. _____
  _____
  e. _____
  _____
  f. _____
  _____
  g. _____
  _____
  h. _____
  _____

IMPLEMENTATION

- Surgery cannot be performed until a client understands the _____, _____, _____, and _____.

- The primary responsibility for informing the client rests with the _____ _____.

- A client's signature on a consent form implies _____ _____.

- Describe five ways in which structured preoperative teaching may influence a client's postoperative recovery.
  a. _____
  _____
  b. _____
  _____
  c. _____
  _____
  d. _____
  _____
  e. _____
  _____

- Describe the criteria developed by the Association of Operating Room Nurses (AORN) that may be used in determining the client's understanding of the surgical procedure.

a. _____

b. _____

c. _____

d. _____

e. _____

f. _____

g. _____

h. _____

- Every preoperative teaching program includes explanations and demonstrations of the following five postoperative exercises. Briefly explain the rationale for each.

a. Diaphragmatic breathing: _____

b. Incentive spirometry: _____

c. Controlled coughing: _____

d. Turning: _____

e. Leg exercises: _____

Physical Preparation
- Briefly describe the following preoperative preparation.

a. Maintenance of normal fluid and electrolyte balance: _____

b. Reduction of risk of surgical wound infection: _____

c. Prevention of bowel and bladder incontinence: _____

d. Promotion of rest and comfort: _____

Day of Surgery

- List the eleven responsibilities of a nurse caring for a client the morning of surgery.

  a. _____

  b. _____

  c. _____

  d. _____

  e. _____

  f. _____

  g. _____

  h. _____

  i. _____

  j. _____

  k. _____

- The signs and symptoms of a latex reaction are _____ .

EVALUATION

Client Care

- The admitting nurse and the nurse in the preoperative area are the sources to evaluate client outcomes.

- List three expected outcomes for a preoperative client.

  a. _____

  b. _____

  c. _____

Client Expectations

- Explain the difficulty in determining a client's expectations regarding preoperative teaching. _____

TRANSPORT TO THE OPERATING ROOM

- List ten pieces of equipment that should be present in the postoperative bedside unit.

  a. _____

  b. _____

  c. _____

  d. _____

  e. _____

  f. _____

  g. _____

  h. _____

  i. _____

  j. _____

INTRAOPERATIVE SURGICAL PHASE

PREOPERATIVE (HOLDING) AREA

- In the holding areas, the nursing responsibilities include: _____

ADMISSION TO THE OPERATING ROOM

- Describe the responsibilities of the nurse in the operating room. _____
  _____
  _____
  _____
  _____

INTRODUCTION OF ANESTHESIA

- Briefly explain the four stages of general anesthesia.
  a. Stage 1: _____
  _____
  b. Stage 2: _____
  _____
  c. Stage 3: _____
  _____
  d. Stage 4: _____
  _____

- Identify the risks of general anesthesia.
  _____
  _____
  _____
  _____
  _____
  _____

- *Regional anesthesia* is _____
  _____.

- Identify and briefly explain the four types of regional induction methods:
  a. _____
  _____
  b. _____
  _____
  c. _____
  _____
  d. _____
  _____

- Local anesthesia involves _____
  _____.

- Define *conscious sedation* and identify its advantages. _____
  _____
  _____
  _____
  _____

POSITIONING THE CLIENT FOR SURGERY

- Explain the principles of positioning the client for surgery. _____
  _____
  _____
  _____
  _____

NURSE'S ROLE DURING SURGERY

- Describe the responsibilities of the nurse during the surgical procedure in the following roles.
  a. Scrub nurse: _____
  _____
  _____
  _____

  b. Circulating nurse: _____
  _____
  _____
  _____

- During the intraoperative phase, the nursing staff continues the preoperative plan. Documentation of intraoperative care provides useful data for the nurse who cares for the client postoperatively.

POSTOPERATIVE SURGICAL PHASE

- Identify the two phases of the postoperative period and describe the usual time frame for ambulatory and hospitalized clients.
  a. _____
  _____
  _____
  _____
  _____
  _____

b. _____
_____
_____
_____
_____
_____

IMMEDIATE POSTOPERATIVE RECOVERY

- Describe the responsibilities of the nurse in the PACU. _____
_____
_____
_____
_____
_____

DISCHARGE FROM THE PACU

- Identify the criteria for discharge from the PACU. _____
_____
_____
_____
_____
_____

RECOVERY IN AMBULATORY SURGERY

- Describe the usual time spent by the client in the following phases of recovery and the reasons for it.
  a. Phase I: _____
  _____
  b. Phase II: _____
  _____

POSTOPERATIVE CONVALESCENCE

- Identify the criteria for discharging ambulatory surgical clients. _____
_____
_____
_____
_____

THE NURINS PROCESS IN POSTOPERATIVE CARE

☙ ASSESSMENT

- Explain the frequency of assessments needed during the postoperative period. _____
_____
_____
_____
_____
_____

- List three major causes of airway obstruction in the postoperative client.
  a. _____
  _____
  b. _____
  _____
  c. _____
  _____
  d. _____
  _____

- List four measures that will maintain airway patency.
  a. _____
  _____
  b. _____
  _____
  c. _____
  _____
  d. _____
  _____

- List four areas to assess in order to determine a postoperative client's circulatory status.
  a. _____
  _____
  b. _____
  _____
  c. _____
  _____
  d. _____
  _____

- Describe the characteristic findings associated with postoperative hemorrhage. _____
  _____
  _____
  _____
  _____
  _____

- Define the following terms related to temperature:
  a. *Shivering:* _____
  _____
  b. *Malignant hyperthermia:* _____
  _____

- List three areas the nurse assesses to determine fluid and electrolyte alterations.
  a. _____
  _____
  b. _____
  _____
  c. _____
  _____

- List the areas of assessment that help to determine a postoperative client's neurological status.
  a. _____
  _____
  b. _____
  _____
  c. _____
  _____
  d. _____
  _____

- The nurse assesses the condition of the skin for _____,
  _____,
  _____,
  and _____.

- Describe how the nurse would assess the amount of drainage from a wound. _____
  _____
  _____
  _____
  _____

- The client may regain voluntary control over urinary function in _____ hours after anesthesia.

- Normally during the immediate recovery phase, bowel sounds are auscultated in all four quadrants.

- Distention may occur in the client who develops a _____.

- List three nursing measures used to minimize nausea in the immediate postoperative period.
  a. _____
  _____
  b. _____
  _____
  c. _____
  _____

- Postoperative pain can be perceived when _____ is regained.

- Assessment of the client's discomfort and evaluation of pain relief therapies are essential nursing functions.

- Acute incisional pain causes clients to become _____
  and _____.

NURSING DIAGNOSIS
- Identify two actual or potential nursing diagnoses that are appropriate for a postoperative client.
  a. _____
  _____
  b. _____
  _____

PLANNING
- List the typical postoperative orders prescribed by surgeons.
  a. _____
  _____
  b. _____
  _____

c. _____

_____

d. _____

_____

e. _____

_____

f. _____

_____

g. _____

_____

h. _____

_____

i. _____

_____

- Identify the goals of care for the postoperative client.

a. _____

_____

b. _____

_____

c. _____

_____

d. _____

_____

IMPLEMENTATION

- Complete the grid on the next page. Identify three nursing interventions for each area of need in the postoperative client.

EVALUATION

Client Care

- The nurse evaluates the effectiveness of care provided to the surgical client on the basis of expected outcomes following nursing interventions.

- Describe how the nurse would evaluate the ambulatory surgical client. _____

_____

_____

_____

_____

Client Expectations

- With short hospital stays and ambulatory surgery, it is important to evaluate the client's expectations early in the postoperative process.

REVIEW QUESTIONS

The student should select the appropriate answer and cite the rationale for choosing that particular answer.

1. Mrs. Young, a 45-year-old diabetic client, is having a hysterectomy in the morning. Because of her history, the nurse would expect:
   a. An increased risk of hemorrhaging
   b. Fluid and electrolyte imbalances
   c. Altered elimination of anesthetic agents
   d. Impaired wound healing

   Answer:_____ Rationale: _____

   _____

   _____

2. The purposes of the nursing history for the client who is to have surgery include all of the following *except*:
   a. Identifying the client's perception and expectations about surgery
   b. Obtaining information about the client's past experience with surgery
   c. Deciding whether or not surgery is indicated
   d. Understanding the impact surgery has on the client's and family's emotional health

   Answer:_____ Rationale: _____

   _____

   _____

Area of Need	Nursing intervention
Maintaining respiratory function	
Preventing circulatory status	
Promoting normal bowel elimination	
Promoting adequate nutrition	
Promoting urinary elimination	
Promoting wound healing	
Promoting rest and comfort	
Maintaing self-concept	

3. All of the following clients are at risk for developing serious fluid and electrolyte imbalances during and after surgery *except:*
   a. Client E, who is 81 years old and having emergency surgery for a bowel obstruction following four days of vomiting and diarrhea
   b. Client F, who is 1 year old and having a cleft palate repair
   c. Client G, who is 55 years old and has a history of chronic respiratory disease
   d. Client H, who is 79 years old and has a history of congestive heart failure

Answer:_____   Rationale: _____
_____
_____

4. The purpose of postoperative leg exercises is to:
   a. Promote venous return
   b. Maintain muscle tone
   c. Assess range of motion
   d. Exercise fatigued muscles

Answer:_____   Rationale: _____
_____
_____

5. The PACU nurse notices that the client is shivering. This is most commonly caused by:
   a. The use of a reflective blanket on the operating room table
   b. Side effects of certain anesthetic agents
   c. Cold irrigations used during surgery
   d. Malignant hypothermia, a serious condition

Answer:_____   Rationale: _____
_____
_____

SYNTHESIS MODEL FOR NURSING CARE PLAN FOR KNOWLEDGE DEFICIT REGARDING PREOPERATIVE AND POSTOPERATIVE CARE

Imagine that you are Joe, the nurse in the Care Plan on page 1677 of your text. Complete the *evaluation phase* of the synthesis model by writing your answers in the appropriate boxes of the model shown. Think about the following:

- What **knowledge** did Joe apply in evaluating Mrs. Campana's care?

- In what way might Joe's previous **experience** influence his evaluation of Mrs. Campana's care?

- During evaluation, what intellectual and professional **standards** were applied to Mrs. Campana's care?

- In what way does critical thinking **attitudes** play a role in how you approach evaluation of Mrs. Cambana's care?

- How might Joe adjust Mrs. Cambana's care?

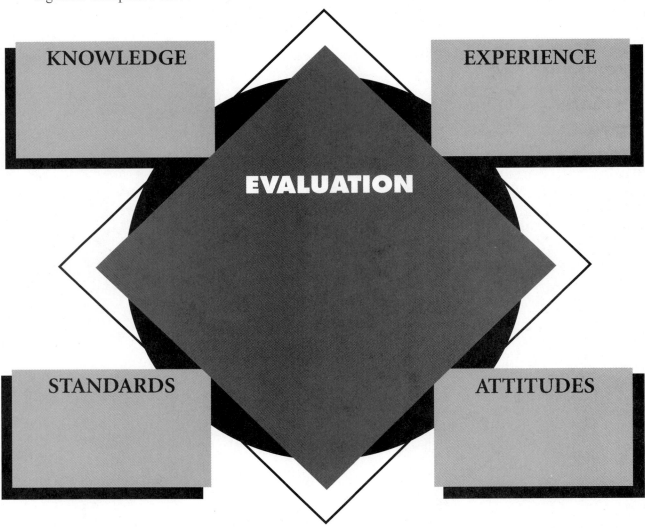

KNOWLEDGE

EXPERIENCE

EVALUATION

STANDARDS

ATTITUDES

Chapter 49 *Synthesis Model for Nursing Care Plan for* Knowledge Deficit Regarding Pre and Postoperative Care.

See answers on page 573.

PROCEDURE PERFORMANCE CHECKLIST
Skill 31-1 Measuring Body Temperature

	S	U	NP	Comments

Measuring Body Temperature

1. Assess for temperature alterations and factors that influence body temperature. ____ ____ ____ _____

2. Determine any activity that may interfere with accuracy of temperature measurement. ____ ____ ____ _____

3. Determine appropriate site and measurement device to be used. ____ ____ ____ _____

4. Explain to client how temperature will be taken and importance of maintaining proper position. ____ ____ ____ _____

5. Wash hands. ____ ____ ____ _____

6. Assist client to a comfortable position. ____ ____ ____ _____

7. Obtain temperature reading:

  A. Oral temperature measurement with glass thermometer:

    (1) Apply disposable gloves. ____ ____ ____ _____

    (2) Hold end (blue tip) of glass thermometer with fingertips. ____ ____ ____ _____

    (3) Read mercury level while gently rotating thermometer at eye level. If mercury is above desired level, grasp tip of thermometer securely and flick wrist downward until reading is below 35.5° C. ____ ____ ____ _____

    (4) Insert thermometer into plastic sleeve cover. ____ ____ ____ _____

    (5) Ask client to open mouth, then place thermometer under tongue in posterior sublingual pocket lateral to center of lower jaw.

    (6) Ask client to hold thermometer with lips closed. Caution client against biting down on thermometer. ____ ____ ____ _____

    (7) Leave thermometer in place for 3 minutes or per agency policy. ____ ____ ____ _____

    (8) Remove thermometer from client's mouth, remove and discard plastic sleeve cover, and read thermometer at eye level. Rotate thermometer until scale appears. ____ ____ ____ _____

    (9) Cleanse thermometer with clean, soft tissue. Dispose of tissue. Store thermometer in appropriate container. ____ ____ ____ _____

Continued

	S	U	NP	Comments

(10) Remove and dispose of gloves. ____ ____ ____ _____

(11) Wash hands. ____ ____ ____ _____

B. Oral temperature measurement with electronic thermometer:

   (1) Apply disposable gloves (optional). ____ ____ ____ _____

   (2) Remove thermometer pack from charging unit. Attach oral probe (blue tip) to thermometer unit. Grasp top of probe stem, being careful not to apply pressure on the ejection button. ____ ____ ____ _____

   (3) Slide disposable plastic probe cover over thermometer probe until it locks in place. ____ ____ ____ _____

   (4) Ask client to open mouth, then place thermometer probe under tongue in posterior sublingual pocket lateral to center of jaw. ____ ____ ____ _____

   (5) Ask client to hold thermometer probe with lips closed. ____ ____ ____ _____

   (6) Leave thermometer probe in place until audible signal occurs and temperature appears on digital display. Remove thermometer probe from client's mouth. ____ ____ ____ _____

   (7) Push ejection button on thermometer stem to discard plastic probe cover into appropriate receptacle. ____ ____ ____ _____

   (8) Return thermometer stem to storage well of recording unit. ____ ____ ____ _____

   (9) If gloves worn, remove and dispose of them in appropriate receptacle. ____ ____ ____ _____

 (10) Wash hands. ____ ____ ____ _____

C. Rectal temperature measurement with glass thermometer:

   (1) Provide privacy. ____ ____ ____ _____

   (2) Assist client to Sims' position with upper leg flexed. Expose client's anal area only. ____ ____ ____ _____

   (3) Apply disposable gloves. ____ ____ ____ _____

   (4) Read mercury level of thermometer while rotating thermometer at eye level. If mercury is above desired level, grasp tip of thermometer securely and flick wrist downward until reading is below 35.5° C. ____ ____ ____ _____

   (5) Insert thermometer into plastic sleeve cover. ____ ____ ____ _____

Continued

	S	U	NP	Comments

(6) Squeeze lubricant onto tissue. Dip thermometer's blunt end into lubricant and cover 2.5 to 3.5 cm for adult clients.

(7) With nondominant hand, separate client's buttocks to expose anus. Ask client to breathe slowly and relax.

(8) Gently insert thermometer into client's anus (3.5 cm for adult client) in direction of umbilicus. Do not force thermometer.

(9) If resistance is felt during insertion, withdraw thermometer immediately.

(10) Hold thermometer in place for 2 minutes or per agency policy.

(11) Remove thermometer, discard plastic sleeve, and wipe off any secretions on thermometer with clean tissue. Dispose of tissue.

(12) Read thermometer at eye level. Rotate thermometer until scale appears.

(13) Wipe client's anal area with soft tissue and discard tissue. Assist client to a comfortable position.

(14) Store thermometer in appropriate protective storage container.

(15) Remove and dispose of gloves.

(16) Wash hands.

D. Rectal temperature measurement with electronic thermometer:

(1) Follow steps 7C(1) and 7C(2).

(2) Remove thermometer pack from charging unit. Attach rectal probe (red tip) to thermometer unit. Grasp top of probe stem.

(3) Slide disposable plastic probe cover over thermometer probe until it locks in place.

(4) Follow steps 7C(6) through 7C(9).

(5) Leave thermometer probe in place until audible signal occurs and temperature appears on digital display. Remove thermometer probe from client's anus.

(6) Push ejection button on thermometer stem to discard plastic probe cover.

(7) Return thermometer stem to storage well of recording unit.

Continued

	S	U	NP	Comments

(8) Wipe client's anal area with soft tissue and discard tissue. Assist client to a comfortable position. _____ _____ _____ _____

(9) Remove and dispose of gloves. _____ _____ _____ _____

(10) Wash hands. _____ _____ _____ _____

(11) Return thermometer to charger. _____ _____ _____ _____

E. Axillary temperature measurement with glass thermometer:

   (1) Wash hands. _____ _____ _____ _____

   (2) Provide privacy. _____ _____ _____ _____

   (3) Assist client to supine or sitting position. _____ _____ _____ _____

   (4) Move client's clothing or gown away from his or her shoulder and arm. _____ _____ _____ _____

   (5) Prepare glass thermometer according to steps 7A(2) and 7A(3). _____ _____ _____ _____

   (6) Insert thermometer into center of client's axilla, lower arm over thermometer, and place arm across chest. _____ _____ _____ _____

   (7) Hold thermometer in place for 3 minutes or per agency policy. _____ _____ _____ _____

   (8) Remove thermometer, discard plastic sleeve, and wipe off any secretions on thermometer with clean tissue. Dispose of tissue. _____ _____ _____ _____

   (9) Read thermometer at eye level. _____ _____ _____ _____

   (10) Store thermometer at client's bedside in protective storage container. _____ _____ _____ _____

   (11) Assist client with replacing clothing or gown. _____ _____ _____ _____

   (12) Wash hands. _____ _____ _____ _____

F. Axillary temperature measurement with electronic thermometer:

   (1) Assist client to supine or sitting position. _____ _____ _____ _____

   (2) Move client's clothing or gown away from his or her shoulder and arm. _____ _____ _____ _____

   (3) Remove thermometer pack from charging unit. Be sure oral probe (blue tip) is attached to thermometer unit. Grasp top of probe stem. _____ _____ _____ _____

   (4) Slide disposable plastic probe cover over thermometer probe until it locks in place. _____ _____ _____ _____

Continued

372

	S	U	NP	Comments
(5) Raise client's arm away from torso and inspect for skin lesions and excessive perspiration. Insert probe into center of client's axilla, lower arm over probe, and place arm across chest.	_____	_____	_____	_____
(6) Leave probe in place until audible signal occurs and temperature appears on digital display.	_____	_____	_____	_____
(7) Remove probe from axilla.	_____	_____	_____	_____
(8) Push ejection button on probe to discard plastic probe cover.	_____	_____	_____	_____
(9) Return probe to storage well of recording unit.	_____	_____	_____	_____
(10) Assist client to a comfortable position.	_____	_____	_____	_____
(11) Wash hands.	_____	_____	_____	_____
(12) Return thermometer to charger.	_____	_____	_____	_____
G. Tympanic membrane temperature with electronic thermometer:				
(1) Assist client to a comfortable position with head turned toward side, away from nurse.	_____	_____	_____	_____
(2) Remove handheld thermometer unit from charging base, being careful to not apply pressure on the ejection button.	_____	_____	_____	_____
(3) Slide disposable speculum cover over tip until it locks into place.	_____	_____	_____	_____
(4) Insert speculum into ear canal following manufacturer's instructions for tympanic probe positioning:	_____	_____	_____	_____
(a) Pull ear pinna upward and back for adult.	_____	_____	_____	_____
(b) Move thermometer in a figure-eight pattern.	_____	_____	_____	_____
(c) Fit probe gently in ear canal and do not move it.	_____	_____	_____	_____
(d) Point probe toward client's nose.	_____	_____	_____	_____
(5) Depress scan button on handheld unit. Leave thermometer probe in place until audible signal occurs and client's temperature appears on digital display.	_____	_____	_____	_____
(6) Carefully remove speculum from client's auditory canal.	_____	_____	_____	_____
(7) Push ejection button on handheld unit to discard plastic probe cover.	_____	_____	_____	_____
(8) If second reading required, replace probe cover and wait 2 to 3 minutes.	_____	_____	_____	_____

Continued

	S	U	NP	Comments
(9) Return handheld unit to charging base.	_____	_____	_____	_____
(10) Assist client to a comfortable position.	_____	_____	_____	_____
(11) Wash hands.	_____	_____	_____	_____
8. Discuss findings with client as needed.	_____	_____	_____	_____
9. If temperature is being assessed for the first time, establish temperature as baseline if within normal range.	_____	_____	_____	_____
10. Compare temperature reading with previous baseline and normal temperature range for client's age group.	_____	_____	_____	_____
11. Record temperature and report abnormal findings.	_____	_____	_____	_____

PROCEDURE PERFORMANCE CHECKLIST
Skill 31-2 Radial and Apical Pulses

	S	U	NP	Comments
Radial and Apical Pulses				
1. Determine need to assess radial or apical pulse.	____	____	____	_____
2. Assess for factors that influence pulse rate.	____	____	____	_____
3. Determine previous baseline apical rate (if available) from client's record.	____	____	____	_____
4. Explain that pulse or heart rate is to be assessed. Encourage client to relax and not speak.	____	____	____	_____
5. Wash hands.	____	____	____	_____
6. Provide privacy.	____	____	____	_____
7. Obtain pulse measurement:				
A. Radial pulse:				
(1) Assist client to supine or sitting position.	____	____	____	_____
(2) If client is supine, place client's forearm straight alongside or across lower chest or upper abdomen with wrist extended straight. If client is sitting, bend client's elbow 90 degrees and support his or her lower arm on a chair or on your arm. Slightly flex client's wrist, with palm down.	____	____	____	_____
(3) Place tips of first two fingers of hand over groove along radial or thumb side of client's inner wrist.	____	____	____	_____
(4) Lightly compress against client's radius, obliterate pulse initially, then relax pressure.	____	____	____	_____
(5) Determine strength of pulse.	____	____	____	_____
(6) After pulse can be felt regularly, look at watch's second hand and begin to count rate.	____	____	____	_____
(7) If pulse is regular, count rate for 30 seconds and multiply total by 2.	____	____	____	_____
(8) If pulse is irregular, count rate for 60 seconds. Assess frequency and pattern of irregularity.	____	____	____	_____
B. Apical pulse:				
(1) Assist client to supine or sitting position. Expose client's sternum and left side of chest.	____	____	____	_____
(2) Locate anatomical landmarks to identify the point of maximal impulse.	____	____	____	_____

Continued

	S	U	NP	Comments
(3) Place diaphragm of stethoscope in palm of hand for 5 to 10 seconds.	_____	_____	_____	_____
(4) Place diaphragm of stethoscope over point of maximal impulse at the fifth intercostal space at the left midclavicular line and auscultate for normal S_1 and S_2 heart sounds.	_____	_____	_____	_____
(5) When S_1 and S_2 are heard with regularity, look at watch's second hand and begin to count rate.	_____	_____	_____	_____
(6) If apical rate is regular, count for 30 seconds and multiply by 2.	_____	_____	_____	_____
(7) If rate is irregular or client is receiving cardiovascular medication, count for 60 seconds.	_____	_____	_____	_____
(8) Note regularity of any dysrhythmia.	_____	_____	_____	_____
(9) Replace client's gown and bed linen.	_____	_____	_____	_____
(10) Assist client in returning to a comfortable position.	_____	_____	_____	_____
(11) Clean earpieces and diaphragm of stethoscope with alcohol swab as needed.	_____	_____	_____	_____
8. Discuss findings with client as needed.	_____	_____	_____	_____
9. Wash hands.	_____	_____	_____	_____
10. Compare readings with client's previous baseline and/or acceptable range of heart rate for client's age group.	_____	_____	_____	_____
11. Compare peripheral pulse rate with apical rate and note discrepancy.	_____	_____	_____	_____
12. Compare radial pulse equality and note discrepancy.	_____	_____	_____	_____
13. Correlate pulse rate with data obtained from blood pressure and related signs and symptoms.	_____	_____	_____	_____
14. Record pulse rate with assessment site and report abnormal findings.	_____	_____	_____	_____

STUDENT: _____ DATE: _____

INSTRUCTOR: _____ DATE: _____

Skill 31-3 Assessing Respirations

	S	U	NP	Comments
Assessing Respirations				
1. Determine need to assess client's respirations.	_____	_____	_____	_____
2. Assess pertinent laboratory values.	_____	_____	_____	_____
3. Determine previous baselines respiratory rate (if available) from client's record.	_____	_____	_____	_____
4. Assist client to a comfortable position, preferably sitting or lying with the head of the bed elevated 45 to 60 degrees.	_____	_____	_____	_____
5. Provide privacy.	_____	_____	_____	_____
6. Wash hands.	_____	_____	_____	_____
7. Be sure client's chest is visible. If necessary, move client's bed linen or gown.	_____	_____	_____	_____
8. Place client's arm in relaxed position across the abdomen or lower chest, or place nurse's hand directly over client's upper abdomen.	_____	_____	_____	_____
9. Observe complete respiratory cycle (one inspiration and one expiration).	_____	_____	_____	_____
10. After cycle is observed, look at watch's second hand and begin to count rate.	_____	_____	_____	_____
11. If rhythm is regular, count number of respirations in 30 seconds and multiply by 2.	_____	_____	_____	_____
12. If rhythm is irregular, less than 12, or greater than 20, count respirations for 60 seconds.	_____	_____	_____	_____
13. Note depth of respirations.	_____	_____	_____	_____
14. Note rhythm of ventilatory cycle.	_____	_____	_____	_____
15. Replace client's bed linen and gown.	_____	_____	_____	_____
16. Wash hands.	_____	_____	_____	_____
17. Discuss findings with client as needed.	_____	_____	_____	_____
18. If respirations are being assessed for the first time, establish rate, rhythm, and depth as baseline if within normal range.	_____	_____	_____	_____
19. Compare respirations with client's previous baseline and normal rate, rhythm, and depth.	_____	_____	_____	_____
20. Record respiratory rate and character and any use of oxygen, and report abnormal findings.	_____	_____	_____	_____

STUDENT: _____ DATE: _____

INSTRUCTOR: _____ DATE: _____

PROCEDURE PERFORMANCE CHECKLIST
Skill 31-4 Measuring Oxygen Saturation (Pulse Oximetry)

	S	U	NP	Comments
Measuring Oxygen Saturation (Pulse Oximetry)				
1. Determine need to measure client's oxygen saturation.	____	____	____	_____
2. Assess for factors that influence measurement of SpO_2.	____	____	____	_____
3. Review client's record for prescriber's order.	____	____	____	_____
4. Determine previous baseline SpO_2 (if available) from client's record.	____	____	____	_____
5. Explain purpose of procedure to client. Instruct client to breathe normally.	____	____	____	_____
6. Assess site for sensor probe placement.	____	____	____	_____
7. Wash hands.	____	____	____	_____
8. Assist client to a comfortable position. If client's finger is chosen as monitoring site, support client's lower arm.	____	____	____	_____
9. Instruct client to breathe normally.	____	____	____	_____
10. Use acetone to remove any fingernail polish from digit to be assessed.	____	____	____	_____
11. Attach sensor probe to monitoring site. Tell client that clip-on probe will feel like a clothespin on the finger and will not hurt.	____	____	____	_____
12. Turn on oximeter by activating power. Observe pulse waveform/intensity display and audible beep. Correlate oximeter pulse rate with client's radial pulse.	____	____	____	_____
13. Leave probe in place until oximeter readout reaches constant value and pulse display reaches full strength during each cardiac cycle. Read SpO_2 on digital display.	____	____	____	_____
14. Inform client that oximeter alarm will sound if probe falls off or is moved.	____	____	____	_____
15. Verify SpO_2 alarm limits and alarm volume for continuous monitoring. Verify that alarms are on. Assess skin integrity under sensor probe and relocate sensor probe at least every 4 hours.				
16. Discuss findings with client as needed.	____	____	____	_____
17. Remove probe and turn oximeter power off after intermittent measurements. Store probe in appropriate location.	____	____	____	_____
18. Assist client in returning to a comfortable position.	____	____	____	_____

Continued

	S	U	NP	Comments
19. Wash hands.				
20. Compare SpO_2 reading with client baseline and acceptable values.	_____	_____	_____	_____
21. Correlate SpO_2 reading with SaO_2 reading obtained from arterial blood gas measurements, if available.	_____	_____	_____	_____
22. Correlate SpO_2 reading with data obtained from respiratory assessment.	_____	_____	_____	_____
23. Report and record SpO_2 readings, respiratory status, oxygen therapy, and client's responses.	_____	_____	_____	_____

PROCEDURE PERFORMANCE CHECKLIST
Skill 31-5 Measuring Blood Pressure (BP)

	S	U	NP	Comments
Measuring Blood Pressure (BP)				
1. Determine need to assess client's BP.	____	____	____	_____
2. Determine best site for BP assessment and cuff size.	____	____	____	_____
3. Determine previous baseline BP (if available) from client's record.	____	____	____	_____
4. Encourage client to avoid exercise and smoking for 30 minutes before assessment of BP.	____	____	____	_____
5. Assist client to sitting or lying position. Make sure room is warm, quiet, and relaxing.	____	____	____	_____
6. Explain to client that BP is to be assessed and have client rest at least 5 minutes before measurement is taken. Ask client not to speak while BP is being measured.	____	____	____	_____
7. Wash hands.	____	____	____	_____
8. With client sitting or lying, position client's forearm or thigh and provide support if needed.	____	____	____	_____
9. Expose extremity by removing constricting clothing.	____	____	____	_____
10. Palpate brachial artery or popliteal artery. Position cuff 2.5 cm above site of pulsation. Center bladder of cuff above artery. With cuff fully deflated, wrap cuff evenly and snugly around upper arm.	____	____	____	_____
11. Position manometer vertically at eye level, no more than 1 m away from client.	____	____	____	_____
12. To determine baseline BP, palpate brachial or radial artery with fingertips of one hand while inflating cuff rapidly to pressure 30 mm Hg above point at which pulse disappears. Slowly deflate cuff and note point when pulse reappears.	____	____	____	_____
13. Deflate cuff fully and wait 30 seconds.	____	____	____	_____
14. Using a stethoscope, make sure that sounds are clear, not muffled.	____	____	____	_____
15. Relocate brachial or popliteal artery and place bell or diaphragm chestpiece of stethoscope over it.	____	____	____	_____
16. Close valve of pressure bulb clockwise until tight.	____	____	____	_____
17. Inflate cuff to 30 mm Hg above palpate systolic pressure.	____	____	____	_____

Continued

	S	U	NP	Comments
18. Slowly release valve and allow mercury to fall at rate of 2 to 3 mm Hg/sec.	_____	_____	_____	_____
19. Note point on manometer when first clear sound is heard.	_____	_____	_____	_____
20. Continue to deflate cuff, noting point at which muffled or dampened sound appears.	_____	_____	_____	_____
21. Continue to deflate cuff gradually, noting point at which sound disappears. Note pressure to nearest 2 mm Hg.	_____	_____	_____	_____
22. Deflate cuff rapidly and completely. Remove cuff from client's arm unless measurement must be repeated.	_____	_____	_____	_____
23. If this is the first assessment of the client, repeat procedure on other arm.	_____	_____	_____	_____
24. Assist client in returning to a comfortable position and cover upper arm if previously clothed.	_____	_____	_____	_____
25. Discuss findings with client as needed.	_____	_____	_____	_____
26. Wash hands.	_____	_____	_____	_____
27. Compare reading with previous baseline and/or acceptable BP for client's age group.	_____	_____	_____	_____
28. Compare BP in both of client's arms or legs.	_____	_____	_____	_____
29. Correlate BP with data obtained from pulse assessment and related cardiovascular signs and symptoms.	_____	_____	_____	_____
30. Inform client of value of and need for periodic reassessment of BP.	_____	_____	_____	_____
31. Record BP and report abnormal findings.	_____	_____	_____	_____

STUDENT: _____ DATE: _____

INSTRUCTOR: _____ DATE: _____

Skill 33-1 Hand Washing

	S	U	NP	Comments
Hand Washing				
1. Inspect surfaces of hands for breaks or cuts in skin or cuticles. Report and cover lesions before providing client care.	_____	_____	_____	_____
2. Inspect hands for heavy soiling.	_____	_____	_____	_____
3. Inspect nails for length.	_____	_____	_____	_____
4. Push wristwatch and long uniform sleeves above wrists. Remove rings during washing.	_____	_____	_____	_____
5. Stand in front of sink, keeping hands and uniform away from sink surface.	_____	_____	_____	_____
6. Turn on water. Turn faucet on or push knee pedals laterally or press foot pedals to regulate water flow and temperature.	_____	_____	_____	_____
7. Avoid splashing water onto uniform.	_____	_____	_____	_____
8. Regulate flow of water so that temperature is warm.	_____	_____	_____	_____
9. Wet hands and wrists thoroughly under running water. Keep hands and forearms lower than elbows during washing.	_____	_____	_____	_____
10. Apply a small amount of soap or antiseptic, lathering thoroughly.	_____	_____	_____	_____
11. Wash hands using plenty of lather and friction for at least 10 to 15 seconds. Interlace fingers and rub palms and back of hands with circular motion at least 5 times each. Keep fingertips down.	_____	_____	_____	_____
12. Clean fingernails of both hands with additional soap or clean orangewood stick.	_____	_____	_____	_____
13. Rinse hands and wrists thoroughly, keeping hands down and elbows up.	_____	_____	_____	_____
14. Optional: Repeat steps 5 through 13 and extend period of washing if hands are heavily soiled.	_____	_____	_____	_____
15. Dry hands thoroughly from fingers to wrists and forearms with paper towel, single-use cloth, or warm air dryer.	_____	_____	_____	_____
16. Discard paper towel, if used, in proper receptacle.	_____	_____	_____	_____
17. Turn off water with foot or knee pedals. To turn off hand faucet, use clean, dry paper towel. Avoid touching handles with hands.	_____	_____	_____	_____

Continued

	S	U	NP	Comments
18. If hands are dry or chapped, a small amount of lotion or barrier cream can be applied.	____	____	____	_____
19. Inspect surfaces of hands for obvious signs of soil or other contaminants.	____	____	____	_____
20. Inspect hands for dermatitis or cracked skin.	____	____	____	_____

STUDENT: _____ DATE: _____

INSTRUCTOR: _____ DATE: _____

Skill 33-2 Preparing a Sterile Field

	S	U	NP	Comments
Preparing a Sterile Field				
1. Select clean work surface above waist level.	_____	_____	_____	_____
2. Assemble equipment and check dates on supplies.	_____	_____	_____	_____
3. Wash hands.	_____	_____	_____	_____
4. Place pack with sterile drape on work surface and open pack.	_____	_____	_____	_____
5. Pick up folded top of drape with one hand; let it unfold. Discard outer cover of pack.	_____	_____	_____	_____
6. Hold drape up and away from the body with both hands.	_____	_____	_____	_____
7. Position bottom half of drape over work surface.	_____	_____	_____	_____
8. Allow top half of drape to be placed over work surface last, positioning as needed.	_____	_____	_____	_____
9. Add sterile items:				
A. Open sterile item.	_____	_____	_____	_____
B. Peel wrapper; do not allow it to touch sterile field.	_____	_____	_____	_____
C. Place item onto field at an angle. Do not hold arm over field.	_____	_____	_____	_____
D. Dispose of wrapper.	_____	_____	_____	_____
10. Perform procedure using sterile technique.	_____	_____	_____	_____

STUDENT: _____ DATE: _____

INSTRUCTOR: _____ DATE: _____

PROCEDURE PERFORMANCE CHECKLIST
Skill 33-3 Surgical Hand Washing

	S	U	NP	Comments

Surgical Hand Washing
1. Consult institutional policy for length of time for hand washing. _____ _____ _____ _____
2. Keep fingernails short, clean, and healthy. Remove artificial nails. _____ _____ _____ _____
3. Inspect hands for presence of abrasions, cuts, or open lesions. _____ _____ _____ _____
4. Apply surgical shoe covers, cap or hood, face mask, and protective eyewear. _____ _____ _____ _____
5. Turn on water using knee or foot controls, and adjust water to comfortable temperature. _____ _____ _____ _____
6. Wet hands and arms under running lukewarm water and later with detergent to 5 cm above elbows. Keep hands above elbows. _____ _____ _____ _____
7. Rinse hands and arms thoroughly under running water. _____ _____ _____ _____
8. Under running water, clean under nails of both hands with nail pick. Discard nail pick after use. _____ _____ _____ _____
9. Wet clean brush and apply antimicrobial detergent. Scrub the nails of one hand with 15 strokes. Holding brush perpendicular, scrub the palm, each side of the thumb and all fingers, and the posterior side of the hand with 10 strokes each. Scrub each section of the arm 10 times. Continue to scrub for at least 5 to 10 minutes. _____ _____ _____ _____
10. Discard brush and rinse hands and arms thoroughly. Turn off water with foot or knee controls and back into room entrance with hands elevated in front of and away from the body. _____ _____ _____ _____
11. Bend slightly forward at the waist, and use a sterile towel to dry one hand thoroughly, moving from fingers to elbow. Dry in a rotating motion. _____ _____ _____ _____
12. Repeat drying method for other hand, using a different area of the towel or a new sterile towel. _____ _____ _____ _____
13. Inspect hands for dermatitis or cracked skin. _____ _____ _____ _____

STUDENT: _____ DATE: _____

INSTRUCTOR: _____ DATE: _____

Skill 33-4 Applying a Sterile Gown and Performing Closed Gloving

	S	U	NP	Comments

Applying a Sterile Gown and Performing Closed Gloving

1. Apply sterile gown:
   A. Apply cap, face mask, eyewear, and foot covers. ___ ___ ___ _____
   B. Perform surgical handwashing and dry hands. ___ ___ ___ _____
   C. Have circulating nurse open pack containing sterile gown. ___ ___ ___ _____
   D. Have circulating nurse prepare glove package. ___ ___ ___ _____
   E. Pick up gown at neckline without touching outside of gown. ___ ___ ___ _____
   F. Hold gown at arm's length; allow it to unfold by itself. ___ ___ ___ _____
   G. Insert each hand through armholes simultaneously. ___ ___ ___ _____
   H. Have circulating nurse bring gown over shoulders, leaving sleeves covering hands. ___ ___ ___ _____
   I. Have circulating nurse tie back of gown at neck and waist. ___ ___ ___ _____

2. Closed gloving procedure:
   A. With hands covered by sleeves, open glove package. ___ ___ ___ _____
   B. With hands covered by sleeves, pick up glove for dominant hand. ___ ___ ___ _____
   C. Place glove palm side down on palm of sleeve-covered hand, with glove fingers pointing toward elbow. ___ ___ ___ _____
   D. Using sleeve-covered nondominant hand, pull glove cuff over dominant hand and gown cuff. ___ ___ ___ _____
   E. Grasping top of glove with nondominant hand, extend fingers of dominant hand. ___ ___ ___ _____
   F. Repeat steps 11 through 14 to glove nondominant hand. ___ ___ ___ _____
   G. Adjust fingers until fully extended into both gloves. ___ ___ ___ _____
   H. For wraparound sterile gowns, release front fastener. ___ ___ ___ _____
   I. Handing tie to stationary team member, turn 360 degrees to left and secure tie to gown. ___ ___ ___ _____

STUDENT: _____ DATE: _____

INSTRUCTOR: _____ DATE: _____

PROCEDURE PERFORMANCE CHECKLIST
Skill 33-5 Open Gloving

	S	U	NP	Comments
Open Gloving				
1. Perform thorough handwashing.	____	____	____	_____
2. Peel apart sides of outer package of glove wrapper.	____	____	____	_____
3. Lay inner package on clean, flat surface just above waist level.	____	____	____	_____
4. Open package, keeping gloves on inside surface of wrapper.	____	____	____	_____
5. If gloves are not prepowdered, apply powder lightly to hands over sink or wastebasket.	____	____	____	_____
6. Identify right and left gloves.	____	____	____	_____
7. Start by applying glove to dominant hand. With thumb and first two fingers of nondominant hand, grasp edge of cuff of glove of dominant hand, touching only inside surface.	____	____	____	_____
8. Carefully pull glove over dominant hand, ensuring cuff does not roll up wrist.	____	____	____	_____
9. With gloved dominant hand, slip fingers underneath second glove's cuff to pick it up.	____	____	____	_____
10. Carefully pull second glove over nondominant hand, and do not allow gloved hand to touch any part of exposed nondominant hand.	____	____	____	_____
11. When both gloves are on, interlock fingers of both hands to secure gloves in position, being careful to touch only sterile sides.	____	____	____	_____
12. Dispose of gloves:				
A. Without touching wrist, grasp outside of one cuff with other gloved hand.	____	____	____	_____
B. Pull glove off, turning it inside out. Discard in receptacle.	____	____	____	_____
C. Tuck fingers of bare hand inside remaining glove cuff. Peel glove off, inside out. Discard in receptacle.	____	____	____	_____
D. Wash hands.	____	____	____	_____

STUDENT: _____ DATE: _____

INSTRUCTOR: _____ DATE: _____

PROCEDURE PERFORMANCE CHECKLIST
Skill 34-1 Administering Oral Medications

	S	U	NP	Comments
Administering Oral Medications				
1. Assess for any contraindications to client receiving oral medication.	_____	_____	_____	_____
2. Assess client's medical history, history of allergies, medication history, and diet history.	_____	_____	_____	_____
3. Review assessment and laboratory data that may influence drug administration.	_____	_____	_____	_____
4. Assess client's knowledge regarding health and medication usage.	_____	_____	_____	_____
5. Assess client's preferences for fluids.	_____	_____	_____	_____
6. Check accuracy and completeness of each record with prescriber's written medication order.	_____	_____	_____	_____
7. Prepare medications:				
A. Wash hands.	_____	_____	_____	_____
B. Arrange medication tray and cups in medication preparation area or move medication cart to position outside client's room.	_____	_____	_____	_____
C. Unlock medicine drawer or cart.	_____	_____	_____	_____
D. Prepare medications for one client at a time. Keep all pages of records for one client together.	_____	_____	_____	_____
E. Select correct drug from stock supply or unit-dose drawer.	_____	_____	_____	_____
F. Calculate drug dose as necessary. Double-check calculation.	_____	_____	_____	_____
G. To prepare tablets or capsules from a floor stock bottle, pour required number into bottle cap and transfer medication to medication cup. Do not touch medication with fingers. Extra tablets or capsules may be returned to bottle. Break prescored medications using a gloved hand or a pill-cutting device.	_____	_____	_____	_____
H. To prepare unit-dose tablets or capsules, place packaged tablet or capsule directly into medicine cup. (Do not remove wrapper.)	_____	_____	_____	_____
I. Place tablets or capsules to be given to client at the same time in one medicine cup unless client requires preadministration assessments.	_____	_____	_____	_____

Continued

	S	U	NP	Comments

J. If client has difficulty swallowing and the pill may be crushed, use a pill-crushing device. If a pill-crushing device is not available, place tablet between two medication cups and grind with a blunt instrument. Mix ground tablet in small amount of soft food (e.g., custard or applesauce).

K. Prepare liquids:

   (1) Remove bottle cap from container and place cap upside down.

   (2) Hold bottle with label against palm of hand while pouring.

   (3) Hold medication cup at eye level and fill to desired level on scale.

   (4) Discard any excess liquid into sink. Wipe lip and neck of bottle with paper towel.

   (5) Draw up volumes of liquid medication of less than 10 ml in syringe without needle.

L. When preparing narcotics, check narcotic record for previous drug count and compare with supply available.

M. Check expiration date on all medications.

N. Compare record with prepared drug and container.

O. Return stock containers or unused unit-dose medications to shelf or drawer and read label again.

P. Do not leave drugs unattended.

8. Administering medications:

A. Take medications to client at correct time.

B. Identify client by comparing name on record with name on client's identification bracelet. Ask client to state name.

C. Explain to client the purpose of each medication and its action. Allow client to ask any questions about drugs he or she is receiving.

D. Assist client to sitting position or to side-lying position if sitting is contraindicated.

E. Administer drugs properly:

   (1) Allow client to hold solid medications in hand or cup before placing in mouth.

   (2) Offer water or juice to help client swallow medications. Give client cold carbonated water if available and not contraindicated.

Continued

394

	S	U	NP	Comments

(3) For drugs administered sublingually, instruct client to place medication under tongue and allow it to dissolve completely. Caution client against swallowing tablet. ____ ____ ____ _____

(4) For drugs administered buccally, instruct client to place medication in mouth against mucous membranes of the cheek until it dissolves. Avoid administering liquids until medication has dissolved. ____ ____ ____ _____

(5) Mix powdered medications with liquids at bedside and give to client to drink. ____ ____ ____ _____

(6) Caution client against chewing or swallowing lozenges. ____ ____ ____ _____

(7) Give effervescent powders and tablets to client immediately after they have dissolved. ____ ____ ____ _____

F. If client is unable to hold medications, place medication cup to client's lips and gently introduce each drug into the mouth, one at a time. ____ ____ ____ _____

G. If tablet or capsule falls to the floor, discard it and repeat preparation. ____ ____ ____ _____

H. Stay in room until client has completely swallowed each medication. Ask client to open mouth if you are uncertain whether medication has been swallowed. ____ ____ ____ _____

I. When administering highly acidic medications, offer client a nonfat snack if not contraindicated. ____ ____ ____ _____

J. Assist client in returning to a comfortable position. ____ ____ ____ _____

K. Dispose of soiled supplies. ____ ____ ____ _____

L. Wash hands. ____ ____ ____ _____

9. Return to client's room within 30 minutes to evaluate client's response to medication. ____ ____ ____ _____

10. Ask client or family member to identify drug name and explain purpose, action, dosage schedule, and potential side effects of drug. ____ ____ ____ _____

11. Notify prescriber if the client exhibits a toxic effect or allergic reaction or if there is an onset of side effects. If either of these occur, withhold further doses of medication. ____ ____ ____ _____

12. Record administration (or withholding) of oral medications. ____ ____ ____ _____

STUDENT: _____ DATE: _____

INSTRUCTOR: _____ DATE: _____

	S	U	NP	Comments
Administering Nasal Instillations				
1. For nasal drops, determine which of client's sinuses is affected.	____	____	____	_____
2. Assess client's history of hypertension, heart disease, diabetes mellitus, and hyperthyroidism.	____	____	____	_____
3. Inspect condition of client's nose and sinuses. Palpate sinuses for tenderness.	____	____	____	_____
4. Assess client's knowledge regarding use of and technique for instillation and willingness to learn self-administration.	____	____	____	_____
5. Explain procedure to client regarding positioning and sensations to expect.	____	____	____	_____
6. Wash hands.	____	____	____	_____
7. Arrange supplies and medications at bedside.	____	____	____	_____
8. Instruct client to clear or blow nose gently, unless contraindicated.	____	____	____	_____
9. Administer nasal drops:				
A. Assist client to supine position.	____	____	____	_____
B. Position client's head properly:				
(1) For access to posterior pharynx, tilt client's head backward.	____	____	____	_____
(2) For access to ethmoid or sphenoid sinus, tilt client's head back over edge of bed or place small pillow under client's shoulder and tilt head back.	____	____	____	_____
(3) For access to frontal and maxillary sinuses, tilt client's head back over edge of bed or pillow with head turned toward side to be treated.	____	____	____	_____
C. Support client's head with nondominant hand.	____	____	____	_____
D. Instruct client to breathe through mouth.	____	____	____	_____
E. Hold dropper 1 cm above client's nares and instill prescribed number of drops toward midline of ethmoid bone.	____	____	____	_____
F. Have client remain in supine position 5 minutes.	____	____	____	_____
G. Offer facial tissue to client to blot runny nose, but caution client against blowing nose for several minutes.	____	____	____	_____
10. Assist client to a comfortable position after drug is absorbed.	____	____	____	_____

Continued

	S	U	NP	Comments
11. Dispose of soiled supplies in proper container.	___	___	___	_____
12. Wash hands.	___	___	___	_____
13. Observe client for onset of side effects for 15 to 30 minutes after administration.	___	___	___	_____
14. Ask if client is able to breathe through nose after decongestant administration.	___	___	___	_____
15. Reinspect condition of nasal passages between instillations.	___	___	___	_____
16. Ask client to review risks of overuse of decongestants and methods for administration.	___	___	___	_____
17. Have client demonstrate self-medication.	___	___	___	_____
18. Record medication administration and client's response.	___	___	___	_____
19. Report any unusual systemic effects.	___	___	___	_____

PROCEDURE PERFORMANCE CHECKLIST
Skill 34-3 Administering Ophthalmic Medications

	S	U	NP	Comments
Administering Ophthalmic Medications				
1. Review prescriber's medication order.	____	____	____	_____
2. Assess condition of client's external eye structures.	____	____	____	_____
3. Determine whether client has any known allergies to eye medications. Ask if client is allergic to latex.	____	____	____	_____
4. Determine whether client has any symptoms of visual alterations.	____	____	____	_____
5. Assess client's level of consciousness and ability to follow directions.	____	____	____	_____
6. Assess client's knowledge regarding drug therapy and desire to self-administer medication.	____	____	____	_____
7. Assess client's ability to manipulate and hold eye dropper.	____	____	____	_____
8. Explain procedure to client.	____	____	____	_____
9. Wash hands.	____	____	____	_____
10. Arrange supplies at client's bedside.	____	____	____	_____
11. Apply clean gloves.	____	____	____	_____
12. Ask client to lie supine or to sit back in chair with head slightly hyperextended.	____	____	____	_____
13. Wash away any crusts or drainage along client's eyelid margins or inner canthus. Soak any crusts that are dried and difficult to remove by applying a damp washcloth or cotton ball over eye for a few minutes.	____	____	____	_____
14. Hold cotton ball or clean tissue in nondominant hand on client's cheekbone just below lower eyelid.	____	____	____	_____
15. With tissue or cotton ball resting below lower lid, gently press downward with thumb or forefinger against bony orbit.	____	____	____	_____
16. Ask client to look at ceiling.	____	____	____	_____
17. Instill eye drops while explaining steps to client:				
A. With dominant had resting on client's forehead, hold filled medication eye dropper or ophthalmic solution approximately 1 to 2 cm above conjunctival sac.	____	____	____	_____
B. Drop prescribed number of medication drops into conjunctival sac.	____	____	____	_____

Continued

	S	U	NP	Comments

C. If client blinks or closes eye or if drops land on outer lid margins, repeat procedure. ____ ____ ____ _____

D. For drugs that cause systemic effects, with a clean tissue apply gentle pressure with your finger and clean tissue on the client's naso-lacrimal duct for 30 to 60 seconds. ____ ____ ____ _____

E. After instilling drops, ask client to close eye gently. ____ ____ ____ _____

18. Instill eye ointment:

A. Ask client to look at ceiling. ____ ____ ____ _____

B. Holding ointment applicator above lower lid margin, apply thin stream of ointment evenly along inner edge of lower eyelid on conjunctiva from inner canthus to outer canthus. ____ ____ ____ _____

C. Have client close eye and rub lid gently in circular motion with cotton ball, if rubbing is not contraindicated. ____ ____ ____ _____

19. Intraocular disk procedures:

A. Application:

(1) Wash hands. ____ ____ ____ _____

(2) Put on gloves. ____ ____ ____ _____

(3) Open package containing disk. Gently press fingertip against disk so it adheres to finger. Position convex side of disk on fingertip. ____ ____ ____ _____

(4) With other hand, gently pull client's lower eyelid away from the eye. Ask client to look up. ____ ____ ____ _____

(5) Place disk in the conjunctival sac so that it floats on the sclera between the iris and lower eyelid. ____ ____ ____ _____

(6) Pull client's lower eyelid out and over disk. ____ ____ ____ _____

B. Removal:

(1) Wash hands. ____ ____ ____ _____

(2) Put on gloves. ____ ____ ____ _____

(3) Explain procedure to client. ____ ____ ____ _____

(4) Gently pull on client's lower eyelid to expose disk. ____ ____ ____ _____

(5) Using forefinger and thumb of opposite hand, pinch disk and lift it out of client's eye. ____ ____ ____ _____

20. If excess medication is on eyelid, gently wipe eyelid from inner to outer canthus. ____ ____ ____ _____

Continued

	S	U	NP	Comments
21. If client had an eye patch, apply clean patch by placing it over affected eye so entire eye is covered. Tape securely without applying pressure to eye.	_____	_____	_____	_____
22. Remove gloves.	_____	_____	_____	_____
23. Dispose of soiled supplies in proper receptacle.	_____	_____	_____	_____
24. Wash hands.	_____	_____	_____	_____
25. Note client's response to instillation. Ask if any discomfort was felt.	_____	_____	_____	_____
26. Observe client's response to medication by assessing visual changes and noting any side effects.	_____	_____	_____	_____
27. Ask client to discuss drug's purpose, action, side effect, and technique of administration.	_____	_____	_____	_____
28. Have client demonstrate self-administration of next dose.	_____	_____	_____	_____
29. Record drug administration and appearance of client's eye.	_____	_____	_____	_____
30. Record and report and undesirable side effects.	_____	_____	_____	_____

PROCEDURE PERFORMANCE CHECKLIST

Skill 34-4 Administering Vaginal Medications

	S	U	NP	Comments
Administering Vaginal Medications				
1. Check medication order.	___	___	___	_____
2. Wash hands.	___	___	___	_____
3. Prepare equipment and supplies.	___	___	___	_____
4. Identify client.	___	___	___	_____
5. Inspect client's external genitalia and vaginal canal.	___	___	___	_____
6. Assess client's ability to manipulate applicator and position herself.	___	___	___	_____
7. Explain procedure to client.	___	___	___	_____
8. Arrange supplies at client's bedside.	___	___	___	_____
9. Provide privacy.	___	___	___	_____
10. Assist client to dorsal recumbent position.	___	___	___	_____
11. Keep client's abdomen and lower extremities draped.	___	___	___	_____
12. Apply disposable gloves.	___	___	___	_____
13. Provide adequate lighting.	___	___	___	_____
14. Insert suppository:				
A. Take suppository from wrapper and lubricate smooth or rounded end.	___	___	___	_____
B. Lubricate gloved finger of dominant hand.	___	___	___	_____
C. Retract client's labial folds with nondominant gloved hand.	___	___	___	_____
D. Insert rounded end of suppository 7.5 to 10 cm along posterior wall of vaginal canal.	___	___	___	_____
E. Withdraw finger and wipe away lubricant from client's orifice and labia.	___	___	___	_____
15. Apply cream or foam:				
A. Fill applicator as directed.	___	___	___	_____
B. Retract client's labial folds with nondominant gloved hand.	___	___	___	_____
C. With dominant gloved hand, insert applicator 5 to 7.5 cm; push plunger.	___	___	___	_____
D. Withdraw applicator and place it on paper towel. Wipe away lubricant from client's orifice and labia.	___	___	___	_____
E. Wash applicator and store for future use.	___	___	___	_____
16. Remove and discard gloves.	___	___	___	_____
17. Wash hands.	___	___	___	_____
18. Instruct client to remain flat on her back for at least 10 minutes.	___	___	___	_____

Continued

	S	U	NP	Comments
19. Offer client perineal pad.	_____	_____	_____	_____
20. Inspect condition of client's vaginal canal and external genitalia between applications.	_____	_____	_____	_____
21. Record medication administration.	_____	_____	_____	_____

PROCEDURE PERFORMANCE CHECKLIST

Skill 34-5 Administering Rectal Suppositories

	S	U	NP	Comments
Administering Rectal Suppositories				
1. Check medication order.	____	____	____	_____
2. Review client's medical record for rectal surgery/bleeding.	____	____	____	_____
3. Wash hands.	____	____	____	_____
4. Prepare needed equipment and supplies.	____	____	____	_____
5. Apply disposable gloves.	____	____	____	_____
6. Identify client.	____	____	____	_____
7. Explain procedure to client.	____	____	____	_____
8. Arrange supplies at client's bedside.	____	____	____	_____
9. Provide privacy.	____	____	____	_____
10. Position client in Sims' position.	____	____	____	_____
11. Keep client draped, except for anal area.	____	____	____	_____
12. Examine external condition of client's anus. Palpate rectal walls.	____	____	____	_____
13. Dispose of gloves, if soiled, and reapply new gloves.	____	____	____	_____
14. Remove suppository from wrapper and lubricate rounded end.	____	____	____	_____
15. Lubricate gloved finger of dominant hand.	____	____	____	_____
16. Ask client to take slow, deep breaths through mouth and to relax anal sphincter.	____	____	____	_____
17. Retract client's buttocks with nondominant hand.	____	____	____	_____
18. With index finger of dominant hand, gently insert suppository through anus, past the internal sphincter, and place against rectal wall, 10 cm for adults or 5 cm for children and infants.	____	____	____	_____
19. Withdraw finger and wipe client's anal area clean.	____	____	____	_____
20. Remove and dispose of gloves.	____	____	____	_____
21. Wash hands.	____	____	____	_____
22. If suppository contains a laxative or fecal softener, be sure that client will receive help to reach bedpan or toilet.	____	____	____	_____
23. Keep client flat on back or on side for 5 minutes.	____	____	____	_____
24. Return in 5 minutes to determine if suppository has been expelled.	____	____	____	_____
25. Observe client for effects of suppository 30 minutes after administration.	____	____	____	_____
26. Record medication administration.	____	____	____	_____

PROCEDURE PERFORMANCE CHECKLIST

Skill 34-6 Instructing Client in the Use of Metered-Dose Inhalers

	S	U	NP	Comments
Instructing Client in the Use of Metered-Dose Inhalers				
1. Assess client's ability to hold, manipulate, and depress canister and inhaler.	___	___	___	_____
2. Assess client's readiness and ability to learn.	___	___	___	_____
3. Assess client's knowledge and understanding of his or her disease and purpose of the action of prescribed medications.	___	___	___	_____
4. Assess drug schedule and number of inhalations prescribed for each dose.	___	___	___	_____
5. Assess client's technique for using an inhaler if he or she has been previously instructed in self-medication.	___	___	___	_____
6. Instruct client in a comfortable environment.	___	___	___	_____
7. Provide adequate time for teaching session.	___	___	___	_____
8. Wash hands.	___	___	___	_____
9. Arrange necessary equipment.	___	___	___	_____
10. Allow client the opportunity to manipulate inhaler, canister, and spacer device. Explain and demonstrate how canister fits into inhaler.	___	___	___	_____
11. Explain what metered dose is and warn client about overuse of the inhaler, including drug side effects.	___	___	___	_____
12. Explain and demonstrate steps for administering inhaled dose of medication:				
A. Remove mouthpiece cover from inhaler.	___	___	___	_____
B. Shake inhaler well.	___	___	___	_____
C. Have client take a deep breath and exhale.	___	___	___	_____
D. Instruct the client to position the inhaler in one of two ways:				
(1) Open lips and place inhaler in mouth with opening toward back of throat.	___	___	___	_____
(2) Position the device 3.5 to 5 cm from the mouth.	___	___	___	_____
E. With the inhaler properly positioned, have client hold it with thumb at the mouthpiece and the index and middle fingers at the top.	___	___	___	_____
F. Instruct client to tilt head back slightly, inhale deeply and slowly through mouth, and depress medication canister fully.	___	___	___	_____
G. Instruct client to hold breath for approximately 10 seconds.	___	___	___	_____

Continued

	S	U	NP	Comments

   H. Have client exhale through pursed lips. ____ ____ ____ _____

13. Explain and demonstrate steps to administer inhaled dose of medication using a spacer such as an aerochamber:

   A. Remove mouthpiece cover from inhaler and mouthpiece of aerochamber. ____ ____ ____ _____

   B. Insert inhaler into end of aerochamber. ____ ____ ____ _____

   C. Shake inhaler well. ____ ____ ____ _____

   D. Have client place aerochamber mouthpiece in mouth and close lips. Tell client not to insert mouthpiece beyond raised lip and to avoid covering small exhalation slots with lips.

   E. Instruct client to breathe normally through aerochamber mouthpiece. ____ ____ ____ _____

   F. Have client depress medication canister, spraying one puff into aerochamber. ____ ____ ____ _____

   G. Instruct client to breathe slowly and fully for 5 seconds. ____ ____ ____ _____

   H. Have client hold a full breath for 5 to 10 seconds. ____ ____ ____ _____

14. Instruct client to wait 2 to 5 minutes between inhalations or as ordered by prescriber. ____ ____ ____ _____

15. Instruct client against repeating inhalations before next scheduled dose. ____ ____ ____ _____

16. Explain that client may feel gagging sensation in throat caused by droplets of medication. ____ ____ ____ _____

17. Instruct client in removing medication canister and cleaning inhaler in warm water. ____ ____ ____ _____

18. Have client explain and demonstrate steps in use of inhaler. ____ ____ ____ _____

19. Ask client to explain drug schedule. ____ ____ ____ _____

20. Ask client to describe side effects of medication and criteria for calling physician. ____ ____ ____ _____

21. Ask if client has any questions and answer them. ____ ____ ____ _____

22. After medication instillation, assess client's respirations and auscultate lungs. ____ ____ ____ _____

23. Record client education and client's ability to perform self-administration of medication. ____ ____ ____ _____

PROCEDURE PERFORMANCE CHECKLIST
Skill 34-7 Preparing Injections

	S	U	NP	Comments

Preparing Injections

1. Check medication order. _____ _____ _____ _____

2. Review pertinent information related to medication. _____ _____ _____ _____

3. Assess client's body build, muscle size, and weight. _____ _____ _____ _____

4. Prepare medication:

   A. Ampule preparation:

   (1) Tap top of ampule lightly and quickly with finger until fluid moves from neck of ampule. _____ _____ _____ _____

   (2) Place small gauze pad around neck of ampule. _____ _____ _____ _____

   (3) Snap neck of ampule quickly and firmly while pointing it away from your body. _____ _____ _____ _____

   (4) Draw up medication quickly. _____ _____ _____ _____

   (5) Hold ampule upside down or set it on a flat surface. Insert syringe or filter needle into center of ampule opening. Do not allow needle tip or shaft to touch rim of ampule. _____ _____ _____ _____

   (6) Aspirate medication into syringe by gently pulling back on plunger. _____ _____ _____ _____

   (7) Keep needle tip under surface of liquid. Tip ampule to bring all fluid within reach of needle. _____ _____ _____ _____

   (8) If air bubbles are aspirated, do not expel air into ampule. _____ _____ _____ _____

   (9) To expel excess air bubbles, remove needle from ampule. Hold syringe with needle pointing up. Tap side of syringe to cause bubbles to rise toward needle. Draw back slightly on plunger, then push plunger upward to eject air. Do not eject fluid. _____ _____ _____ _____

   (10) If syringe contains excess fluid, use sink for disposal. Hold syringe vertically with needle tip up and slanted slightly toward sink. Slowly eject excess fluid into sink. Recheck fluid level in syringe by holding it vertically. _____ _____ _____ _____

Continued

	S	U	NP	Comments

(11) Cover needle with its safety sheath or cap. Change needle on syringe or use filter needle if you suspect medication is on needle shaft. _____ _____ _____ _____

B. Vial containing a solution:

(1) Remove cap covering top of unused vial to expose sterile rubber seal, keeping rubber seal sterile. If using a multidose vial that has been used before, firmly and briskly wipe surface of rubber seal with alcohol swab and allow it to dry. _____ _____ _____ _____

(2) Pick up syringe and remove needle cap. Pull back on plunger to draw amount of air into syringe equivalent to volume of medication to be aspirated from vial. _____ _____ _____ _____

(3) With vial on flat surface, insert tip of needle with beveled tip entering first through center of rubber seal. Apply pressure to tip of needle during insertion. _____ _____ _____ _____

(4) Inject air into vial's airspace, holding on to plunger. Hold plunger with firm pressure; plunger may be forced backward by air pressure within the vial. _____ _____ _____ _____

(5) Invert vial while keeping firm hold on syringe and plunger. Hold vial between thumb and middle fingers of nondominant hand. Grasp end of syringe barrel and plunger with thumb and forefinger of dominant hand to counteract pressure in vial. _____ _____ _____ _____

(6) Keep tip of needle below fluid level. _____ _____ _____ _____

(7) Allow air pressure from vial to fill syringe gradually with medication. Pull back slightly on plunger to obtain correct amount of solution. _____ _____ _____ _____

(8) When desired volume has been obtained, position needle into vial's airspace. Tap side of syringe barrel carefully to dislodge any air bubbles. Eject any air remaining at top of syringe into vial. _____ _____ _____ _____

(9) Remove needle from vial by pulling back on barrel of syringe. _____ _____ _____ _____

Continued

	S	U	NP	Comments

(10) Hold syringe at a 90-degree angle at eye level to ensure correct volume and absence of air bubbles. Remove any remaining air by tapping barrel to dislodge any air bubbles. Draw back slightly on plunger, then push plunger upward to eject air. Do not eject fluid.

(11) If medication is to be injected into client's tissue, change needle to appropriate guage and length according to route of medication.

(12) For multidose vial, make label that includes date of mixing, concentration of drug per milliliter, and your initials.

C. Vial containing a powder (reconstituting medications):

(1) Remove cap covering vial of powdered medication and cap covering vial of proper diluent.

(2) Draw up diluent into syringe by following steps 4B(2) through 4B(10).

(3) Insert tip of needle through center of rubber seal of powdered medication. Inject diluent into vial. Remove needle.

(4) Mix medication thoroughly. Roll vial in palms, Do not shake.

(5) Read label carefully to determine dose after reconstitution.

5. Dispose of soiled supplies. Place broken ampule and/or used vials and used needle in puncture-proof and leak-proof container.

6. Clean work area.

7. Wash hands.

STUDENT: _____ DATE: _____

INSTRUCTOR: _____ DATE: _____

PROCEDURE PERFORMANCE CHECKLIST
Skill 34-8 Administering Injections

	S	U	NP	Comments

Administering Injections
1. Review prescriber's medication order. _____ _____ _____ _____
2. Assess client's history of allergies. _____ _____ _____ _____
3. Check expiration date of vial or ampule. _____ _____ _____ _____
4. Observe client's verbal and nonverbal responses _____ _____ _____ _____
   to receiving an injection.
5. Assess for contraindications to subcutaneous or _____ _____ _____ _____
   intramuscular injections.
6. Prepare correct medication dose from ampule or _____ _____ _____ _____
   vial. Check carefully. Be sure all air is expelled.
7. Identify client by checking identification arm-
   band and asking client's name. Compare with _____ _____ _____ _____
   record.
8. Explain steps of procedure to client and tell _____ _____ _____ _____
   client injection will cause a slight burning or
   sting.
9. Provide privacy. _____ _____ _____ _____
10. Wash hands. _____ _____ _____ _____
11. Keep sheet or gown draped over client's body _____ _____ _____ _____
    parts not requiring exposure.
12. Select appropriate injection site. Inspect skin sur-
    face of site for bruises, inflammation, or edema:
    A. For subcutaneous (SQ) injections: Palpate _____ _____ _____ _____
       sites for masses or tenderness. Avoid these
       areas. For daily insulin injections, rotate site
       daily. Check that needle is correct size by
       grasping skinfold at site with thumb and
       forefinger. Measure fold from top to bottom.
    B. For intramuscular (IM) injections: Note _____ _____ _____ _____
       integrity and size of muscle and palpate for
       tender or hard areas. Avoid these areas. If
       injections are given frequently, rotate sites.
    C. For intradermal (ID) injections: Note lesions _____ _____ _____ _____
       or discoloration of forearm. Select site three
       to four fingerwidths below antecubital space
       and a handwidth above wrist.
13. Assist client to a comfortable position:
    A. For SQ injections: Have client relax arm, leg, _____ _____ _____ _____
       or abdomen, depending on site chosen.
    B. For IM injections: Have client lie flat, on _____ _____ _____ _____
       side, or prone, depending on site chosen.

Continued

	S	U	NP	Comments
C. For ID injections: Have client extend elbow and support it and forearm on flat surface.	_____	_____	_____	_____
D. Talk with client about subject of interest.	_____	_____	_____	_____
14. Relocate site using anatomical landmarks.	_____	_____	_____	_____
15. Cleanse site with an antiseptic swab. Apply swab at center of site and rotate outward in a circular direction for about 5 cm.	_____	_____	_____	_____
16. Hold swab or gauze between third and fourth fingers of nondominant hand.	_____	_____	_____	_____
17. Remove needle cap or sheath from needle by pulling it straight off.	_____	_____	_____	_____
18. Hold syringe between thumb and forefinger of dominant hand:				
A. For SQ and IM injections: Hold as dart, with palm down.	_____	_____	_____	_____
B. For ID injections: Hold with bevel of needle pointing up.	_____	_____	_____	_____
19. Administer injection:				
A. SQ injection:				
(1) For average-size client, spread skin tightly across injection site or pinch skin with nondominant hand.	_____	_____	_____	_____
(2) Inject needle quickly and firmly at a 45- to 90-degree angle, then release skin, if pinched.	_____	_____	_____	_____
(3) For obese client, pinch skin at site and inject needle at 90-degree angle below tissue fold.	_____	_____	_____	_____
(4) After needle enters site, grasp lower end of syringe barrel with nondominant hand. Move dominant hand to end of plunger. Avoid moving syringe while slowly pulling back on plunger to aspirate drug. If blood appears in syringe, remove needle, discard medication and syringe, and repeat procedure. Do not aspirate when giving heparin.	_____	_____	_____	_____
(5) Inject medication slowly.	_____	_____	_____	_____
B. IM injection:				
(1) Position nondominant hand at proper anatomical landmarks and pull skin down to administer in a Z-track. Inject needle quickly into muscle at a 90-degree angle.	_____	_____	_____	_____
(2) If client's muscle mass is small, grasp body of muscle between thumb and fingers.	_____	_____	_____	_____
(3) Aspirate as in step 19A(4).	_____	_____	_____	_____

Continued

414

	S	U	NP	Comments

    (4) Inject medication slowly.   _____ _____ _____ _____

    (5) Wait 10 seconds, then smoothly and steadily withdraw needle while placing antiseptic swab or dry gauze gently above or over injection site.   _____ _____ _____ _____

 C. ID injection:

    (1) With nondominant hand, stretch skin across injection site with forefinger or thumb.   _____ _____ _____ _____

    (2) Place needle against client's skin and insert it slowly at a 5- to 15-degree angle until resistance is felt. Advance needle through epidermis approximately 3 mm below skin surface so that needle tip can be seen through skin.   _____ _____ _____ _____

    (3) Inject medication slowly. Remove needle and begin again if no resistance is felt.   _____ _____ _____ _____

    (4) While injecting medication, notice that a small bleb approximately 6 mm in diameter appears on skin's surface.   _____ _____ _____ _____

20. Withdraw needle while applying alcohol swab or gauze gently over site.   _____ _____ _____ _____

21. Do no massage site after SQ injection of heparin or insulin or after ID injection. Apply bandage over ID site.   _____ _____ _____ _____

22. Assist client to a comfortable position.   _____ _____ _____ _____

23. Discard uncapped needle or needle enclosed in safety shield and attached syringe into puncture- and leak-proof receptacle. If unable to leave client's bedside, use a one-handed technique to recap needle.   _____ _____ _____ _____

24. Remove and dispose of gloves.   _____ _____ _____ _____

25. Wash hands.   _____ _____ _____ _____

26. Stay with client and observe for any immediate reactions.   _____ _____ _____ _____

27. Return to room in 10 to 30 minutes to evaluate client's response to injection and medication. Inspect injection site and ask about client's sensations.   _____ _____ _____ _____

28. Ask client to explain purpose and effects of medication.   _____ _____ _____ _____

29. For ID injections, use skin pencil and draw circle around perimeter of injection site. Check site within 48 to 72 hours of injection.   _____ _____ _____ _____

Continued

	S	U	NP	Comments
30. Record medication administration.	____	____	____	_____
31. Record and report client's response to injection and any undesirable effects caused by the medication.	____	____	____	_____

STUDENT: _____ DATE: _____

INSTRUCTOR: _____ DATE: _____

PROCEDURE PERFORMANCE CHECKLIST

Skill 34-9 Adding Medications to Intravenous Fluid Containers

	S	U	NP	Comments
Adding Medications to Intravenous Fluid Containers				
1. Check prescriber's order to determine type of intravenous (IV) solution to use and type of medication and dosage.	____	____	____	_____
2. Collect necessary information for safe administration of the drug.	____	____	____	_____
3. Assess for the compatibility of multiple medications in a single IV solution.	____	____	____	_____
4. Assess client's systemic fluid balance.	____	____	____	_____
5. Assess client's history of allergies.	____	____	____	_____
6. Assess IV insertion site for signs of infiltration or phlebitis.	____	____	____	_____
7. Assess client's understanding of the purpose of the drug therapy.	____	____	____	_____
8. Wash hands.	____	____	____	_____
9. Assemble supplies in medication room.	____	____	____	_____
10. Prepare prescribed medication from vial or ampule.	____	____	____	_____
11. Add medication to new container:				
A. Locate injection port:				
(1) *Solutions in bags*: Locate medication injection port on plastic IV solution bag.	____	____	____	_____
(2) *Solutions in bottles:* Locate injection site on IV solution bottle, which is often covered by a metal or plastic cap.	____	____	____	_____
B. Wipe off port or injection site with alcohol or antiseptic swab.	____	____	____	_____
C. Remove needle cap or sheath from syringe and insert needle through center of injection port or site.	____	____	____	_____
D. Inject medication.	____	____	____	_____
E. Withdraw syringe from bag or bottle.	____	____	____	_____
F. Mix medication and IV solution by holding bag or bottle and turning it gently end to end.	____	____	____	_____
G. Complete medication label with name, dose of medication, date, time, and initials. Stick label on bottle or bag.	____	____	____	_____
12. Bring assembled items to client's bedside.	____	____	____	_____
13. Identify client.	____	____	____	_____
14. Explain procedure to client and alert client to expected sensations.	____	____	____	_____

Continued

	S	U	NP	Comments

15. Regulate infusion at ordered rate. _____ _____ _____ _____
16. Add medication to existing container:
   A. Prepare vented IV bottle or plastic bag:
      (1) Check volume of solution remaining in _____ _____ _____ _____
          bottle or bag.
      (2) Close off IV infusion clamp. _____ _____ _____ _____
      (3) Wipe off medication port with an alco- _____ _____ _____ _____
          hol or antiseptic swab.
      (4) Insert syringe needle through injection _____ _____ _____ _____
          port and inject medication.
      (5) Lower bag or bottle from IV pole and _____ _____ _____ _____
          gently mix. Rehang bag.
   B. Complete medication label and stick it to bag _____ _____ _____ _____
      or bottle.
   C. Regulate infusion to desired rate. _____ _____ _____ _____
17. Properly dispose of equipment and supplies. Do _____ _____ _____ _____
   not cap needle of syringe. Discard sheathed nee-
   dles as a unit with needle covered.
18. Wash hands. _____ _____ _____ _____
19. Observe client for signs and symptoms of drug _____ _____ _____ _____
   reaction.
20. Observe client for signs and symptoms of fluid _____ _____ _____ _____
   volume excess.
21. Periodically return to client's room to assess IV _____ _____ _____ _____
   insertion site and rate of infusion.
22. Observe client for signs or symptoms of IV infil- _____ _____ _____ _____
   tration.
23. Record solution and medication added to par- _____ _____ _____ _____
   enteral fluid on appropriate form and report any
   side effects observed.

STUDENT: _____ DATE: _____

INSTRUCTOR: _____ DATE: _____

PROCEDURE PERFORMANCE CHECKLIST

Skill 34-10 Administering Medications by IV Bolus

	S	U	NP	Comments
Administering Medications by IV Bolus				
1. Check medication order.	____	____	____	_____
2. Assess IV or heparin (saline) lock site for infiltration or phlebitis.	____	____	____	_____
3. Assemble and prepare equipment and supplies.	____	____	____	_____
4. Prepare medication from vial or ampule. Check dilution instructions. Apply a small-gauge needle to syringe.	____	____	____	_____
5. Wash hands.	____	____	____	_____
6. Apply disposable gloves.	____	____	____	_____
7. Identify client.	____	____	____	_____
8. Determine that IV fluids are infusing at proper rate.	____	____	____	_____
9. Procedure for existing line:				
A. Select injection port of tubing closest to needle insertion site.	____	____	____	_____
B. Cleanse injection port with antiseptic swab. Allow port to dry.	____	____	____	_____
C. Connect syringe to IV line: Insert small-gauge needle into port or remove cap on port and attach tip of syringe directly to needleless system.	____	____	____	_____
D. Occlude IV line by pinching tubing above port. Aspirate for blood return.	____	____	____	_____
E. Continue to occlude tubing while injecting medication slowly. Time administration.	____	____	____	_____
F. Release tubing. Withdraw syringe and recheck IV rate.	____	____	____	_____
G. Replace needleless injection port cap with new cap.	____	____	____	_____
10. Procedure for IV lock or needleless system:				
A. Prepare flush solutions per agency policy.	____	____	____	_____
B. Cleanse lock's rubber diaphragm with antiseptic swab.	____	____	____	_____
C. Insert small-gauge needle through center of rubber diaphragm.	____	____	____	_____
D. Aspirate for blood return.	____	____	____	_____
E. Flush reservoir with 1 ml saline.	____	____	____	_____
F. Remove needle and saline syringe.	____	____	____	_____
G. Cleanse lock's diaphragm with antiseptic swab again.	____	____	____	_____

Continued

	S	U	NP	Comments

H. Insert needle of medication syringe into diaphragm. _____ _____ _____ _____

I. Inject prepared medication slowly. Time administration. _____ _____ _____ _____

J. Withdraw needle and syringe. _____ _____ _____ _____

K. Cleanse diaphragm again. _____ _____ _____ _____

L. Flush reservoir with 1 ml saline or heparin (or per agency policy). _____ _____ _____ _____

M. For needleless valve cap: Remove protective cap; flush with saline; inject prepared medication; withdraw syringe; repeat flush; and replace sterile cap over valve. _____ _____ _____ _____

11. Procedure for IV push by epidural route (given by specially prepared nurses only):

A. Check medication order. _____ _____ _____ _____

B. Prepare equipment and supplies. _____ _____ _____ _____

C. Draw up the narcotic using a 5 ml syringe or larger. (Verify agency policy for use of filter needle when aspirating medication from an ampule.) _____ _____ _____ _____

D. Identify client. _____ _____ _____ _____

E. Assess level of client sedation using standardized scale. _____ _____ _____ _____

F. Swab client's injection cap with povidone-iodine. Swab cap with sterile gauze. _____ _____ _____ _____

G. With 3 ml syringe and small-gauge needle, insert needle into injection cap and aspirate. Terminate procedure if more than 1 ml of clear or bloody fluid returns, and notify anesthetist. Continue procedure if less than 1/2 ml of fluid returns on aspiration. _____ _____ _____ _____

H. Insert medication syringe into injection cap and inject drug slowly. Reduce rate of injection if client complains of pain. _____ _____ _____ _____

12. Dispose of all equipment properly. _____ _____ _____ _____

13. Remove and dispose of gloves. _____ _____ _____ _____

14. Wash hands. _____ _____ _____ _____

15. Observe client closely for adverse reactions during and for several minutes after administration. _____ _____ _____ _____

16. Record medication administration. _____ _____ _____ _____

PROCEDURE PERFORMANCE CHECKLIST

Skill 34-11 Administering Intravenous Medications by Piggyback, Intermittent Intravenous Infusion Sets, and Miniinfusion Pumps

Administering Intravenous Medications by
Piggyback, Intermittent Intravenous Infusion Sets,
and Miniinfusion Pumps

1. Check prescriber's order to determine type of IV solution to be used, type of medication, and dose, route, and time of administration.

2. Collect necessary information for safe administration of the drug.

3. Assess patency of client's existing IV infusion line by noting infusion rate of main IV line.

4. Asses IV insertion site for signs of infiltration or phlebitis.

5. Assess client's history of allergies.

6. Assess client's understanding of the purpose of the drug therapy.

7. Assemble supplies at client's bedside. Prepare client by informing him or her that medication will be given through IV equipment.

8. Wash hands.

9. Apply disposable gloves.

10. Identify client by looking at armband and asking client's name.

11. Explain purpose of medication and side effects to client. Encourage client to report symptoms of discomfort at site.

12. Administer infusion:

A. Piggyback or tandem infusion:

    (1) Connect infusion tubing to medication bag. Allow solution to fill tubing by opening regulator flow clamp.

    (2) Hang piggyback medication bag above level of primary fluid bag. Hang tandem infusion at same level as primary fluid bag.

    (3) Connect tubing of piggyback or tandem infusion to appropriate connector on primary infusion line:

        (a) Stopcock: Wipe off stopcock port with alcohol swab and connect tubing. Turn stopcock to open position.

Continued

	S	U	NP	Comments

(b) Needleless system: Wipe off needleless port and insert tip of piggyback or tandem infusion tubing.

| | ____ | ____ | ____ | _____ |

(c) Tubing port: Connect sterile needle to end of piggyback or tandem infusion tubing, remove cap, cleanse injection port on main IV line, and insert needle through center of port.

| | ____ | ____ | ____ | _____ |

(4) Regulate flow rate of medication solution by adjusting regulator clamp.

(5) After medication has infused, check flow regulator on primary infusion.

(6) Regulate main infusion line to desired rate, if necessary.

(7) Leave secondary bag and tubing in place for future drug administration or discard in appropriate containers.

B. Volume-control administration set:

(1) Assemble supplies in medication room.

(2) Prepare medication from vial or ampule.

(3) Explain procedure to client. Encourage client to report symptoms of discomfort at site.

(4) Fill volume-control set with desired amount of fluid (50 to 100 ml) by opening clamp between volume-control set and main IV bag.

(5) Close clamp and check to be sure clamp on air vent of volume-control set chamber is open.

(6) Clean injection port with antiseptic swab.

(7) Remove needle cap or sheath and insert syringe needle through port, then inject medication. Gently rotate volume-control set between hands.

(8) Regulate IV infusion rate to allow medication to infuse in 30 to 90 minutes.

(9) Label volume-control set with name of drug, dosage, total volume including diluent, and time of administration.

(10) Dispose of uncapped needle or needle enclosed in safety shield and syringe in proper container.

C. Miniinfusor administration:

Continued

	S	U	NP	Comments
(1) Connect prefilled syringe to miniinfusion tubing.	___	___	___	_____
(2) Carefully apply pressure to syringe plunger, allowing tubing to fill with medication.	___	___	___	_____
(3) Place syringe into miniinfusor pump. Be sure syringe is secure.	___	___	___	_____
(4) Connect miniinfusion tubing to main IV line. (See 12A(3).)	___	___	___	_____
(5) Explain purpose of medication and side effects to client. Ask client to report symptoms of discomfort at site.	___	___	___	_____
(6) Hang infusion pump with syringe on IV pole alongside main IV bag. Press button on pump to begin infusion.	___	___	___	_____
(7) After medication has infused, check flow regulator on primary infusion. Regulate main infusion line to desired rate as needed. (Note: If stopcock is used, turn off miniinfusion line.)	___	___	___	_____
(8) Remove disposable gloves.	___	___	___	_____
(9) Wash hands.	___	___	___	_____
13. Observe client for signs of adverse reactions.	___	___	___	_____
14. During 30 to 90 minutes of infusion, periodically check infusion rate and condition of IV site.	___	___	___	_____
15. Ask client to explain purpose and side effects of medication.	___	___	___	_____
16. Record medication administration and IV infusion.	___	___	___	_____
17. Report any adverse reactions.	___	___	___	_____

STUDENT: _____ DATE: _____

INSTRUCTOR: _____ DATE: _____

PROCEDURE PERFORMANCE CHECKLIST
Skill 37-1 Use of Restraints

	S	U	NP	Comments

Use of Restraints
1. Assess client's need for restraint.
2. Review agency policies regarding restraints. Check physician's order for purpose and type of restraint.
3. Review restraint manufacturer's instructions before entering client's room.
4. Assess the area of the client's body where the restraint is to be placed.
5. Explain to client and family the need for restraint. Attempt to obtain consent.
6. Place client in proper body alignment.
7. Pad bony prominences before applying restraints.
8. Apply restraint, making sure it is not over an IV line or other device.
9. Attach restraints to bed frame, not side rails.
10. When client is in a chair, secure jacket restraint by placing ties under armrests and securing them at the back of the chair.
11. Secure restraints with a quick-release tie.
12. Make sure two fingers will fit under secured restraint.
13. Assess proper placement of restraint and condition of client's restrained body part at least every 30 minutes or per agency policy.
14. Remove restraints for 30 minutes every 2 hours. Do not leave restrained client unattended. Initiate special precautions for a violent or noncompliant client.
15. Secure call bell or intercom within client's reach.
16. Leave client's bed or chair with wheels locked. Bed should be in lowest position.
17. Wash hands.
18. Inspect client for any injury.
19. Observe IV catheters and urinary catheters to determine that they are positioned correctly and that therapy remains uninterrupted.
20. Record client behaviors that may place client at risk for injury.
21. Document client's response and expected or unexpected outcomes after restraint is applied.

STUDENT: _____ DATE: _____

INSTRUCTOR: _____ DATE: _____

PROCEDURE PERFORMANCE CHECKLIST
Skill 37-2 Seizure Precautions

	S	U	NP	Comments
Seizure Precautions				
1. Assess client's history and related medical/surgical conditions.	___	___	___	_____
2. Inspect client's environment for safety hazards.	___	___	___	_____
3. Prepare needed equipment and supplies.	___	___	___	_____
4. Position client safely if seizure begins. Guide the sitting or standing client to the floor. Cradle client's head in lap or place pillow beneath it. Clear area of furniture. Lower bed and raise side rails (padded) for client in bed.	___	___	___	_____
5. Provide privacy.	___	___	___	_____
6. Turn client on side, if possible, with head flexed slightly forward.	___	___	___	_____
7. Do not restrain client. Loosen client's clothing.	___	___	___	_____
8. Do not place anything in client's mouth.	___	___	___	_____
9. Observe sequence and timing of seizure activity. Note aura, level of consciousness, mobility, incontinence, sleep patterns, or confusion afterward.	___	___	___	_____
10. Stay with client, explain occurrence, and offer support.	___	___	___	_____
11. For status epilepticus:				
A. Insert airway when client's jaw is relaxed between seizure activity.	___	___	___	_____
B. Obtain oxygen and suction equipment. Prepare for IV insertion.	___	___	___	_____
C. Pad side rails and headboard.	___	___	___	_____
12. Record and report seizure activity and interventions.	___	___	___	_____

PROCEDURE PERFORMANCE CHECKLIST
Skill 38-1 Bathing a Client

	S	U	NP	Comments
Bathing a Client				
1. Assess client's tolerance for activity, discomfort level, cognitive ability and musculoskeletal function.	____	____	____	_____
2. Review orders for specific precautions concerning client's movement or positioning.	____	____	____	_____
3. Explain procedure to client and ask client about bathing preferences.	____	____	____	_____
4. Prepare room for comfort and privacy.	____	____	____	_____
5. Prepare equipment and supplies.	____	____	____	_____
6. Bathe client:	____	____	____	_____
A. Complete or partial bed bath:				
(1) Offer client bedpan or urinal. Provide towel and washcloth.	____	____	____	_____
(2) Wash hands.	____	____	____	_____
(3) Apply disposable gloves as needed.	____	____	____	_____
(4) Lower side rail closest to you, and assist client in assuming a comfortable position that maintains body alignment. Bring client toward side of bed closest to you. Place bed in high position.	____	____	____	_____
(5) Loosen top covers at foot of bed. Place bath blanket over top sheet. Fold and remove top sheet from under blanket.	____	____	____	_____
(6) If top sheet is to be reused, fold it for later replacement. If not, place it in laundry bag.	____	____	____	_____
(7) Remove client's gown or pajamas.	____	____	____	_____
(8) Pull side rail up. Fill washbasin two thirds full with warm water. Have client test temperature. Place plastic container of lotion in bath water to warm, if desired.	____	____	____	_____
(9) Remove pillow if allowed and raise head of bed 30 to 45 degrees. Place bath towel under client's head. Place second bath towel over client's chest.	____	____	____	_____
(10) Fold washcloth around fingers of your hand to form mitt. Immerse mitt in water and wring thoroughly.	____	____	____	_____

Continued

	S	U	NP	Comments

(11) Wash client's eyes with plain warm water. Inquire if client is wearing contact lenses. Use different section of mitt for each eye. Move mitt from inner to outer canthus. Soak any crusts on eyelid for 2 to 3 minutes with damp cloth before attempting removal. Dry eye thoroughly but gently. _____ _____ _____ _____

(12) As if client prefers to have soap used on face. Wash, rinse, and dry well client's forehead, cheeks, nose, neck, and ears. _____ _____ _____ _____

(13) Remove bath blanket from client's arm that is closest to you. Place bath towel lengthwise under arm. Raise side rail and move to other side to wash arm, if desired. _____ _____ _____ _____

(14) Bathe client's arm with soap and water using long, firm strokes from distal to proximal areas. Raise and support client's arm above head (if possible) while washing axilla. _____ _____ _____ _____

(15) Rinse and dry arm and axilla thoroughly. Apply deodorant or talcum powder, if used. _____ _____ _____ _____

(16) Fold bath towel in half and lay it on bed beside client. Place basin on towel. Immerse client's hand in water. Allow hand to soak for 3 to 5 minutes before washing hand and fingernails. Remove hand from basin and dry well. _____ _____ _____ _____

(17) Raise side rail and move to other side of bed. Lower side rails and repeat steps 13 through 16 for other arm. _____ _____ _____ _____

(18) Check temperature of bath water, and change water if necessary. _____ _____ _____ _____

(19) Cover client's chest with bath towel, and fold bath blanket down to umbilicus. Lift edge of towel away from client's chest. Bathe client's chest using long, firm strokes with mitted hand. Wash skinfolds under female clients' breasts. Keep client's chest covered between washing and rinsing. Dry well. _____ _____ _____ _____

(20) Place bath towel(s) lengthwise over client's chest and abdomen. Fold blanket down to just above client's pubic region. _____ _____ _____ _____

Continued

430

	S	U	NP	Comments

(21) Lift bath towel. Bathe client's abdomen with mitted hand. Stroke from side to side. Keep client's abdomen covered between washing and rinsing. Dry well. _____ _____ _____ _____

(22) Help client put on clean gown or paja-ma top. _____ _____ _____ _____

(23) Cover client's chest and abdomen with top of bath blanket. Expose client's nearer leg by folding blanket toward midline. Drape client's perineum. _____ _____ _____ _____

(24) Bend client's leg at knee by positioning your arm under client's leg. Elevate leg from mattress slightly while grasping client's heel, and slide bath towel lengthwise under leg. Ask client to hold foot still. Place bath basin on towel on bed, and secure its position next to the foot to be washed. _____ _____ _____ _____

(25) Allow client's feet to soak after the bath, unless contraindicated. _____ _____ _____ _____

(26) Use long, firm strokes in washing from client's ankle to knee and from knee to thigh, unless contraindicated. Dry well. _____ _____ _____ _____

(27) Cleanse client's foot, making sure to bathe between toes. Clean and clip nails as needed. Dry well. Apply lotion to dry skin. Do not massage any reddened area on client's skin. _____ _____ _____ _____

(28) Raise side rail and move to other side of bed. Lower side rail and repeat steps 23 through 27 for client's other leg and foot. _____ _____ _____ _____

(29) Cover client with bath blanket, raise side rail for client's safety, and change bath water. _____ _____ _____ _____

(30) Lower side rail. Assist client in assum-ing a prone or side-lying position (as applicable). Place towel lengthwise along client's side. _____ _____ _____ _____

(31) Keep client draped by sliding bath blanket over his or her shoulders and thighs. Wash, rinse, and dry back from neck to buttocks using long, firm strokes. Give client a back rub. _____ _____ _____ _____

(32) Apply disposable gloves if not done previously. _____ _____ _____ _____

Continued

	S	U	NP	Comments

(33) Assist client in assuming a side-lying or supine position. Cover client's chest and upper extremities with towel and lower extremities with bath blanket. Expose client's genitalia only. Wash, rinse, and dry perineum. Apply water-repellent ointment to area exposed to moisture. _____ _____ _____ _____

(34) Dispose of gloves in receptacle. _____ _____ _____ _____

(35) Apply additional body lotion or oil to client as desired. _____ _____ _____ _____

(36) Assist client in dressing. Comb client's hair. _____ _____ _____ _____

(37) Make client's bed. _____ _____ _____ _____

(38) Remove soiled linen and place it in laundry bag. Clean and replace bathing equipment. Replace call light and client's personal possessions. Leave room as clean and comfortable as possible. _____ _____ _____ _____

(39) Wash hands. _____ _____ _____ _____

B. Tub bath or shower:

(1) Consider client's condition, and review orders for precautions. _____ _____ _____ _____

(2) Schedule use of tub or shower. _____ _____ _____ _____

(3) Check tub or shower for cleanliness. If necessary, use cleaning techniques outlined in agency policy. Place rubber mat on tub or shower bottom. Place disposable bath mat or towel on floor in front of tub or shower. _____ _____ _____ _____

(4) Collect all hygienic aids, toiletry items, and linens requested by client. Place within easy reach of tub or shower. _____ _____ _____ _____

(5) Assist client to bathroom if necessary. Have client wear robe and slippers to bathroom. _____ _____ _____ _____

(6) Demonstrate how to use call signal for assistance. _____ _____ _____ _____

(7) Place "Occupied" sign on bathroom door. _____ _____ _____ _____

Continued

	S	U	NP	Comments

(8) Fill bathtub halfway with warm water. Ask client to test water, and adjust temperature if needed. Show client which faucet controls hot water. If client is taking a shower, turn shower on and adjust temperature before client enters shower stall. Provide tub chair or shower seat if needed. _____ _____ _____ _____

(9) Instruct client to use safety bars when getting in and out of tub or shower. Caution client against use of bath oil in tub water. _____ _____ _____ _____

(10) Instruct client not to remain in tub longer than 20 minutes. Check on client every 5 minutes. _____ _____ _____ _____

(11) Return to bathroom when client signals, and knock before entering. _____ _____ _____ _____

(12) Drain tub before client attempts to get out of it. Place bath towel over client's shoulders. Assist client as needed. _____ _____ _____ _____

(13) Assist client in donning clothing, if necessary. _____ _____ _____ _____

(14) Assist client to room and to a comfortable position in bed or chair. _____ _____ _____ _____

(15) Clean tub or shower according to agency policy. Remove soiled linen and place it in laundry bag. Discard disposable equipment in proper receptacle. Place "Unoccupied" sign on bathroom door. Return supplies to storage area. _____ _____ _____ _____

(16) Wash hands. _____ _____ _____ _____

7. Observe client's skin, paying particular attention to areas that were previously soiled, reddened, or that showed early signs of breakdown. _____ _____ _____ _____

8. Observe client's range of motion during the bath. _____ _____ _____ _____

9. Ask client to rate level of comfort. _____ _____ _____ _____

10. Record bath on flow sheet. Note level of assistance required. _____ _____ _____ _____

11. Record condition of client's skin and any significant findings. _____ _____ _____ _____

12. Report evidence of alterations in client's skin integrity. _____ _____ _____ _____

PROCEDURE PERFORMANCE CHECKLIST
Skill 38-2 Providing Perineal Care

	S	U	NP	Comments

Providing Perineal Care

1. Assess client's risk for developing infection of genitalia, urinary tract, or reproductive tract.

2. Assess client's cognitive and musculoskeletal function.

3. Assess client's genitalia for signs of inflammation, skin breakdown, or infection.

4. Assess client's knowledge of the importance of perineal hygiene.

5. Explain procedure and purpose to client.

6. Prepare necessary equipment and supplies.

7. Provide privacy.

8. Raise bed to comfortable working position. Lower side rail, and assist client in assuming a side-lying position. Place towel lengthwise along client's side and keep client covered with bath blanket.

9. Apply disposable gloves.

10. Remove any fecal matter in a fold of underpad or toilet tissue. Cleanse client's buttocks and anus, washing from front to back. Clean, rinse, and dry area thoroughly. Place an absorbent pad under client's buttocks. Remove and discard underpad and replace with clean pad.

11. Change gloves when they are soiled.

12. Fold top bed linen down toward foot of bed. Raise client's gown so genital area is exposed:
    A. "Diamond" drape client.
    B. Raise side rail. Fill washbasin with warm water.
    C. Place washbasin and toilet tissue on overbed table. Place washcloths in basin.

13. Provide perineal care:
    A. Female perineal care:
       (1) Assist client to dorsal recumbent position.
       (2) Lower side rails, and help client flex knees and spread legs. Note limitations in client's positioning.
       (3) Fold lower corner of bath blanket up between client's legs onto abdomen. Wash and dry client's upper thighs.

Continued

	S	U	NP	Comments

(4) Wash client's labia majora. Use non-dominant hand to gently retract labia from thigh. With dominant hand, carefully wash in skinfolds. Wipe from perineum to rectum. Repeat on opposite side using a different section of the washcloth. Rinse and dry area thoroughly.

(5) Separate labia with nondominant hand to expose urethral meatus and vaginal orifice. Wash downward from pubic area toward rectum in one smooth stroke. Use separate section of cloth for each stroke. Cleanse thoroughly around labia minora, clitoris, and vaginal orifice.

(6) Pour warm water over perineal area if client uses bedpan. Dry perineal area thoroughly, using front-to-back method.

(7) Fold lower corner of bath blanket back between client's legs and over perineum. Ask client to lower legs and assume comfortable position.

B. Male perineal care:

(1) Lower side rails, and assist client to supine position. Note any restriction in client's mobility.

(2) Fold top half of bath blanket below client's penis. Wash and dry client's upper thighs.

(3) Gently raise client's penis and place bath towel underneath it. Gently grasp shaft of penis. Retract foreskin if client is uncircumcised. Defer procedure until later if client has an erection.

(4) Wash tip of client's penis at urethral meatus first. Using circular motion, cleanse from meatus outward. Discard washcloth and repeat with clean cloth until penis is clean. Rinse and dry area gently.

(5) Return foreskin to its natural position.

(6) Wash shaft of penis with gentle but firm downward strokes. Pay special attention to underlying surface. Rinse and dry penis thoroughly. Instruct client to spread legs apart slightly.

Continued

	S	U	NP	Comments

(7) Gently cleanse scrotum. Lift it carefully and wash underlying skin folds. Rinse and dry.

(8) Fold bath blanket back over client's perineum, assist client to a side-lying position, and cleanse client's anal area.

14. Apply thin layer of skin barrier containing petrolatum or zinc oxide over anal and perineal skin of incontinent clients.

15. Remove gloves and dispose of them in proper receptacle.

16. Assist client in assuming a comfortable position, and cover client with sheet.

17. Remove bath blanket and dispose of all soiled bed linen. Return unused equipment to storage area.

18. Inspect surface of client's external genitalia and surrounding skin after cleansing.

19. Ask if client feels a sense of cleanliness.

20. Observe for abnormal drainage or discharge from client's genitalia.

21. Report and record procedure, appearance of suture line (if present), and the presence of any abnormal findings.

STUDENT: _____ DATE: _____

INSTRUCTOR: _____ DATE: _____

Skill 38-3 Administering a Back Rub

	S	U	NP	Comments

Administering a Back Rub

1. Assess client for contraindications.
2. Assess client's pulse and blood pressure, if necessary.
3. Explain procedure and position to client.
4. Prepare needed equipment and supplies.
5. Adjust bed to high, comfortable position.
6. Adjust light, temperature, and sound within room.
7. Lower side rail and position client in a prone or side-lying position, with back toward you.
8. Provide privacy.
9. Expose client's back, shoulders, upper arms, and buttocks.
10. Wash hands in warm water.
11. Warm lotion in hands or under warm water.
12. Explain that lotion will feel cool and wet.
13. Apply lotion to sacral area and stroke upward from buttocks to shoulders, over upper arms, and back to buttocks, using a continuous, firm stroke and keeping hands on skin.
14. Continue for at least 3 minutes.
15. Knead client's skin by grasping it between thumb and fingers, moving upward along one side of the spine from buttocks to shoulders and nape of neck, the kneading or stroking down and repeating on other side.
16. End massage with long stroking movements, and tell client you are ending.
17. Have client turn to opposite side, and massage client's other hip.
18. Wipe excess lubricant from client's back with bath towel.
19. Assist client in redressing, if necessary.
20. Help client to a comfortable position and raise side rails as needed. Lower bed.
21. Properly dispose of soiled towel.
22. Wash hands.
23. Ask if client feels comfortable or has any areas of pain or tension.

Continued

	S	U	NP	Comments
24. Reassess client's pulse and blood pressure.	_____	_____	_____	_____
25. Record client's response to massage and condition of client's skin.	_____	_____	_____	_____

STUDENT: _____ DATE: _____

INSTRUCTOR: _____ DATE: _____

Skill 38-4 Performing Nail and Foot Care

	S	U	NP	Comments

Performing Nail and Foot Care

1. Inspect all areas of client's fingers, toes, feet, and nails. _____ _____ _____ _____

2. Assess circulation to client's toes, feet, and fingers. _____ _____ _____ _____

3. Observe client's walking gait. _____ _____ _____ _____

4. Ask female clients whether they frequently use nail polish and polish remover. _____ _____ _____ _____

5. Assess type of footwear worn by client. _____ _____ _____ _____

6. Assess client's risk for foot or nail problems. _____ _____ _____ _____

7. Assess types of home remedies client has used for existing foot problems. _____ _____ _____ _____

8. Assess client's ability to care for nails or feet. _____ _____ _____ _____

9. Assess client's knowledge of foot and nail care practices. _____ _____ _____ _____

10. Explain procedure to client. _____ _____ _____ _____

11. Obtain physician's order for cutting client's nails if agency policy requires it. _____ _____ _____ _____

12. Wash hands. _____ _____ _____ _____

13. Arrange equipment on overbed table. _____ _____ _____ _____

14. Provide privacy. _____ _____ _____ _____

15. Assist ambulatory client to sit in bedside chair. Help bed-bound client to supine position with head of bed elevated. Place disposable bath mat on floor under client's feet, or place towel on mattress. _____ _____ _____ _____

16. Fill washbasin with warm water. Test temperature. _____ _____ _____ _____

17. Place basin on bath mat or towel, and help client place feet in basin. Place call light within client's reach. _____ _____ _____ _____

18. Adjust overbed table to low position, and place it over client's lap. _____ _____ _____ _____

19. Fill emesis basin with warm water, and place basin on paper towels on overbed table. _____ _____ _____ _____

20. Instruct client to place fingers in emesis basin and to place arms in a comfortable position. _____ _____ _____ _____

21. Allow client's feet and fingernails to soak for 10 to 20 minutes unless contraindicated. Rewarm water after 10 minutes.

Continued

	S	U	NP	Comments
22. Clean gently under client's fingernails with orange stick while fingers are immersed. Remove emesis basin, and dry client's fingers thoroughly.	_____	_____	_____	_____
23. Clip client's fingernails straight across and even with tops of fingers unless contraindicated. Shape nails with emery board or file.	_____	_____	_____	_____
24. Push client's cuticles back gently with orange stick.	_____	_____	_____	_____
25. Move overbed table away from client.	_____	_____	_____	_____
26. Put on disposable gloves.	_____	_____	_____	_____
27. Scrub callused areas of client's feet with wash-cloth.	_____	_____	_____	_____
28. Clean gently under client's toenails with orange stick. Remove client's feet from basin and dry thoroughly.	_____	_____	_____	_____
29. Clean and trim toenails using the procedures described in steps 22 and 23. Do not file corners of toenails.	_____	_____	_____	_____
30. Apply lotion to client's feet and hands, and assist client back to bed and into a comfortable position.	_____	_____	_____	_____
31. Remove disposable gloves and place in receptacle.	_____	_____	_____	_____
32. Clean and return equipment and supplies to proper place.	_____	_____	_____	_____
33. Dispose of soiled linen in hamper.	_____	_____	_____	_____
34. Wash hands.	_____	_____	_____	_____
35. Inspect client's nails and surrounding skin surfaces after soaking and nail trimming.	_____	_____	_____	_____
36. Ask client to explain or demonstrate nail care.	_____	_____	_____	_____
37. Observe client's walk after toenail care.	_____	_____	_____	_____
38. Record and report procedure and observations.	_____	_____	_____	_____

STUDENT: _____ DATE: _____

INSTRUCTOR: _____ DATE: _____

PROCEDURE PERFORMANCE CHECKLIST
Skill 38-5 Providing Oral Hygiene

	S	U	NP	Comments
Providing Oral Hygiene				
1. Wash hands.	____	____	____	_____
2. Apply disposable gloves.	____	____	____	_____
3. Inspect integrity of client's lips, teeth, buccal mucosa, gums, palate, and tongue.	____	____	____	_____
4. Identify presence of common oral problems.	____	____	____	_____
5. Remove gloves.	____	____	____	_____
6. Wash hands.	____	____	____	_____
7. Assess client's risk for oral hygiene problems.	____	____	____	_____
8. Determine client's oral hygiene practices.	____	____	____	_____
9. Assess client's ability to grasp and manipulate a toothbrush.	____	____	____	_____
10. Prepare equipment at bedside.	____	____	____	_____
11. Explain procedure to client and discuss preferences regarding use of hygienic aids.	____	____	____	_____
12. Place paper towels on overbed table, and arrange other equipment within easy reach.	____	____	____	_____
13. Raise bed to comfortable working position. Raise head of bed (if allowed) and lower side rail. Move client, or help client move closer. The client can also be in a side-lying position.	____	____	____	_____
14. Place towel over client's chest.	____	____	____	_____
15. Apply gloves.	____	____	____	_____
16. Apply toothpaste to toothbrush while holding brush over emesis basin. Pour small amount of water over toothpaste.	____	____	____	_____
17. Hold toothbrush bristles at a 45-degree angle to client's gumline. Brush inner and outer surfaces of client's upper and lower teeth. Clean biting surfaces of teeth, and brush sides of teeth.	____	____	____	_____
18. Have client hold brush at a 45-degree angle and lightly brush over surface and sides of tongue. Instruct client to avoid initiating gag reflex.	____	____	____	_____
19. Allow client to rinse mouth thoroughly.	____	____	____	_____
20. Allow client to gargle to rinse mouth with mouthwash as desired.	____	____	____	_____
21. Assist in wiping client's mouth.	____	____	____	_____
22. Allow client to floss.	____	____	____	_____
23. Allow client to rinse mouth thoroughly with cool water and spit into emesis basin. Assist in wiping client's mouth.	____	____	____	_____

Continued

	S	U	NP	Comments
24. Assist client to a comfortable position, remove emesis basin and bedside table, raise side rail, and lower bed to original position.	_____	_____	_____	_____
25. Wipe off overbed table.	_____	_____	_____	_____
26. Discard soiled linens and paper towels in appropriate containers.	_____	_____	_____	_____
27. Remove and dispose of soiled gloves.	_____	_____	_____	_____
28. Return equipment to proper place.	_____	_____	_____	_____
29. Wash hands.	_____	_____	_____	_____
30. Ask client if any area of the oral cavity feels uncomfortable or irritated.	_____	_____	_____	_____
31. Apply gloves and inspect condition of client's oral cavity.	_____	_____	_____	_____
32. Ask client to describe proper oral hygiene techniques.	_____	_____	_____	_____
33. Observe client brushing his or her teeth.	_____	_____	_____	_____
34. Record and report procedure and observations.	_____	_____	_____	_____

PROCEDURE PERFORMANCE CHECKLIST

Skill 38-6 Performing Mouth Care for an Unconscious or Debilitated Client

	S	U	NP	Comments
Performing Mouth Care for an Unconscious or Debilitated Client				
1. Wash hands.	___	___	___	_____
2. Apply disposable gloves.	___	___	___	_____
3. Test client for presence of gag reflex.	___	___	___	_____
4. Inspect condition of client's oral cavity.	___	___	___	_____
5. Remove gloves.	___	___	___	_____
6. Wash hands.	___	___	___	_____
7. Assess client's risk for oral hygiene problems.	___	___	___	_____
8. Position client on side, with head turned well toward dependent side and head of bed lowered. Raise side rail.	___	___	___	_____
9. Explain procedure to client.	___	___	___	_____
10. Wash hands.	___	___	___	_____
11. Apply disposable gloves.	___	___	___	_____
12. Place paper towels on overbed table and arrange equipment. If needed, prepare suction.	___	___	___	_____
13. Provide privacy.	___	___	___	_____
14. Raise bed to its highest horizontal level. Lower side rail.	___	___	___	_____
15. Position client close to side of bed. Turn client's head toward mattress.	___	___	___	_____
16. Place towel under client's head and place emesis basin under client's chin.	___	___	___	_____
17. Separate client's upper and lower teeth with padded tongue blade. Insert blade when client is relaxed, if possible. Do not use force.	___	___	___	_____
18. Clean client's mouth using toothbrush or sponge toothettes moistened with peroxide and water. Clean chewing and inner tooth surfaces first. Clean outer tooth surfaces. Swab roof of mouth, gums, and insides of cheeks. Gently swab or brush tongue, but avoid stimulating the gag reflex. Rinse client's mouth with a clean swab, toothette, or bulb syringe. Repeat rinse several times.	___	___	___	_____
19. Suction secretions as they accumulate, if necessary.	___	___	___	_____
20. Apply thin layer of water-soluble jelly to client's lips.	___	___	___	_____
21. Inform client that procedure is complete.	___	___	___	_____

Continued

	S	U	NP	Comments
22. Remove gloves and dispose of them in proper receptacle.	_____	_____	_____	_____
23. Reposition client comfortably, raise side rail, and return bed to original position.	_____	_____	_____	_____
24. Clean equipment and return it to its proper place.	_____	_____	_____	_____
25. Place soiled linen in proper receptacle.	_____	_____	_____	_____
26. Wash hands.	_____	_____	_____	_____
27. Apply gloves and inspect client's oral cavity.	_____	_____	_____	_____
28. Ask debilitated client if mouth feels clean.	_____	_____	_____	_____
29. Assess client's respirations on an ongoing basis.	_____	_____	_____	_____
30. Record and report procedure and pertinent observations.	_____	_____	_____	_____

PROCEDURE PERFORMANCE CHECKLIST

Skill 38-7 Caring for the Client with Contact Lenses

	S	U	NP	Comments
Caring for the Client with Contact Lenses				
1. Place towel just below client's face.	____	____	____	_____
2. Stand at client's side. Inspect client's eyes or ask client if contact lenses are in place.	____	____	____	_____
3. Ask if client feels any eye discomfort, and assess length of time client normally wears lenses.	____	____	____	_____
4. Ask if client is able to manipulate and hold contact lens.	____	____	____	_____
5. Assess client for any unusual visual signs/symptoms.	____	____	____	_____
6. Assess types of medications prescribed for client.	____	____	____	_____
7. After lenses are removed (see step 11), inspect eyes for signs of corneal irritation and redness.	____	____	____	_____
8. Discuss procedure with client.	____	____	____	_____
9. Have client assume supine or sitting position in bed or chair.	____	____	____	_____
10. Assemble supplies at client's bedside.	____	____	____	_____
11. Remove contact lenses:				
A. Soft lenses:				
(1) Wash hands.	____	____	____	_____
(2) Apply disposable gloves if necessary.	____	____	____	_____
(3) Place towel just below client's face.	____	____	____	_____
(4) Add a few drops of sterile saline solution to client's eye.	____	____	____	_____
(5) Tell client to look straight ahead.	____	____	____	_____
(6) Retract client's lower eyelid with middle finger.	____	____	____	_____
(7) Slide lens off cornea and onto white of eye with pad of index finger.	____	____	____	_____
(8) Pull upper eyelid down gently with thumb of other hand and compress lens slightly between thumb and index finger.	____	____	____	_____
(9) Gently pinch lens and lift it out of the eye.	____	____	____	_____
(10) Clean and rinse lens. Place lens in proper storage case compartment: R for right lens and L for left lens.	____	____	____	_____
(11) Repeat steps 11A(4) through 11A(10) for other lens.	____	____	____	_____

Continued

	S	U	NP	Comments

(12) Secure cover over storage case. Label with client's name and room number. _____ _____ _____ _____

(13) Assess appearance and condition of client's eyes after lenses are removed. _____ _____ _____ _____

(14) Place soiled towel in proper receptacle. _____ _____ _____ _____

(15) Remove and dispose of gloves. _____ _____ _____ _____

(16) Wash hands. _____ _____ _____ _____

B. Rigid lenses:

  (1) Wash hands. _____ _____ _____ _____

  (2) Apply disposable gloves if necessary. _____ _____ _____ _____

  (3) Place towel just below client's face. _____ _____ _____ _____

  (4) Be sure lens is positioned directly over cornea. _____ _____ _____ _____

  (5) Place index finger on outer corner of client's eye, and draw skin gently back toward client's ear. _____ _____ _____ _____

  (6) Tell client to blink. Do not release pressure on eyelid until blink is completed. _____ _____ _____ _____

  (7) Gently retract eyelid beyond edges of lens if lens does not pop out. Press lower eyelid gently against lower edge of lens. _____ _____ _____ _____

  (8) Allow both of client's eyelids to close slightly, and grasp lens as it rises from the eye. Cup lens in hand. _____ _____ _____ _____

  (9) Clean and rinse lens. Place lens in proper storage compartment: R for right lens and L for left lens. Center lens in storage case, convex side down. _____ _____ _____ _____

(10) Repeat steps 11B(4) through 11B(9) for other lens. _____ _____ _____ _____

(11) Secure cover over storage case. Label with client's name and room number. _____ _____ _____ _____

(12) Place soiled towel in proper receptacle. _____ _____ _____ _____

(13) Remove and dispose of gloves. _____ _____ _____ _____

(14) Wash hands. _____ _____ _____ _____

12. Clean and disinfect contact lenses:

A. Wash hands. _____ _____ _____ _____

B. Assemble supplies at client's bedside. Place towel over work area. _____ _____ _____ _____

C. Open lens container carefully. Do not flip lens caps open suddenly. Remove lens. _____ _____ _____ _____

D. Apply one or two drops of cleaning solution to lens in palm of hand. _____ _____ _____ _____

Continued

	S	U	NP	Comments

E. Rub lens gently but thoroughly on both sides for 20 to 30 seconds. Use index finger (soft lenses) or little finger or cotton-tipped applicator soaked with cleaning solution (rigid lenses) to clean inside lens. Be careful not to damage lens. _____ _____ _____ _____

F. Hold lens over emesis basin and rinse thoroughly with manufacturer-recommended rinsing solution (soft lenses) or cold tap water (rigid lenses). _____ _____ _____ _____

G. Place lens in proper storage case compartment and fill with storage solution. _____ _____ _____ _____

H. Repeat steps 12C through 12G for other lens. _____ _____ _____ _____

13. Insert lenses:

A. Soft lenses:

(1) Wash hands thoroughly with mild non-cosmetic soap, rinse well, and dry with clean lint-free towel or paper towel. _____ _____ _____ _____

(2) Apply gloves if needed. _____ _____ _____ _____

(3) Place towel over client's chest. _____ _____ _____ _____

(4) Remove right lens from storage case and rinse with recommended rinsing solution. Inspect lens for foreign materials, tears, and other damage. _____ _____ _____ _____

(5) Check that lens is not inverted. _____ _____ _____ _____

(6) Use middle or index finger of hand not holding lens to retract client's upper eyelid until iris is exposed. _____ _____ _____ _____

(7) Use middle finger of hand holding lens to pull down client's lower eyelid. _____ _____ _____ _____

(8) Instruct client to look straight ahead, then place lens directly on cornea and release lids slowly, starting with lower lid. _____ _____ _____ _____

(9) Tell client to slowly close eye and roll it toward the lens if the lens is not on the cornea. _____ _____ _____ _____

(10) Tell client to blink a few times. _____ _____ _____ _____

(11) Center lens properly over the cornea. _____ _____ _____ _____

(12) Repeat steps 13A(4) through 13A(11) for left eye. _____ _____ _____ _____

(13) Assist client to a comfortable position. _____ _____ _____ _____

(14) If client's vision is blurred, do the following:

(a) Retract client's eyelids. _____ _____ _____ _____

(b) Locate position of lens. _____ _____ _____ _____

Continued

	S	U	NP	Comments

(c) Ask client to look in direction opposite of lens, and with index finger, apply pressure to lower eyelid margin and position lens over cornea. ____ ____ ____ _____

(d) Have client look slowly toward lens. ____ ____ ____ _____

(15) Discard soiled supplies and solution from storage case. ____ ____ ____ _____

(16) Rinse case thoroughly and allow to air dry. ____ ____ ____ _____

(17) Wash hands. ____ ____ ____ _____

B. Rigid lenses:

(1) Wash and dry hands. ____ ____ ____ _____

(2) Apply disposable gloves if needed. ____ ____ ____ _____

(3) Place towel over client's chest. ____ ____ ____ _____

(4) Remove right lens from storage case. Attempt to lift lens straight up. ____ ____ ____ _____

(5) Rinse lens with cold tap water. ____ ____ ____ _____

(6) Wet lens on both sides using prescribed wetting solution. ____ ____ ____ _____

(7) Place lens concave side up on tip of index finger of dominant hand. ____ ____ ____ _____

(8) Instruct client to look straight ahead while retracting lower eyelid. Place lens gently over center of client's cornea. ____ ____ ____ _____

(9) Ask client to close eyes briefly and avoid blinking. ____ ____ ____ _____

(10) Center lens properly over the cornea. ____ ____ ____ _____

(11) Repeat steps 13B(4) through 13B(10) for left eye. ____ ____ ____ _____

(12) Assist client to a comfortable position. ____ ____ ____ _____

(13) Discard soiled supplies and solution from storage case. ____ ____ ____ _____

(14) Rinse case thoroughly and allow to air dry. ____ ____ ____ _____

(15) Wash hands. ____ ____ ____ _____

14. Ask client if lens feels comfortable after removal and reinsertion of lenses. ____ ____ ____ _____

15. Inspect client's eye (over time) for signs of ocular infection.

16. Assess client's visual acuity. ____ ____ ____ _____

17. Observe client for signs of eye injury. ____ ____ ____ _____

18. Record and report lens insertion or removal and any signs or symptoms of visual alteration noted during procedure. ____ ____ ____ _____

PROCEDURE PERFORMANCE CHECKLIST
Skill 38-8 Making an Occupied Bed

	S	U	NP	Comments

Making an Occupied Bed

	S	U	NP	Comments
1. Determine if client is incontinent or has excess drainage on bed linen.	___	___	___	_____
2. Check cart for orders or specific precautions for movement and positioning of client.	___	___	___	_____
3. Explain procedure to client.	___	___	___	_____
4. Prepare needed equipment and supplies.	___	___	___	_____
5. Wash hands.	___	___	___	_____
6. Assemble and arrange equipment on bedside chair or table.	___	___	___	_____
7. Provide privacy.	___	___	___	_____
8. Lower side rail on near side of bed. Remove call light.	___	___	___	_____
9. Adjust bed height to comfortable working position.	___	___	___	_____
10. Loosen top linen sheet at foot of bed.	___	___	___	_____
11. Remove bedspread and blanket separately by folding them into squares and placing them in linen bag (if not to be reused). Do not allow linen to contact uniform. Do not fan or shake linen.	___	___	___	_____
12. Fold blanket and spread if they will be reused. Fold them into neat squares and place them over back of chair.	___	___	___	_____
13. Cover client with bath blanket in following manner: Unfold bath blanket over top sheet. Ask client to hold top edge of bath blanket, or tuck top of bath blanket under client's shoulder. Grasp top sheet under bath blanket at client's shoulders, and bring sheet down to foot of bed. Remove sheet and discard it in linen bag.	___	___	___	_____
14. With assistance, slide mattress toward head of bed.	___	___	___	_____
15. Position client on his or her side on the far side of the bed, facing away. Adjust pillow under client's head, and raise farthest side rail.	___	___	___	_____
16. Loosen bottom bed linens, moving from head to foot of bed.	___	___	___	_____
17. Fanfold first drawsheet and then bottom sheet toward client. Tuck edges of linen just under client's buttocks, back, and shoulders.	___	___	___	_____

Continued

	S	U	NP	Comments

18. Wipe off moisture on mattress with towel and appropriate disinfectant. _____ _____ _____ _____

19. Apply clean linen to exposed half of bed:

   A. Place clean mattress pad on bed by folding it lengthwise with center crease in middle of bed. Fanfold top layer over mattress. _____ _____ _____ _____

   B. Unfold bottom sheet lengthwise so center crease is situated lengthwise along center of bed. Fanfold sheet's top layer toward center of bed alongside client. Smooth bottom layer of sheet over mattress, near side. Allow sheet's edge to hang about 25 cm over mattress edge. Lower hem of bottom sheet should lie seam down and even with bottom edge of mattress. _____ _____ _____ _____

20. Miter bottom sheet at head of bed:

   A. Face head of bed diagonally. Place hand away from head of bed under top cover of mattress, near mattress edge, and lift. _____ _____ _____ _____

   B. Tuck top edge of bottom sheet smoothly under mattress. _____ _____ _____ _____

   C. Face side of bed and pick up top edge of sheet at approximately 45 cm down from top of mattress. _____ _____ _____ _____

   D. Lift sheet and lay it on top of mattress to form neat triangular fold, with lower base of triangle even with mattress side edge. _____ _____ _____ _____

   E. Tuck lower edge of sheet, which is hanging free below mattress, under mattress. Tuck with palms down without pulling triangular fold. _____ _____ _____ _____

   F. Hold portion of sheet covering side edge of mattress in place with one hand. Pick up top of triangular linen fold and bring it down over side of mattress. Tuck this portion of sheet under mattress. _____ _____ _____ _____

21. Tuck remaining portion of sheet under mattress, moving toward foot of bed. Keep linen smooth. _____ _____ _____ _____

22. Open drawsheet so it unfolds in half. Lay center fold along middle of bed lengthwise, and position sheet so it will be under client's buttocks and torso. Fanfold top layer toward client with edge alongside client's back. Smooth bottom layer out over mattress and tuck excess edge under mattress. _____ _____ _____ _____

23. Place waterproof pad under drawsheet with center fold against client's side. Fanfold far half toward client. _____ _____ _____ _____

Continued

452

	S	U	NP	Comments

24. Raise side rail on working side of bed and go to other side. _____ _____ _____ _____

25. Lower side rail. Assist client to roll slowly onto other side, onto the folds of linen. _____ _____ _____ _____

26. Loosen edges of soiled linen from underneath mattress. _____ _____ _____ _____

27. Remove soiled linen by folding it into a bundle or squares, with soiled side turned in. Discard in linen bag. _____ _____ _____ _____

28. Spread clean, fanfolded linen smoothly over edge of mattress from head to foot of bed. _____ _____ _____ _____

29. Assist client in rolling back into supine position. Reposition pillow. _____ _____ _____ _____

30. Miter top corner of bottom sheet (see step 20). When tucking corner, be sure sheet is smooth and free of wrinkles. _____ _____ _____ _____

31. Grasp remaining edge of bottom sheet. Keep back straight and pull as excess linen is tucked under mattress. Proceed from head to foot of bed. _____ _____ _____ _____

32. Smooth fanfolded drawsheet over bottom sheet. Grasp edge of sheet with palms down, lean back, and tuck sheet under mattress. Tuck from middle to top and to bottom. _____ _____ _____ _____

33. Place top sheet over client, with center fold lengthwise down middle of bed. Open sheet from head to foot, and unfold it over client. _____ _____ _____ _____

34. Ask client to hold clean top sheet, or tuck sheet around client's shoulders. Remove bath blanket and discard in linen bag. _____ _____ _____ _____

35. Place blanket on bed, unfolding it so that crease runs lengthwise along middle of bed. Unfold blanket to cover client. Top edge of blanket should be parallel with edge of top sheet and 15 to 20 cm down from top sheet's edge. _____ _____ _____ _____

36. Place spread over bed according to step 31. Be sure top edge of spread extends about 2.5 cm above blanket's edge. Tuck top edge of spread over and under top edge of blanket. _____ _____ _____ _____

37. Make cuff by turning edge of top sheet down over edge of blanket and spread. _____ _____ _____ _____

38. Lift mattress corner slightly with one hand and tuck top linens under mattress. Top sheet and blanket are tucked under together. Allow for movement of client's feet. _____ _____ _____ _____

39. Make modified mitered corner with top sheet, blanket, and spread:

Continued

	S	U	NP	Comments

A. Pick up side edge of top sheet, blanket, and spread approximately 45 cm up from foot of mattress. Lift linens to form triangular fold, and lay it on bed. ___ ___ ___ _____

B. Tuck lower edge of sheet, which is hanging free below mattress, under mattress. Do not pull triangular fold. ___ ___ ___ _____

C. Pick up triangular fold and bring it down over mattress while holding linen in place along side of mattress. Do not tuck tip of triangle. ___ ___ ___ _____

40. Raise side rail. Make other side of bed. Spread sheet, blanket, and bedspread out evenly. Fold top edge of spread over blanket, and make cuff with top sheet (see step 37). Make modified corner at foot of bed (see step 39). ___ ___ ___ _____

41. Change pillowcase:

A. Have client raise head. Remove pillow while supporting client's neck. ___ ___ ___ _____

B. Remove soiled pillowcase and discard in linen bag. ___ ___ ___ _____

C. Grasp clean pillowcase at center of closed end. Gather case, turning it inside out over hand holding it. Pick up middle of one end of pillow. Pull pillowcase down over pillow with other hand. ___ ___ ___ _____

D. Fit pillow corners evenly in corners of pillowcase. ___ ___ ___ _____

42. Support client's head under neck and place pillow under head. ___ ___ ___ _____

43. Place call light within client's reach. Return bed to comfortable position. ___ ___ ___ _____

44. Open room curtains. Rearrange furniture. Place personal items easily within client's reach on overbed table or bedside stand. Return bed to comfortable height. ___ ___ ___ _____

45. Discard dirty linen in linen hamper or chute. ___ ___ ___ _____

46. Wash hands. ___ ___ ___ _____

STUDENT: _____ DATE: _____

INSTRUCTOR: _____ DATE: _____

PROCEDURE PERFORMANCE CHECKLIST
Skill 39-1 Pulse Oximetry

	S	U	NP	Comments
Pulse Oximetry				
1. Explain procedure to client.	___	___	___	_____
2. Wash hands.	___	___	___	_____
3. Determine best site for measurement.	___	___	___	_____
4. Prepare selected site.	___	___	___	_____
5. Assist client to a comfortable position. Instruct client to breathe normally.	___	___	___	_____
6. Apply probe and activate oximeter. Observe pulse waveform/intensity display and audible beep. Correlate oximeter with client's radial pulse.	___	___	___	_____
7. Ensure alarm limits are set and turned on.	___	___	___	_____
8. Read saturation level.	___	___	___	_____
9. Move finger sensor every 4 hours and spring tension sensor every 2 hours.	___	___	___	_____
10. Record use of pulse oximetry and oxygen saturation.	___	___	___	_____
11. Correlate oxygen saturation with blood gas measurements (if available).	___	___	___	_____
12. Record and report oxygen saturation, client responses, and abnormal findings.	___	___	___	_____

PROCEDURE PERFORMANCE CHECKLIST
Skill 39-2 Suctioning

	S	U	NP	Comments
Suctioning				
1. Assess client for signs and symptoms of airway obstruction.	____	____	____	_____
2. Determine factors that influence upper or lower airway functioning.	____	____	____	_____
3. Assess client's understanding of procedure.	____	____	____	_____
4. Obtain prescriber's order (if indicated).	____	____	____	_____
5. Explain purpose of procedure and expected sensations to client.	____	____	____	_____
6. Assist client to a comfortable position.	____	____	____	_____
7. Place towel across client's chest.	____	____	____	_____
8. Wash hands.	____	____	____	_____
9. Apply face shield if splashing is likely.	____	____	____	_____
10. Connect one end of connecting tubing to suction machine, and place other end in convenient location near client. Turn suction device on, and set vacuum regulator to appropriate negative pressure.	____	____	____	_____
11. Increase supplemental oxygen therapy to 100% as indicated or ordered. Encourage client to breathe deeply.	____	____	____	_____
12. Prepare suction catheter with following sterile technique:				
A. Open suction kit or catheter with use of aseptic technique. Place sterile drape (if available) across client's chest or on overbed table.	____	____	____	_____
B. Unwrap or open sterile basin and place on bedside table. Fill with about 100 ml of sterile normal saline solution or water.	____	____	____	_____
C. Open lubricant. Squeeze small amount onto open sterile catheter package.	____	____	____	_____
13. Apply sterile glove to each hand, or apply nonsterile glove to nondominant hand and sterile glove to dominant hand.	____	____	____	_____
14. Pick up suction catheter with dominant hand without touching nonsterile surfaces. Pick up connecting tubing with nondominant hand. Secure catheter to tubing.	____	____	____	_____
15. Suction small amount of normal saline solution from basin.	____	____	____	_____

Continued

	S	U	NP	Comments

16. Coat distal 6 to 8 cm of catheter with water-soluble lubricant. Do not lubricate for oral suction. _____ _____ _____ _____

17. Suction airway:

   A. Insert catheter appropriate distance for child or adult. _____ _____ _____ _____

   B. Nasopharyngeal and nasotracheal:

     (1) Remove client's oxygen delivery device, if applicable. Gently but quickly insert catheter into client's naris during inhalation. Insert it at a slight downward slant or through mouth, without applying suction. Do not force catheter through naris. Position client's head to right or left. Pull catheter back 1 cm if resistance is felt. _____ _____ _____ _____

     (2) Apply intermittent suction for up to 10 to 15 seconds, withdrawing catheter while rotating it back and forth between dominant thumb and forefinger. Encourage client to cough. Replace oxygen device, if applicable. _____ _____ _____ _____

     (3) Rinse catheter and connecting tubing with normal saline or water until cleared. _____ _____ _____ _____

     (4) Assess for need to repeat suctioning procedure. Allow adequate time between suction passes. Ask client to breathe deeply and cough. _____ _____ _____ _____

     (5) Perform oropharyngeal suctioning when secretions have been cleared. Do not suction nose again after suctioning mouth. _____ _____ _____ _____

   C. Oropharyngeal:

     (1) Insert catheter into client's mouth along gumline to pharynx. Move catheter around mouth until secretions are cleared. Encourage client to cough. Replace oxygen mask. Do not dislodge any oral tubing. _____ _____ _____ _____

     (2) Rinse catheter with water in cup or basin until connecting tubing is cleared of secretions. Turn off suction. Wash face if secretions are present on client's skin. _____ _____ _____ _____

   D. Endotracheal or tracheal tube:

     (1) Hyperinflate and/or hyperoxygenate client before suctioning. _____ _____ _____ _____

Continued

458

	S	U	NP	Comments

(2) Open swivel adapter or remove oxygen or humidity delivery device with non-dominant hand. ____ ____ ____ _____

(3) Insert catheter (without applying suction) into artificial airway with thumb and forefinger of dominant hand until resistance is met or client coughs; then pull catheter back 1 cm. ____ ____ ____ _____

(4) Apply intermittent suction, and slowly withdraw catheter while rotating it back and forth between dominant thumb and forefinger. Encourage client to cough. Watch for respiratory distress. ____ ____ ____ _____

(5) Close swivel adapter or replace oxygen delivery device. Encourage client to breathe deeply if able. ____ ____ ____ _____

(6) Rinse catheter and connecting tubing with normal saline until clear. Use continuous suction. ____ ____ ____ _____

(7) Assess client's cardiopulmonary status. ____ ____ ____ _____

(8) Repeat steps 17C(1) through 17C(7) once or twice more to clear secretions. Allow adequate time between suction passes. ____ ____ ____ _____

(9) Perform nasopharyngeal and oropharyngeal suctioning. Do not reinsert catheter into endotracheal or tracheostomy tube. ____ ____ ____ _____

18. Roll catheter around fingers of dominant hand. Pull glove off inside out so that catheter remains coiled in glove. Pull off other glove over first glove. Discard in appropriate receptacle. Turn off suction device. ____ ____ ____ _____

19. Remove towel, place in laundry or appropriate receptacle, and reposition client. ____ ____ ____ _____

20. Readjust oxygen to original level, if indicated. ____ ____ ____ _____

21. Reposition client as indicated by condition. Reapply clean gloves for client's personal care. ____ ____ ____ _____

22. Discard remainder of normal saline into appropriate receptacle. Discard or clean and replace basin. ____ ____ ____ _____

23. Remove and discard face shield. ____ ____ ____ _____

24. Wash hands. ____ ____ ____ _____

25. Place unopened suction kit on suction machine or at head of bed according to institution preference. ____ ____ ____ _____

26. Compare client's respiratory assessments before and after suctioning. ____ ____ ____ _____

Continued

	S	U	NP	Comments
27. Ask client if breathing is easier and if congestion is decreased.	_____	_____	_____	_____
28. Observe airway secretions.	_____	_____	_____	_____
29. Record and report the amount and characteristics of secretions, respiratory status, and client's response to procedure.	_____	_____	_____	_____

STUDENT: _____ DATE: _____

INSTRUCTOR: _____ DATE: _____

Skill 39-3 Care of Clients with Chest Tubes

	S	U	NP	Comments
Care of Clients with Chest Tubes				
1. Assess client for respiratory distress and chest pain, breath sounds over affected lung area, and stable vital signs.	_____	_____	_____	_____
2. Observe client for increased respiratory distress.	_____	_____	_____	_____
3. Observe the following:				
A. Chest tube dressing	_____	_____	_____	_____
B. Tubing, for kinks, dependent loops, or clots	_____	_____	_____	_____
C. Chest drainage system	_____	_____	_____	_____
4. Provide two shodded hemostats for each chest tube, and attach them to top of client's bed with adhesive tape.	_____	_____	_____	_____
5. Position client in one of the following ways:	_____	_____	_____	_____
A. Semi-Fowler's position to evacuate air (pneumothorax)	_____	_____	_____	_____
B. High Fowler's position to drain fluid (hemo-thorax)	_____	_____	_____	_____
6. Maintain tube connection between chest and drainage tubes. Make sure it is intact and taped.	_____	_____	_____	_____
7. Coil excess tubing on mattress next to client. Secure with rubber band and safety pin or system's clamp.	_____	_____	_____	_____
8. Adjust tubing to hang in straight line from top of mattress to drainage chamber. Indicate time that drainage began.	_____	_____	_____	_____
9. Strip or milk chest tube only if indicated.	_____	_____	_____	_____
10. Wash hands.	_____	_____	_____	_____
11. Observe the following:				
A. Chest tube dressing, tubing, and drainage system	_____	_____	_____	_____
B. Water seal for fluctuations with client's inspiration and expiration	_____	_____	_____	_____
C. Bubbling in water-seal bottle or chamber	_____	_____	_____	_____
D. Type and amount of fluid drainage	_____	_____	_____	_____
E. Client vital signs and skin color	_____	_____	_____	_____
F. Bubbling in the suction-control chamber	_____	_____	_____	_____
12. Record and report status of chest tubes, dressing, and client's responses.	_____	_____	_____	_____

STUDENT: _____ DATE: _____

INSTRUCTOR: _____ DATE: _____

PROCEDURE PERFORMANCE CHECKLIST
Skill 39-4 Applying a Nasal Cannula

	S	U	NP	Comments
Applying a Nasal Cannula				
1. Assess client's respiratory status.	____	____	____	_____
2. Explain procedure and purpose to client and family.	____	____	____	_____
3. Prepare needed equipment and supplies.	____	____	____	_____
4. Wash hands.	____	____	____	_____
5. Attach nasal cannula to humidified oxygen source.	____	____	____	_____
6. Adjust oxygen flow to prescribed rate.	____	____	____	_____
7. Place tips of cannula into nares.	____	____	____	_____
8. Adjust band until cannula fits snugly and comfortably.	____	____	____	_____
9. Secure oxygen tubing to clothes, maintaining sufficient slack.	____	____	____	_____
10. Check cannula every 8 hours.	____	____	____	_____
11. Keep humidification jar filled at all times.	____	____	____	_____
12. Assess nares and external nose for skin breakdown.	____	____	____	_____
13. Check oxygen flow rate and physician's orders every 8 hours.	____	____	____	_____
14. Wash hands.	____	____	____	_____
15. Inspect client for relief of symptoms.	____	____	____	_____
16. Record procedure and observations.	____	____	____	_____
17. Report on therapy and client's response.	____	____	____	_____

PROCEDURE PERFORMANCE CHECKLIST
Skill 39-5 Using Home Liquid Oxygen Equipment

	S	U	NP	Comments
Using Home Liquid Oxygen Equipment				
1. Assess client's need for and client's/family's ability to use equipment.	_____	_____	_____	_____
2. Assess client's or family's ability to observe for hypoxia.	_____	_____	_____	_____
3. Explain procedure to client and family.	_____	_____	_____	_____
4. Prepare equipment.	_____	_____	_____	_____
5. Wash hands.	_____	_____	_____	_____
6. Demonstrate steps for oxygen therapy.	_____	_____	_____	_____
7. Prepare primary and portable oxygen.	_____	_____	_____	_____
8. Have client or family perform each step with guidance.	_____	_____	_____	_____
9. Discuss signs and symptoms of respiratory tract infection and hypoxia.	_____	_____	_____	_____
10. Instruct client and family to notify physician if signs or symptoms of hypoxia or respiration infection occur.	_____	_____	_____	_____
11. Wash hands.	_____	_____	_____	_____
12. Record teaching, information provided, and client's/family's understanding.	_____	_____	_____	_____

PROCEDURE PERFORMANCE CHECKLIST
Skill 39-6 Cardiopulmonary Resuscitation

	S	U	NP	Comments

Cardiopulmonary Resuscitation

1. Assess victim for unresponsiveness. ____ ____ ____ _____

2. Activate emergency services (dial "911" in the community setting). Follow agency policy for cardiopulmonary resuscitation. ____ ____ ____ _____

3. Determine victim's breathlessness and carotid or brachial pulse. ____ ____ ____ _____

4. Place victim supine on a hard surface. ____ ____ ____ _____

5. Assume correct position for one- or two-person rescue. For two-person rescue, one kneels parallel to victim's sternum, second person is positioned at victim's head. ____ ____ ____ _____

6. Apply gloves and face shield, if available. ____ ____ ____ _____

7. Open victim's airway with head tilt/chin lift or jaw thrust maneuver. ____ ____ ____ _____

8. Insert oral airway, if available. ____ ____ ____ _____

9. Prepare for artificial respiration by pinching victim's nose and occluding victim's mouth or nose (or infant's mouth or nose) with your mouth or by using an Ambu bag. ____ ____ ____ _____

10. Properly administer artificial respiration with correct timing. ____ ____ ____ _____

11. Observe for rise and fall of chest wall. If necessary, reposition victim's head and neck and recheck for airway obstruction. ____ ____ ____ _____

12. Suction any secretions or turn client's head to side (unless contraindicated). ____ ____ ____ _____

13. Assess for victim's carotid pulse (or brachial pulse in infant). ____ ____ ____ _____

14. Begin external cardiac compressions on pulseless victim, using proper technique for victim's age:
    A. For adult victims:
       (1) Use proper hand position (one hand on top of the other) over sternum. ____ ____ ____ _____
       (2) Extend or interlace fingers. ____ ____ ____ _____
       (3) Lock elbows, keep arms straight and shoulders directly over victim's sternum, and compress chest 4 to 5 cm at a rate of 80 to 100 compressions per minute. ____ ____ ____ _____

Continued

	S	U	NP	Comments

(4) Ventilate victim's lungs every 5 seconds.

B. For child victims:

(1) Use proper hand position (one hand
over sternum).

(2) Compress sternum 2 to 4 cm at a rate
of 100 compressions per minute.

(3) Ventilate lungs every 3 to 4 seconds.

C. For infant victims:

(1) Use proper hand position (index and
middle fingers over sternum).

(2) Compress chest 1 to 2 cm at a rate of at
least 100 compressions per minute.

(3) Ventilate lungs every 3 seconds.

15. Palpate for pulse with each chest compression
for first minute (two-person rescue).

16. Continue administering cardiopulmonary resuscitation until appropriate or necessary to stop.

17. Assess carotid pulse at 5-minute intervals after
first minute.

18. Do not interrupt cardiopulmonary resuscitation
for more than 5 seconds.

19. Remove and discard gloves and face shield.

20. Record the incident, all treatments and medications given, all procedures performed, and the
victim's response.

STUDENT: _____ DATE: _____

INSTRUCTOR: _____ DATE: _____

PROCEDURE PERFORMANCE CHECKLIST

Skill 40-1 Initiating a Peripheral Intravenous Infusion

	S	U	NP	Comments
Initiating a Peripheral Intravenous Infusion				
1. Review client's medical record for order. Follow "five rights" for administration of medications.	___	___	___	_____
2. Observe client for signs and symptoms indicating fluid or electrolyte imbalances.	___	___	___	_____
3. Assess client's prior experience with intravenous (IV) therapy.	___	___	___	_____
4. Determine if client is to have surgery or blood transfusion.	___	___	___	_____
5. Assess laboratory data and client's allergies.	___	___	___	_____
6. Assess client for risk factors.	___	___	___	_____
7. Explain procedure to client.	___	___	___	_____
8. Assist client to a comfortable sitting or lying position.	___	___	___	_____
9. Wash hands.	___	___	___	_____
10. Organize equipment on bedside stand or overbed table.	___	___	___	_____
11. Change client's gown to a more easily removable gown with snaps at shoulder, if available.	___	___	___	_____
12. Open sterile packages and maintain a sterile technique throughout.	___	___	___	_____
13. Check IV solution. Make sure prescribed additives (e.g., potassium, vitamins) have been added. Check solution for color, clarity, and expiration date. Check bag for leaks.	___	___	___	_____
14. Open infusion set.	___	___	___	_____
15. Place roller clamp about 2 to 4 cm below drip chamber and move roller clamp to "off" position.	___	___	___	_____
16. Remove protective sheath over IV tubing port.	___	___	___	_____
17. Insert infusion set into fluid bag or bottle. Remove protector cap from tubing insertion spike and insert spike into opening of IV bag. Cleanse rubber stopper on bottled solutions with antiseptic, and insert spike into black rubber stopper of IV bottle.	___	___	___	_____
18. Prime infusion tubing by filling with IV solution. Compress drip chamber and release, allowing it to fill one third to one half full.	___	___	___	_____

Continued

	S	U	NP	Comments

19. Remove tubing protector cap and slowly release roller clamp to allow fluid to travel from drip chamber through tubing to needle adapter. Return roller clamp to "off" position after tubing is primed. _____ _____ _____ _____

20. Clear tubing of air bubbles. Firmly tap IV tubing where air bubbles are located. Check entire length of tubing to ensure that all air bubbles are removed. _____ _____ _____ _____

21. Replace tubing cap protector on end of tubing. _____ _____ _____ _____

22. Optional: Prepare heparin or normal saline lock for infusion. Use a sterile technique to connect the IV plug to the loop or short extension tubing. Inject 1 to 3 ml normal saline through the plug and through the loop or short extension tubing. _____ _____ _____ _____

23. Apply disposable gloves. _____ _____ _____ _____

24. Identify site for IV replacement. _____ _____ _____ _____

25. Place tourniquet 10 to 15 cm above insertion site. Check presence of distal pulse. _____ _____ _____ _____

26. Select well-dilated vein. Foster vein dilation with the following techniques:

   A. Stroke the extremity from distal to proximal sites below the proposed venipuncture site. _____ _____ _____ _____

   B. Tell client to open and close the fist of the arm where the site has been selected. _____ _____ _____ _____

   C. Lower the extremity on which the site has been selected. _____ _____ _____ _____

27. Release tourniquet temporarily. Clip excess hair at site, if necessary. _____ _____ _____ _____

28. Cleanse insertion site using firm, circular motion and povidone-iodine solution. Refrain from touching cleansed site. Allow the site to dry for at least 2 minutes. If client is allergic to iodine, use 70% alcohol and allow site to dry for 60 seconds. _____ _____ _____ _____

29. Perform venipuncture. Anchor vein by placing thumb over vein and stretching skin against the direction of insertion 7 to 10 cm distal to the site.

   A. Butterfly needle: Hold needle at 20- to 30-degree angle with bevel up slightly distal to actual site of venipuncture. _____ _____ _____ _____

   B. Over-the needle catheter: Insert over-the-needle catheter with bevel up at 20- to 30-degree angle slightly distal to actual site and in the direction of the vein. _____ _____ _____ _____

Continued

470

	S	U	NP	Comments

C. Needleless IV catheter safety device: Insert using same technique as for over-the-needle catheter. ___ ___ ___ _____

30. Look for blood return through tubing of butterfly needle or flashback chamber of over-the-needle catheter. Lower needle until almost flush with skin. Advance butterfly needle until hub rests at venipuncture site. Advance over-the-needle catheter 1/4 inch into vein and then loosen stylet. Advance catheter into vein until hub rests at venipuncture site. Do not reinsert the stylet once it is loosened. ___ ___ ___ _____

31. Stabilize the catheter with one hand by placing pressure on the hub or on the vein above insertion site. Release tourniquet and remove stylet from over-the-needle catheter. Do not recap the stylet. Slide the catheter off the stylet while gliding the protective guard over the stylet. ___ ___ ___ _____

32. Connect needle adapter of administration set or heparin lock to hub of over-the-needle catheter or butterfly tubing. Do not touch point of entry of needle adapter. ___ ___ ___ _____

33. Bloodless method: Hold pressure over tip of inserted catheter with thumb. With index finger and thumb, remove cap and attach tubing to catheter hub. ___ ___ ___ _____

34. Release roller clamp slowly to begin infusion at a rate to maintain patency of IV line. ___ ___ ___ _____

35. Secure IV catheter or needle:
   A. Place narrow piece of tape under catheter hub with sticky side up and cross tape over catheter. ___ ___ ___ _____
   B. Place second piece of narrow tape directly across hub of catheter. ___ ___ ___ _____

36. Apply sterile dressing over site. ___ ___ ___ _____
   A. Transparent dressing:
      (1) Remove adherent backing. Apply dressing to site. Smooth dressing over site, leaving end of catheter hub uncovered. ___ ___ ___ _____
      (2) Fold a 2-inch by 2-inch piece of gauze in half and cover with tape. Place under the catheter hub. Curl a loop of tubing and tape over the gauze and tubing. ___ ___ ___ _____

37. For IV fluid administration, adjust flow rate to correct drops per minute:
   A. For heparin lock, flush with 1 to 3 ml of heparin (10 to 100 U/ml). ___ ___ ___ _____

Continued

	S	U	NP	Comments

B. For saline lock, flush with 1 to 3 ml of sterile normal saline. _____ _____ _____ _____

38. Write date and time, gauge size and size of catheter, and placement of IV line and dressing. _____ _____ _____ _____

39. Dispose of used needles in appropriate sharps container. _____ _____ _____ _____

40. Discard supplies. _____ _____ _____ _____

41. Remove gloves. _____ _____ _____ _____

42. Wash hands. _____ _____ _____ _____

43. Observe client every hour to determine if fluid is infusing correctly. _____ _____ _____ _____

44. Observe client every hour to determine response to therapy. _____ _____ _____ _____

45. Record peripheral IV insertion. _____ _____ _____ _____

46. Record and report client's response to IV fluid, amount infused, and integrity and patency of system. _____ _____ _____ _____

STUDENT: _____ DATE: _____

INSTRUCTOR: _____ DATE: _____

Skill 40-2 Regulating Intravenous Flow Rate

	S	U	NP	Comments
Regulating Intravenous Flow Rate				
1. Observe for patency of intravenous (IV) line and needle or catheter.	_____	_____	_____	_____
2. Check client's medical record for correct solution, additives, and time of infusion.	_____	_____	_____	_____
3. Check client's knowledge of how positioning of IV site affects flow rate.	_____	_____	_____	_____
4. Verify with client how venipuncture site feels.	_____	_____	_____	_____
5. Calculate flow rate.	_____	_____	_____	_____
6. Check calibration (drop factor) in drops per milliliter (gtt/ml) of infusion set.	_____	_____	_____	_____
7. Select formula to calculate flow rate after determining ml/hr.	_____	_____	_____	_____
8. Read prescriber's orders and follow "five rights" for correct solution and proper additives.	_____	_____	_____	_____
9. Determine hourly rate.	_____	_____	_____	_____
10. Place adhesive or fluid indicator tape on IV bottle or bag next to volume markings.	_____	_____	_____	_____
11. Calculate minute rate based on drop factor of infusion set.	_____	_____	_____	_____
12. Time flow rate by counting drops in drip chamber for 1 minute, then adjust roller clamp to increase or decrease rate of infusion.	_____	_____	_____	_____
13. Follow this procedure for infusion controller or pump:				
A. Place electronic eye on drip chamber below origin of drop and above fluid level in chamber or consult manufacturer's directions for setup of the infusion. If controller is used, ensure that IV bag is 1 m above the IV site.	_____	_____	_____	_____
B. Place IV infusion tubing within ridges of control box in direction of flow or consult manufacturer's directions for use of pump. Select drops per minute or volume per hour. Close door to control chamber. Turn on power and press start button.	_____	_____	_____	_____
C. Open drip regulator while infusion controller or pump is in use.	_____	_____	_____	_____
D. Monitor infusion rates and IV site for infiltration according to agency policy.	_____	_____	_____	_____
E. Assess patency and integrity of system when alarm sounds.	_____	_____	_____	_____

Continued

	S	U	NP	Comments

14. Follow this procedure for volume control device:
   A. Place volume control device between IV bag and insertion spike of infusion set.   _____ _____ _____ _____
   B. Place 2 hours' allotment of fluid into device.   _____ _____ _____ _____
   C. Assess system at least hourly. Add fluid to volume control device as needed. Regulate flow rate.   _____ _____ _____ _____

15. Observe client for signs of overhydration or dehydration.   _____ _____ _____ _____

16. Evaluate client for signs of infiltration: inflammation at site, clot in catheter, kink or knot in infusion tubing.   _____ _____ _____ _____

17. Record and report solutions, infusion rates, use of electronic infusion device, and client's responses.   _____ _____ _____ _____

PROCEDURE PERFORMANCE CHECKLIST

Skill 40-3 Changing Intravenous Solution and Infusion Tubing

	S	U	NP	Comments
Changing Intravenous Solution and Infusion Tubing				
1. Changing intravenous (IV) solution:				
A. Check prescriber's orders.	____	____	____	_____
B. Note date and time solution was last changed.	____	____	____	_____
C. Determine compatibility of IV fluids and additives.	____	____	____	_____
D. Determine client's understanding of need for continued IV therapy.	____	____	____	_____
E. Assess patency of current IV access site.	____	____	____	_____
F. Prepare next solution at least 1 hour before needed. Check that solution is correct and properly labeled. Check solution expiration date.	____	____	____	_____
G. Prepare to change solution when less than 50 ml of fluid remains in bottle or bag.	____	____	____	_____
H. Explain procedure to client.	____	____	____	_____
I. Keep drip chamber at least half full.	____	____	____	_____
J. Wash hands.	____	____	____	_____
K. Prepare new solution for changing. Remove protective cover from IV tubing port.	____	____	____	_____
L. Move roller clamp to stop flow rate.	____	____	____	_____
M. Remove old IV fluid container from IV pole.	____	____	____	_____
N. Remove spike from old solution bag or bottle and, without touching tip, insert spike into new bag or bottle.	____	____	____	_____
O. Hang new bag or bottle of solution.	____	____	____	_____
P. Check for air in tubing. Remove bubbles in tubing: Insert a needle and syringe into a port below the air and aspirate into the syringe. Swab port with alcohol and allow to dry before inserting needle into port.	____	____	____	_____
Q. Keep drip chamber one third to one half full. If the drip chamber is too full, pinch off tubing below the drip chamber, invert the container, squeeze the drip chamber, hang up the bottle, and release the tubing.	____	____	____	_____
R. Regulate flow to prescribed rate.	____	____	____	_____
S. Observe client for signs of overhydration or dehydration.	____	____	____	_____
T. Observe IV system for patency and development of complications.	____	____	____	_____

Continued

	S	U	NP	Comments

2. Changing infusion tubing:

A. Determine when new infusion set is needed. _____ _____ _____ _____

B. Observe for occlusions in tubing. _____ _____ _____ _____

C. Explain procedure to client. _____ _____ _____ _____

D. Wash hands. _____ _____ _____ _____

E. Open new infusion set, keeping protective _____ _____ _____ _____
    coverings over infusion spike and connector
    site for butterfly needle or IV catheter.

F. Apply nonsterile disposable gloves. _____ _____ _____ _____

G. Remove IV dressing. Do not remove tape _____ _____ _____ _____
    securing needle or catheter to skin.

H. For IV infusion:

   (1) Move roller clamp on new IV tubing to _____ _____ _____ _____
    "off" position.

   (2) Slow rate of infusion by regulating drip _____ _____ _____ _____
    rate on old tubing. Maintain keep vein
    open (KVO) rate.

   (3) Compress drip chamber and fill cham- _____ _____ _____ _____
    ber.

   (4) Remove old tubing from solution and _____ _____ _____ _____
    hang or tape drip chamber on IV pole 1
    m above IV site.

   (5) Place insertion spike of new tubing into _____ _____ _____ _____
    old solution bag opening and hang
    solution bag on IV pole.

   (6) Compress and release drip chamber on _____ _____ _____ _____
    new tubing. Slowly fill drip chamber
    one third to one half full.

   (7) Slowly open roller clamp, remove pro- _____ _____ _____ _____
    tective cap from needle adapter, and
    flush tubing with solution. Replace cap.

   (8) Turn roller clamp on old tubing to "off" _____ _____ _____ _____
    position.

I. For heparin lock:

   (1) Use sterile technique to connect the _____ _____ _____ _____
    new injection cap to the loop or tubing.

   (2) Swab injection cap with alcohol. Insert _____ _____ _____ _____
    syringe with 1 to 3 ml saline and inject
    through the injection cap into the loop
    or short extension tubing.

J. Stabilize hub of catheter or needle and apply _____ _____ _____ _____
    pressure over vein just above insertion site.
    Gently pull out old tubing. Maintain stability
    of hub and quickly insert needle adapter of
    new tubing or heparin lock into hub.

K. Open roller clamp on new tubing. Allow _____ _____ _____ _____
    solution to run rapidly for 30 to 60 seconds.

Continued

	S	U	NP	Comments
L. Regulate IV drip according to orders and monitor rate hourly.	_____	_____	_____	_____
M. Apply new dressing if necessary.	_____	_____	_____	_____
N. Discard old tubing in proper container.	_____	_____	_____	_____
O. Remove and dispose of gloves.	_____	_____	_____	_____
P. Wash hands.	_____	_____	_____	_____
Q. Evaluate flow rate and observe connection site for leakage.	_____	_____	_____	_____
R. Record changing of tubing and solution.	_____	_____	_____	_____
S. Place a piece of tape or preprinted label with the date and time of tubing change and attach to tubing below level of drip chamber.	_____	_____	_____	_____

STUDENT: _____ DATE: _____

INSTRUCTOR: _____ DATE: _____

PROCEDURE PERFORMANCE CHECKLIST
Skill 40-4 Changing Peripheral Intravenous Dressing

	S	U	NP	Comments
Changing Peripheral Intravenous Dressing				
1. Determine when dressing was last changed.	___	___	___	_____
2. Observe present dressing for moisture and intact-ness.	___	___	___	_____
3. Palpate the catheter site through the intact dress-ing for inflammation or discomfort.	___	___	___	_____
4. Inspect exposed catheter site for swelling or infiltration.	___	___	___	_____
5. Assess client's understanding of need for contin-ued intravenous (IV) infusion.	___	___	___	_____
6. Explain procedure to client and family.	___	___	___	_____
7. Wash hands.	___	___	___	_____
8. Apply disposable gloves.	___	___	___	_____
9. Remove tape, gauze, and/or transparent dressing from old dressing one layer at a time, leaving tape that secures the IV needle in place or hold-ing that needle in place.	___	___	___	_____
10. Observe insertion site for signs and/or symptoms of infection.	___	___	___	_____
11. Discontinue infusion if necessary.	___	___	___	_____
12. Remove tape securing needle or catheter. Stabilize needle or catheter with one finger. Use adhesive remover to cleanse skin and remove adhesive residue, if needed.	___	___	___	_____
13. Keep one finger over catheter at all times until tape or dressing is replaced.	___	___	___	_____
14. Cleanse peripheral IV insertion site with alcohol and then with povidone-iodine solution starting at insertion site and working outward, creating concentric circles. Allow each solution to dry for 2 minutes.	___	___	___	_____
15. Apply new transparent or gauze dressing (see Skill 40-1).	___	___	___	_____
16. Remove and discard gloves.	___	___	___	_____
17. Anchor IV tubing with additional pieces of tape. Minimize tape placed over polyurethane dress-ing.	___	___	___	_____
18. Write date and time of dressing change and size and gauge of catheter directly on dressing.	___	___	___	_____
19. Discard equipment.	___	___	___	_____
20. Wash hands.	___	___	___	_____

Continued

	S	U	NP	Comments
21. Observe functioning and patency of IV system in response to changing dressing.	_____	_____	_____	_____
22. Monitor client's body temperature.	_____	_____	_____	_____
23. Record appearance of IV site, dressing, and status of IV.	_____	_____	_____	_____

STUDENT: _____ DATE: _____

INSTRUCTOR: _____ DATE: _____

Skill 43-1 Inserting a Small-Bore Nasoenteric Tube for Enteral Feedings

	S	U	NP	Comments
Inserting a Small-Bore Nasoenteric Tube for Enteral Feedings				
1. Assess client for the need for enteral tube feeding.	___	___	___	_____
2. Assess client for appropriate route of administration:				
A. Close each of client's nostrils alternately, and ask client to breathe.	___	___	___	_____
B. Assess for gag reflex.	___	___	___	_____
C. Review client's medical history for nasal problems and risk of aspiration.	___	___	___	_____
3. Review prescriber's order for type of tube and enteral feeding schedule.	___	___	___	_____
4. Wash hands.	___	___	___	_____
5. Explain procedure to client.	___	___	___	_____
6. Stand on same side of bed as nares for insertion. Assist client to high Fowler's position unless contraindicated. Place pillow behind client's head and shoulders.	___	___	___	_____
7. Place bath towel over client's chest. Keep facial tissues within reach.	___	___	___	_____
8. Determine length of tube to be inserted and mark with tape: Measure distance from tip of client's nose to earlobe to xiphoid process of sternum.	___	___	___	_____
9. Prepare nasogastric or nasointestinal tube for intubation:				
A. Do not ice plastic tubes.	___	___	___	_____
B. Inject 10 ml of water from 30-ml or larger Luer-Lok or catheter-tip syringe into the tube.	___	___	___	_____
C. Make certain that guidewire is securely positioned against weighted tip and that both Luer-Lok connections are snugly fitted together.	___	___	___	_____
10. Cut tape 10 cm long.	___	___	___	_____
11. Apply disposable gloves.	___	___	___	_____
12. Dip tube with surface lubricant into glass of water.	___	___	___	_____
13. Insert tube through client's nostril to back of throat. Aim back and down toward ear.	___	___	___	_____
14. Flex client's head toward chest after tube has passed through nasopharynx.	___	___	___	_____

Continued

	S	U	NP	Comments

15. Emphasize client's need to breathe through mouth and swallow during procedure.

16. Advance tube each time client swallows until desired length has been passed. Do not force tube. If resistance is met or client starts to cough, choke, or become cyanotic, stop advancing the tube and pull it back.

17. Check for position of tube in back of throat with penlight and tongue blade.

18. Perform measures to verify placement of tube:
    A. Inject 30 ml of air into tube, and aspirate gastrointestinal contents with a syringe.
    B. Measure pH and observe appearance of gastrointestinal contents.

19. Apply tincture of benzoin or other skin adhesive on tip of client's nose and tube. Allow to dry.

20. Remove gloves and secure tube with tape, avoiding pressure on naris:
    A. Split one end of tape lengthwise 5 cm. Place the intact end of tape over bridge of client's nose. Wrap each of the 5-cm strips around tube as it exits client's nose.
    B. Fasten end of nasogastric tube to client's gown by looping rubber band around tube in slip knot. Pin rubber band to gown.

21. For intestinal placement, position client on right side if possible until confirmation of placement. Otherwise, assist client to a comfortable position.

22. Obtain x-ray film of client's abdomen.

23. Apply gloves.

24. Administer oral hygiene.

25. Cleanse tubing at nostril.

26. Remove gloves.

27. Dispose of equipment.

28. Wash hands.

29. Inspect client's nares and oropharynx for any irritation after insertion.

30. Ask if client feels comfortable.

31. Observe client for gagging or any difficulty breathing.

32. Record and report type and size of tube insertion and position and client's tolerance of procedure.

PROCEDURE PERFORMANCE CHECKLIST

Skill 43-2 Administering Enteral Tube Feedings via Nasoenteric Tubes

	S	U	NP	Comments

Administering Enteral Tube Feedings via
Nasoenteric Tubes

1. Assess client's need for enteral tube feedings. _____ _____ _____ _____

2. Auscultate client for bowel sounds before feeding. _____ _____ _____ _____

3. Obtain client's baselines weight and laboratory values. Assess client for fluid volume excess or deficit and electrolyte and metabolic abnormalities. _____ _____ _____ _____

4. Verify prescriber's order for formula, rate, route, and frequency of feeding. _____ _____ _____ _____

5. Explain procedure to client. _____ _____ _____ _____

6. Wash hands. _____ _____ _____ _____

7. Prepare feeding container to administer formula:

  A. Have formula at room temperature. _____ _____ _____ _____

  B. Connect tubing to container as needed or prepare ready-to-hang container. _____ _____ _____ _____

  C. Shake formula container well and fill container and tubing with formula. _____ _____ _____ _____

8. Place client in high Fowler's position or elevate head of bed 30 degrees. _____ _____ _____ _____

9. Determine tube placement:

  A. Aspirate gastric contents to check for gastric residual. Return aspirated contents to stomach unless the volume exceeds 150 ml. _____ _____ _____ _____

  B. Consider results when assessing tube placement. _____ _____ _____ _____

10. Initiate feeding:

  A. Bolus or intermittent feeding:

    (1) Pinch proximal end of feeding tube. _____ _____ _____ _____

    (2) Remove plunger from syringe and attach barrel of syringe to end of tube. _____ _____ _____ _____

    (3) Fill syringe with measured amount of formula. Release tube and hold syringe high enough to allow it to be emptied gradually by gravity. Refill. Repeat until prescribed amount has been delivered to the client. _____ _____ _____ _____

Continued

	S	U	NP	Comments

(4) If feeding bag is used, hang feeding bag on IV pole. Fill bag with prescribed amount of formula and allow bag to empty gradually over at least 30 minutes.   _____ _____ _____ _____

(5) Flush tubing with water after completion of bolus or intermittent feeding unless contraindicated.   _____ _____ _____ _____

B. Continuous-drip method:

(1) Hang feeding bag and tubing on IV pole.   _____ _____ _____ _____

(2) Connect distal end of tubing to the proximal end of the feeding tube.   _____ _____ _____ _____

(3) Connect tubing through infusion pump and set rate.   _____ _____ _____ _____

11. Advance tube feeding gradually per guidelines.   _____ _____ _____ _____

12. When tubing feedings are not being administered, cap or clamp the proximal end of the feeding tube.   _____ _____ _____ _____

13. Administer water via feeding tube as ordered with diluted formula.   _____ _____ _____ _____

14. Rinse bag and tubing with warm water whenever feedings are interrupted.   _____ _____ _____ _____

15. Measure amount of aspirate every 4 hours.   _____ _____ _____ _____

16. Monitor client's finger-stick blood glucose every 6 hours until maximum administration is reached and maintained for 24 hours.   _____ _____ _____ _____

17. Monitor client's intake and output every 24 hours.   _____ _____ _____ _____

18. Weigh client daily until maximum administration rate is reached and maintained for 24 hours, then weigh client 3 times per week.   _____ _____ _____ _____

19. Observe return of normal laboratory values.   _____ _____ _____ _____

20. Record and report type of feeding, status of feeding tube, client's tolerance, and adverse effects.   _____ _____ _____ _____

STUDENT: _____ DATE: _____

INSTRUCTOR: _____ DATE: _____

PROCEDURE PERFORMANCE CHECKLIST

Skill 43-3 Administering Enteral Feedings via Gastrostomy or Jejunostomy Tube

	S	U	NP	Comments
Administering Enteral Feedings via Gastrostomy or Jejunostomy Tube				
1. Assess client's need for enteral tube feedings.	___	___	___	_____
2. Auscultate client for bowel sounds before feeding. Consult physician if bowel sounds are absent.	___	___	___	_____
3. Obtain client's baseline weight and laboratory values.	___	___	___	_____
4. Verify order for formula, rate, route, and frequency.	___	___	___	_____
5. Explain procedure to client.	___	___	___	_____
6. Prepare feeding container to administer formula:				
A. Have formula at room temperature.	___	___	___	_____
B. Connect tubing to container as needed or prepare ready-to-hang bag.	___	___	___	_____
C. Fill container and tubing with formula.	___	___	___	_____
7. Elevate head of bed 30 to 45 degrees.	___	___	___	_____
8. Verify tube placement:				
A. Gastrostomy tube: Aspirate client's gastric secretions and check appearance and pH. Return aspirated contents unless the volume exceeds 150 ml.	___	___	___	_____
B. Jejunostomy tube: Aspirate client's intestinal secretions and check appearance and pH.	___	___	___	_____
9. Flush tube with 30 ml of water.	___	___	___	_____
10. Initiate feedings:	___	___	___	_____
A. Syringe feedings:				
(1) Pinch proximal end of gastrostomy tube.	___	___	___	_____
(2) Remove plunger and attach barrel of syringe to end of tube, then fill syringe with formula.	___	___	___	_____
(3) Allow syringe to empty gradually. Refill until prescribed amount of formula has been delivered to client.	___	___	___	_____
B. Continuous-drip feedings:				
(1) Fill feeding container with enough formula for 4 hours of feeding.	___	___	___	_____
(2) Hang container on IV pole and clear tubing of air.	___	___	___	_____
(3) Thread tubing on pump according to manufacturer's directions.	___	___	___	_____

Continued

	S	U	NP	Comments
(4) Connect tubing to end of feeding tube.	_____	_____	_____	_____
(5) Begin infusion at prescribed rate.	_____	_____	_____	_____
11. Assess client's skin around tube exit site. Cleanse skin daily with warm water and mild soap. Dressings around the exit site are not recommended.	_____	_____	_____	_____
12. Dispose of supplies.	_____	_____	_____	_____
13. Wash hands.	_____	_____	_____	_____
14. Measure the amount of aspirate every 4 hours.	_____	_____	_____	_____
15. Monitor client's finger-stick blood glucose every 6 hours until maximum administration rate is reached and maintained for 24 hours.	_____	_____	_____	_____
16. Monitor intake and output every 24 hours.	_____	_____	_____	_____
17. Weigh client daily until maximum administration rate is reached and maintained for 24 hours, then weigh client 3 times per week.	_____	_____	_____	_____
18. Observe return of normal laboratory values.	_____	_____	_____	_____
19. Record and report amount and type of feeding, status of tube, client's tolerance, and any adverse effects.	_____	_____	_____	_____

STUDENT: _____ DATE: _____

INSTRUCTOR: _____ DATE: _____

PROCEDURE PERFORMANCE CHECKLIST

Skill 44-1 Collecting a Midstream (Clean-Voided) Urine Specimen

	S	U	NP	Comments
Collecting a Midstream (Clean-Voided) Urine Specimen				
1. Assess client's status.	____	____	____	_____
2. Prepare equipment and supplies.	____	____	____	_____
3. Explain procedure to client.	____	____	____	_____
4. Provide fluids a half hour before collecting specimen, unless contraindicated.	____	____	____	_____
5. Wash hands.	____	____	____	_____
6. Provide privacy.	____	____	____	_____
7. Have client cleanse perineal area, or assist client with this process.	____	____	____	_____
8. Open sterile kit and prepare appropriately.	____	____	____	_____
9. Apply sterile gloves.	____	____	____	_____
10. Open specimen container. Place cap with inside surface facing up.	____	____	____	_____
11. Pour antiseptic over cotton balls or gauze.	____	____	____	_____
12. Assist or allow client to cleanse perineal area and collect specimen:				
A. Male client:				
(1) Cleanse client's penis and rinse.	____	____	____	_____
(2) After client begins urinating, pass container into stream and collect 30 to 60 ml or urine.	____	____	____	_____
B. Female client:				
(1) Cleanse client's perineal area and rinse.	____	____	____	_____
(2) After client begins urinating, pass container into stream and collect 30 to 60 ml or urine.	____	____	____	_____
13. Remove container before urine flow stops.	____	____	____	_____
14. Place cap on container.	____	____	____	_____
15. Cleanse urine from outside of container.	____	____	____	_____
16. Place container in plastic specimen bag.	____	____	____	_____
17. Remove bedpan (if applicable) and assist client to a comfortable position.	____	____	____	_____
18. Label specimen and attach laboratory requisition slip.	____	____	____	_____
19. Remove and dispose of gloves.	____	____	____	_____
20. Wash hands.	____	____	____	_____
21. Take specimen to laboratory within 15 minutes or refrigerate.	____	____	____	_____
22. Record date and time specimen was obtained.	____	____	____	_____

STUDENT: _____ DATE: _____

INSTRUCTOR: _____ DATE: _____

PROCEDURE PERFORMANCE CHECKLIST
Skill 44-2 Inserting a Straight or Indwelling Catheter

	S	U	NP	Comments
Inserting a Straight or Indwelling Catheter				
1. Assess client's status.	___	___	___	_____
2. Review client's medical record.	___	___	___	_____
3. Assess client's knowledge of the purpose of catheterization.	___	___	___	_____
4. Explain procedure to client.	___	___	___	_____
5. Arrange for assistance if necessary.	___	___	___	_____
6. Begin monitoring intake and output.	___	___	___	_____
7. Wash hands.	___	___	___	_____
8. Provide privacy.	___	___	___	_____
9. Raise bed to appropriate working height.	___	___	___	_____
10. Stand on left side of bed if right-handed (or vice versa). Clear bedside table and arrange equipment.	___	___	___	_____
11. Raise side rail on opposite side of bed, and put side rail down on working side.	___	___	___	_____
12. Place waterproof pad under client.	___	___	___	_____
13. Position client:				
A. Female client:				
(1) Assist client to dorsal recumbent position. Ask client to relax thighs so hip joints can be externally rotated.	___	___	___	_____
(2) Position client in side-lying position with upper leg flexed at knee and hip if client cannot be in supine position.	___	___	___	_____
B. Male client: Assist client to supine position with thighs slightly abducted.	___	___	___	_____
14. Drape client:				
A. Female client: Diamond drape client.				
B. Male client: Drape client's upper trunk with bath blanket and cover lower extremities with bed sheets so only genitalia is exposed.				
15. Apply disposable gloves.	___	___	___	_____
16. Wash client's perineal area with soap and water as needed. Dry area thoroughly.	___	___	___	_____
17. Remove gloves.	___	___	___	_____
18. Position light to illuminate perineal area.	___	___	___	_____
19. Open package containing drainage system. Place drainage bag over edge of bottom of bed frame, and bring drainage tube up between side rail and mattress (indwelling catheter only).	___	___	___	_____

Continued

	S	U	NP	Comments

20. Open catheterization kit according to directions, keeping bottom container sterile. _____ _____ _____ _____

21. Apply sterile gloves. _____ _____ _____ _____

22. Organize supplies on sterile field. Open inner sterile package containing catheter. Pour sterile antiseptic solution into correct compartment containing sterile cotton balls. Open packet containing lubricant. Remove specimen container (lid should be loosely placed on top) and prefilled syringe from collection compartment of tray, and set them aside on sterile field. _____ _____ _____ _____

23. Test balloon by injecting fluid from prefilled syringe into balloon port. _____ _____ _____ _____

24. Lubricate 2.5 to 5 cm of catheter for female clients and 12.5 to 17.5 cm for male clients. _____ _____ _____ _____

25. Apply sterile drape:
   A. Female client:
      (1) Allow top edges of drape to form cuff over both hands. Place drape down on bed between client's thighs. Slip cuffed edge just under client's buttocks. _____ _____ _____ _____
      (2) Pick up fenestrated sterile drape and allow it to unfold without touching an unsterile object. Apply drape over client's perineum, exposing labia. _____ _____ _____ _____
   B. Male client:
      (1) First method: Apply drape over client's thighs and under penis without completely opening fenestrated drape. _____ _____ _____ _____
      (2) Second method: Apply drape over client's thighs just below penis. Pick up fenestrated sterile drape, allow it to unfold, and drape it over penis with fenestrated slit resting over penis.

26. Place sterile tray and contents on sterile drape between client's thighs. Open specimen container. _____ _____ _____ _____

27. Cleanse urethral meatus:
   A. Female client:
      (1) Retract client's labia with nondominant hand to fully expose urethral meatus. Maintain position of nondominant hand throughout procedure. _____ _____ _____ _____

Continued

490

	S	U	NP	Comments

(2) With forceps, pick up cotton ball saturated with antiseptic solution and clean perineal area, wiping front to back from clitoris toward anus. Wipe along the far labial fold, near labial fold, and directly over center of urethral meatus.   _____ _____ _____ _____

B. Male client:

(1) Retract foreskin of client's penis with nondominant hand. Grasp penis at shaft just below glans. Retract urethral meatus between thumb and forefinger. Maintain nondominant hand in this position throughout procedure.   _____ _____ _____ _____

(2) With forceps, pick up cotton ball saturated with antiseptic solution and clean penis. Move cotton ball in circular motion from urethral meatus down to base of glans. Repeat cleansing three more times, using clean cotton ball each time.   _____ _____ _____ _____

28. Pick up catheter with gloved dominant hand 7.5 to 10 cm from catheter tip. Hold end of catheter loosely coiled in palm of dominant hand.   _____ _____ _____ _____

29. Insert catheter:

A. Female client:

(1) Ask client to bear down gently as if to void urine, and slowly insert catheter through urethral meatus.   _____ _____ _____ _____

(2) Advance catheter a total of 5 to 7.5 cm in adult or until urine flows out catheter's end. Advance catheter another 2.5 to 5 cm when urine appears. Do not force. Place end of catheter in urine tray receptacle.   _____ _____ _____ _____

(3) Release labia and hold catheter securely with nondominant hand. Inflate balloon of retention catheter.   _____ _____ _____ _____

B. Male client:

(1) Lift client's penis to position perpendicular to client's body and apply light traction.   _____ _____ _____ _____

(2) Ask client to bear down as if to void urine, and slowly insert catheter through urethral meatus.   _____ _____ _____ _____

Continued

	S	U	NP	Comments

(3) Advance cather17 to 22.5 cm in adult or until urine flows out catheter's end. Withdraw catheter if resistance is felt. Advance catheter another 2.5 to 5 cm when urine appears. _____ _____ _____ _____

(4) Lower client's penis and hold catheter securely in nondominant hand. Place end of catheter in urine tray receptacle. Inflate balloon of retention catheter. _____ _____ _____ _____

30. Collect urine specimen as needed. Fill specimen cup or jar to desired level by holding end of catheter in dominant hand over cup. _____ _____ _____ _____

31. Allow client's bladder to empty fully if institution policy permits. _____ _____ _____ _____

32. Remove straight, single-use catheter: Withdraw catheter slowly but smoothly until removed. _____ _____ _____ _____

33. Remove indwelling catheter:
   A. Slowly inflate balloon with fluid from pre-filled syringe. _____ _____ _____ _____
   B. Release catheter with nondominant hand and pull gently to feel resistance. _____ _____ _____ _____

34. Attach end of retention catheter to collecting tube of drainage system. Keep drainage bag below level of bladder. Do not place bag on side rails of bed. _____ _____ _____ _____

35. Anchor catheter, allowing sufficient slack for client movement.
   A. Female client: Secure catheter tubing to client's inner thigh with strip of nonaller-genic tape. _____ _____ _____ _____
   B. Male client: Secure catheter tubing to top of thigh or lower abdomen. _____ _____ _____ _____

36. Assist client to a comfortable position. Wash and dry client's perineal area as needed. _____ _____ _____ _____

37. Remove and dispose of gloves. _____ _____ _____ _____

38. Dispose of equipment, drapes, and urine in proper receptacles. _____ _____ _____ _____

39. Wash hands. _____ _____ _____ _____

40. Palpate client's bladder. _____ _____ _____ _____

41. Ask if client is comfortable. _____ _____ _____ _____

42. Observe character and amount of urine in drainage system. _____ _____ _____ _____

43. Determine that no urine is leaking from catheter or tubing connections. _____ _____ _____ _____

44. Record and report catheterization, characteristics and amount of urine, specimen collection (if performed), and client's response to procedure and teaching concepts. _____ _____ _____ _____

Continued

492

	S	U	NP	Comments
45. Initiate intake and output records.	____	____	____	_____
46. Report absence of urine immediately.	____	____	____	_____

STUDENT: _____ DATE: _____

INSTRUCTOR: _____ DATE: _____

PROCEDURE PERFORMANCE CHECKLIST
Skill 44-3 Indwelling Catheter Care

	S	U	NP	Comments
Indwelling Catheter Care				
1. Assess client for bowel incontinence or discomfort at catheter insertion site.	____	____	____	_____
2. Prepare equipment and supplies.	____	____	____	_____
3. Explain procedure to client.	____	____	____	_____
4. Provide privacy.	____	____	____	_____
5. Wash hands.	____	____	____	_____
6. Position client properly.	____	____	____	_____
7. Place waterproof pad under client.	____	____	____	_____
8. Drape client.	____	____	____	_____
9. Apply disposable gloves.	____	____	____	_____
10. Undo anchor tapes to free catheter tubing.	____	____	____	_____
11. Expose and assess client's urethral meatus.	____	____	____	_____
12. Cleanse client's perineal tissues with soap and water.				
A. Female client: Cleanse each labium majus and labia minora. Clean toward anus. Move down catheter.	____	____	____	_____
B. Male client: Cleanse around catheter, then around meatus and glans in circular motion.	____	____	____	_____
13. Reassess client's meatus for discharge.	____	____	____	_____
14. With soap and water, wipe in a circular motion approximately 10 cm down the length of the catheter.	____	____	____	_____
15. Apply antibiotic ointment (if ordered) at meatus and along catheter.	____	____	____	_____
16. Assist client to a comfortable position.	____	____	____	_____
17. Dispose of supplies and gloves.	____	____	____	_____
18. Wash hands.	____	____	____	_____
19. Record and report client's status.	____	____	____	_____

STUDENT: _____ DATE: _____

INSTRUCTOR: _____ DATE: _____

PROCEDURE PERFORMANCE CHECKLIST
Skill 44-4 Closed and Open Catheter Irrigation

	S	U	NP	Comments
Closed and Open Catheter Irrigation				
1. Verify prescriber's order.	____	____	____	_____
2. Assess appearance and amount of client's urine and type of catheter used.	____	____	____	_____
3. Determine patency of catheter.	____	____	____	_____
4. Measure urine in drainage bag.	____	____	____	_____
5. Explain procedure to client.	____	____	____	_____
6. Wash hands.	____	____	____	_____
7. Apply disposable gloves for closed method (see below).	____	____	____	_____
8. Provide privacy.	____	____	____	_____
9. Assess client for bladder distention.	____	____	____	_____
10. Position client properly.	____	____	____	_____
11. Closed intermittent irrigation:				
A. Prepare solution and draw into syringe.	____	____	____	_____
B. Clamp indwelling catheter below injection port.	____	____	____	_____
C. Cleanse port with swab.	____	____	____	_____
D. Insert syringe at 30-degree angle.	____	____	____	_____
E. Slowly inject fluid into catheter and bladder.	____	____	____	_____
F. Withdraw syringe, remove clamp, and allow solution to drain into bag.	____	____	____	_____
12. Close continuous irrigation:				
A. Using aseptic technique, insert tip of irrigation tubing into bag containing solution.	____	____	____	_____
B. Close clamp on tubing and hang solution on IV pole.	____	____	____	_____
C. Open clamp, allow solution to flow through tubing, and close clamp.	____	____	____	_____
D. Connect to irrigation tubing using a triple lumen catheter or Y connector to double lumen catheter. Connect tubing securely.	____	____	____	_____
E. For intermittent flow, clamp tubing on drainage, open irrigation tubing, allow prescribed amount to enter bladder, close irrigation clamp, and open drainage clamp.	____	____	____	_____
F. For continuous irrigation, calculate drip rate, adjust clamp on tubing, and establish security and patency of system.	____	____	____	_____
13. Open irrigation:				
A. Prepare sterile supplies.	____	____	____	_____
B. Apply sterile gloves.	____	____	____	_____

Continued

	S	U	NP	Comments

C. Position waterproof drape. _____ _____ _____ _____

D. Aspirate 30 ml of solution into sterile irrigating syringe. _____ _____ _____ _____

E. Disconnect catheter from drainage tubing, allow urine to flow into basin, and cover open end of tubing with sterile cap. _____ _____ _____ _____

F. Insert syringe, gently instill solution, and withdraw syringe. _____ _____ _____ _____

G. Allow solution to drain into basin; repeat until drainage is clear. _____ _____ _____ _____

H. When irrigation is completed, reestablish closed drainage system. _____ _____ _____ _____

I. If solution does not return, have client change position, or gently aspirate solution. _____ _____ _____ _____

14. Reanchor catheter to client. _____ _____ _____ _____

15. Assist client to a comfortable position. _____ _____ _____ _____

16. Lower bed and raise side rails, if indicated. _____ _____ _____ _____

17. Dispose of supplies. _____ _____ _____ _____

18. Remove and dispose of gloves. _____ _____ _____ _____

19. Wash hands. _____ _____ _____ _____

20. Calculate irrigation fluid used and subtract from total drainage. _____ _____ _____ _____

21. Record and report type and amount of irrigation, character of drainage, and any unexpected findings. _____ _____ _____ _____

STUDENT: _____ DATE: _____

INSTRUCTOR: _____ DATE: _____

PROCEDURE PERFORMANCE CHECKLIST
Skill 44-5 Applying a Condom Catheter

	S	U	NP	Comments
Applying a Condom Catheter				
1. Assess client's urinary status.	_____	_____	_____	_____
2. Assess client's mental status.	_____	_____	_____	_____
3. Assess condition of client's penis.	_____	_____	_____	_____
4. Assess client's knowledge of the purpose of a condom catheter.	_____	_____	_____	_____
5. Explain procedure to client.	_____	_____	_____	_____
6. Arrange for assistance if moving dependent client.	_____	_____	_____	_____
7. Wash hands.	_____	_____	_____	_____
8. Provide privacy.	_____	_____	_____	_____
9. Raise bed to appropriate working height. Raise side rail on opposite side of bed, and lower side rail on working side.	_____	_____	_____	_____
10. Assist client to a supine position. Place bath blanket over client's upper torso. Fold sheets so client's lower genitalia are covered; only genitalia should be exposed.	_____	_____	_____	_____
11. Prepare urinary drainage collection bag and tubing. Clamp off drainage bag port. Secure collection bag to bed frame. Bring drainage tubing up through side rails and onto bed. Prepare leg bag for connection to condom catheter, if necessary.	_____	_____	_____	_____
12. Apply disposable gloves.	_____	_____	_____	_____
13. Clean client's perineal area and dry thoroughly.	_____	_____	_____	_____
14. Clip hair at base of client's penis.	_____	_____	_____	_____
15. Apply skin preparation to client's penis and allow to dry. If client is uncircumcised, return foreskin to normal position.	_____	_____	_____	_____
16. With nondominant hand, grasp client's penis along shaft. With dominant hand, hold condom sheath and tip of penis and slowly roll sheath onto penis.	_____	_____	_____	_____
17. Spiral wrap client's penile shaft with strip of elastic adhesive. Do not use any tape, because it may impede circulation.	_____	_____	_____	_____
18. Connect drainage tubing to end of condom catheter. Catheter can be connected to large-volume bag or leg bag.	_____	_____	_____	_____
19. Place excess coiling of tubing on bed and secure to bottom sheet.	_____	_____	_____	_____

Continued

	S	U	NP	Comments
20. Place client in safe, comfortable position. Lower bed and place side rails accordingly.	_____	_____	_____	_____
21. Dispose of supplies.	_____	_____	_____	_____
22. Wash hands.	_____	_____	_____	_____
23. Observe client's urinary drainage.	_____	_____	_____	_____
24. Inspect client's penis with condom catheter in place within 30 minutes of application. Ask client if there is any discomfort.	_____	_____	_____	_____
25. Remove and change condom and inspect skin on penile shaft when hygiene is performed and when condom is reapplied.	_____	_____	_____	_____
26. Record and report pertinent client information: condom application, condition of skin, voiding pattern.	_____	_____	_____	_____
27. Monitor intake and output as indicated.	_____	_____	_____	_____

PROCEDURE PERFORMANCE CHECKLIST
Skill 45-1 Administering a Cleansing Enema

	S	U	NP	Comments
Administering a Cleansing Enema				
1. Assess status of client.	___	___	___	_____
2. Assess client for presence of increased intracranial pressure, glaucoma, or recent rectal or prostate surgery.	___	___	___	_____
3. Determine client's understanding of purpose of enema.	___	___	___	_____
4. Check client's medical record.	___	___	___	_____
5. Review prescriber's order for enema.	___	___	___	_____
6. Collect appropriate equipment.	___	___	___	_____
7. Explain procedure to client.	___	___	___	_____
8. Assemble enema bag with appropriate solution and rectal tube.	___	___	___	_____
9. Wash hands.	___	___	___	_____
10. Apply gloves.	___	___	___	_____
11. Provide privacy.	___	___	___	_____
12. Raise bed to appropriate working height and raise side rail on opposite side.	___	___	___	_____
13. Assist client to left side-lying position with right knee flexed.	___	___	___	_____
14. Place waterproof pad under client's hips and buttocks.	___	___	___	_____
15. Cover client with bath blanket so that only rectal area is exposed and anus is clearly visible.	___	___	___	_____
16. Place bedpan or commode in easily accessible position.	___	___	___	_____
17. Administer enema:				
A. Prepackaged disposable container:				
(1) Remove plastic cap from rectal tip.	___	___	___	_____
(2) Gently separate client's buttocks and locate rectum. Instruct client to relax by breathing out slowly through mouth.	___	___	___	_____
(3) Insert tip of bottle gently into rectum (7.5 to 10 cm in adult, 5 to 7.5 cm in child, 2.5 to 3.75 cm in infant).	___	___	___	_____
(4) Squeeze bottle until all of solution has entered client's rectum and colon. Instruct client to retain solution until the urge to defecate occurs.	___	___	___	_____

Continued

	S	U	NP	Comments

B. Enema bag:

(1) Add warmed solution to enema bag: Warm tap water as it flows from faucet, place saline container in basin of hot water before adding saline to enema bag, and check temperature of solution. _____ _____ _____ _____

(2) Raise container, release clamp, and allow solution to flow long enough to fill tubing. _____ _____ _____ _____

(3) Reclamp tubing. _____ _____ _____ _____

(4) Lubricate 6 to 8 cm of tip of rectal tube with lubricating jelly. _____ _____ _____ _____

(5) Gently separate client's buttocks and locate anus. Instruct client to relax by breathing out slowly through mouth. _____ _____ _____ _____

(6) Insert tip of rectal tube slowly by pointing tip in direction of client's umbilicus. _____ _____ _____ _____

(7) Hold tubing in client's rectum constantly until end of fluid instillation. _____ _____ _____ _____

(8) Open regulating clamp, and allow solution to enter slowly, with container at client's hip level. _____ _____ _____ _____

(9) Raise enema container slowly to appropriate level above client's anus. _____ _____ _____ _____

(10) Lower container or clamp tubing if client complains of cramping or if fluid escapes around rectal tube. _____ _____ _____ _____

(11) Clamp tubing after all solution is instilled. _____ _____ _____ _____

18. Place layers of toilet tissue around tube at anus and gently withdraw rectal tube. _____ _____ _____ _____

19. Explain to client that feeling of distention is normal. Ask client to retain solution as long as possible while lying quietly in bed. If client is an infant or young child, gently hold client's buttocks together for a few minutes. _____ _____ _____ _____

20. Discard enema container and tubing in receptacle, or rinse container thoroughly with soap and warm water if it is to be reused. _____ _____ _____ _____

21. Assist client to bathroom or help position client on bedpan. _____ _____ _____ _____

22. Observe character of client's feces and solution (caution client against flushing toilet before inspection). _____ _____ _____ _____

23. Assist client as needed in washing anal area with warm soap and water. _____ _____ _____ _____

24. Remove and discard gloves. _____ _____ _____ _____

Continued

	S	U	NP	Comments
25. Wash hands.	_____	_____	_____	_____
26. Inspect color, consistency, and amount of stool and fluid passed.	_____	_____	_____	_____
27. Assess condition of client's abdomen.	_____	_____	_____	_____
28. Record type and volume of enema given and characteristics of results.	_____	_____	_____	_____
29. Report to physician if client fails to defecate.	_____	_____	_____	_____

PROCEDURE PERFORMANCE CHECKLIST
Skill 45-2 Pouching an Ostomy

	S	U	NP	Comments

Pouching an Ostomy

1. Auscultate client for bowel sounds.
2. Observe client's skin barrier and pouch for leakage and length of time in place.
3. Observe stoma for color, swelling, trauma, and healing.
4. Measure the stoma with each pouching change.
5. Observe client's abdominal incision (if present).
6. Observe effluent from stoma and keep a record of intake and output.
7. Ask client about skin tenderness.
8. When assessing client's skin for irritation, check that the pouching system is not leaking.
9. Avoid unnecessary changing of entire pouching system.
10. Assess client's abdomen for best type of pouching system to use.
11. Assess client's self-care ability.
12. After skin barrier and pouch removal, assess client's skin around stoma.
13. Determine client's emotional response and knowledge and understanding of an ostomy and its care.
14. Explain procedure to client. Encourage client's interaction and questions.
15. Assemble equipment.
16. Provide privacy.
17. Position client either standing or supine.
18. Drape client.
19. Wash hands.
20. Apply disposable gloves.
21. Place towel or disposable waterproof barrier under client.
22. Remove used pouch and skin barrier gently by pushing the skin away from the barrier.
23. Cleanse client's peristomal skin gently with warm tap water using gauze pads or clean washcloth. Do not scrub the skin. Dry area completely by patting the skin with gauze or towel.
24. Measure the stoma for correct size of pouching system needed.

Continued

	S	U	NP	Comments

25. Select appropriate pouch for client based on assessment. With a custom cut-to-fit pouch, use an ostomy guide to cut opening 1/16 to 1/8 of an inch larger than stoma before removing backing. Prepare pouch by removing backing from barrier and adhesive. With ileostomy, apply thin circle of barrier paste around opening in pouch. Allow to dry. _____ _____ _____ _____

26. Apply skin barrier and pouch. If creases occur next to stoma, use barrier paste to fill in; let dry 1 to 2 minutes. _____ _____ _____ _____

   A. For one-piece pouching system:

      (1) Use skin sealant wipes on skin directly under adhesive skin barrier or pouch; allow to dry. Press the adhesive backing of the pouch and/or skin barrier smoothly against the skin, starting from the bottom and working up and around the sides. _____ _____ _____ _____

      (2) Hold pouch by barrier, center over stoma, and press down gently on barrier. Bottom of pouch should point toward client's knees. _____ _____ _____ _____

      (3) Maintain gentle finger pressure around barrier for 1 to 2 minutes. _____ _____ _____ _____

   B. For two-piece pouching system: Apply flange as in steps above for one-piece system, then snap on pouch and maintain finger pressure. _____ _____ _____ _____

27. Apply nonallergenic paper tape around pectin skin barrier using "picture frame" method. A belt may be attached for extra security, rather than tape. _____ _____ _____ _____

28. A small amount of ostomy deodorant may be put in pouch. _____ _____ _____ _____

29. Fold bottom of drainable open-ended pouches up once and close with closure device. _____ _____ _____ _____

30. Properly dispose of old pouch and soiled equipment. Spray room deodorant if necessary. _____ _____ _____ _____

31. Remove gloves.

32. Wash hands. _____ _____ _____ _____

33. Change pouch every 3 to 7 days unless leaking. _____ _____ _____ _____

34. Ask if client feels discomfort around stoma. _____ _____ _____ _____

35. Note appearance of stoma skin and incision (if present). _____ _____ _____ _____

36. Auscultate client for bowel sounds and observe characteristics of stool. _____ _____ _____ _____

Continued

	S	U	NP	Comments
37. Observe client's nonverbal behaviors as pouch is applied.	_____	_____	_____	_____
38. Ask if client has any questions about pouching.	_____	_____	_____	_____
39. Record type of pouch used and skin barrier applied.				
40. Record amount and appearance of client's stool and texture and condition of peristomal skin and sutures.	_____	_____	_____	_____
41. Record and report abdominal distention and excessive tenderness, nature of client's bowel sounds, and any unexpected findings.	_____	_____	_____	_____
42. Record client's level of participation and need for teaching.	_____	_____	_____	_____

PROCEDURE PERFORMANCE CHECKLIST
Skill 45-3 Irrigating a Colostomy

	S	U	NP	Comments
Irrigating a Colostomy				
1. Assess client's stool.				
2. Determine time for irrigation.				
3. Assess client's understanding of procedure.				
4. Explain procedure to client.				
5. Assist client with positioning.				
6. Wash hands.				
7. Apply disposable gloves.				
8. Provide privacy.				
9. Remove appliance and cleanse client's skin.				
10. Apply irrigation sleeve.				
11. Fill container with solution; hang at client's shoulder level.				
12. Attach cone to irrigating tube. Allow fluid to fill length of tube.				
13. Apply lubricant to tube.				
14. Insert cone through top of sleeve and then firmly into stoma.				
15. Begin flow and readjust position of cone as needed.				
16. Adjust flow by raising or lowering container.				
17. Administer 500 to 1000 ml of solution slowly over 15 minutes.				
18. When done, clamp tubing and remove cone.				
19. Clamp top of sleeve.				
20. When most of solution has returned, rinse sleeve with water, fold end up, and fasten it to top. Have client ambulate, unless restricted to bed.				
21. When all feces returns, rinse sleeve with water and special liquid cleanser.				
22. Remove sleeve and wash, rinse, and dry it.				
23. Apply new pouch.				
24. Dispose of equipment and gloves.				
25. Wash hands.				
26. Inspect volume and character of client's fecal material.				
27. Note client's response during infusion.				
28. Palpate and auscultate client's abdomen after return of irrigant.				
29. Assist client to a comfortable position.				

Continued

	S	U	NP	Comments
30. Record pertinent information about procedure, client's ability to perform irrigation, and client's teaching needs.	___	___	___	_____
31. Assess for fecal drainage or distention between irrigations.	___	___	___	_____

PROCEDURE PERFORMANCE CHECKLIST
Skill 45-4 Inserting and Maintaining a Nasogastric Tube

	S	U	NP	Comments
Inserting and Maintaining a Nasogastric Tube				
1. Inspect condition of client's nasal and oral cavities.	____	____	____	_____
2. Ask if client has history of nasal surgery and note if deviated nasal septum is present.	____	____	____	_____
3. Palpate client's abdomen for distention, pain, and rigidity. Auscultate for bowel sounds.	____	____	____	_____
4. Assess client's level of consciousness and ability to follow instructions.	____	____	____	_____
5. Check medical record for prescriber's order, type of nasogastric (NG) tube to be placed, and whether tube is to be attached to suction or drainage bag.	____	____	____	_____
6. Explain procedure to client.	____	____	____	_____
7. Wash hands.	____	____	____	_____
8. Apply disposable gloves.	____	____	____	_____
9. Position client in high Fowler's position with pillow behind client's head and shoulders. Raise bed to a comfortable working level.	____	____	____	_____
10. Provide privacy.	____	____	____	_____
11. Stand on client's right side if you are right-handed and on left side if left-handed.	____	____	____	_____
12. Place bath towel over client's chest. Give facial tissues to client.	____	____	____	_____
13. Instruct client to relax and breathe normally while occluding one naris. Repeat this action for other naris. Select nostril with greater air flow.	____	____	____	_____
14. Measure distance to insert tube using traditional Hanson method.	____	____	____	_____
15. Mark length of tube to be inserted with small piece of tape placed so it can easily be removed.	____	____	____	_____
16. Cut a 10-cm piece of tape. Split one end down the middle lengthwise 5 cm. Place on bed rail or bedside table.	____	____	____	_____
17. Curve 10 to 15 cm of end of tube tightly around index finger, then release.	____	____	____	_____
18. Lubricate 7.5 to 10 cm of end of tube with water-soluble lubricating jelly.	____	____	____	_____
19. Alert client that procedure is to begin.	____	____	____	_____
20. Instruct client to extend neck back against pillow. Insert tube slowly through naris, with curved end pointing downward.	____	____	____	_____

Continued

	S	U	NP	Comments

21. Continue to pass tube along floor of nasal passage, aiming down toward ear. When resistance is felt, apply gentle downward pressure to advance tube (do not force past resistance). ____ ____ ____ _____

22. If resistance is met, try to rotate the tube and see if it advances. If there is still resistance, withdraw tube, allow client to rest, relubricate tube, and insert into client's other naris. ____ ____ ____ _____

23. Continue insertion of tube until just past client's nasopharynx by gently rotating tube toward client's opposite naris.

   A. Stop tube advancement, allow client to relax, and provide tissues. ____ ____ ____ _____

   B. Explain to client that next step requires that client swallow. Give client glass of water, unless contraindicated. ____ ____ ____ _____

24. With tube just above client's oropharynx, instruct client to flex head forward, take a small sip of water, and swallow. Advance tube 2.5 to 5 cm with each swallow of water. If client is not allowed fluids, instruct client to dry swallow or suck air through straw. ____ ____ ____ _____

25. If client begins to cough, gag, or choke, withdraw tube slightly and stop advancement. Instruct client to breathe easily and take sips of water. ____ ____ ____ _____

26. Pull tube back slightly if client continues to cough. ____ ____ ____ _____

27. If client continues to gag, check back of pharynx using flashlight and tongue blade. ____ ____ ____ _____

28. After client relaxes, continue to advance tube desired distance. ____ ____ ____ _____

29. Once tube is correctly advanced, remove tape used to mark length of tube and place the prepared split tape with nonsplit side on client's nose. Anchor tape with one of split ends while checking tube placement. ____ ____ ____ _____

30. Check tube placement:

   A. Ask client to talk. ____ ____ ____ _____

   B. Inspect posterior pharynx for presence of coiled tube. ____ ____ ____ _____

   C. Draw up 10 to 20 ml of air into catheter-tipped syringe and attach to end of tube. Auscultate left upper quadrant of client's abdomen while quickly ejecting air into the tube. ____ ____ ____ _____

   D. Aspirate gently back on syringe to obtain gastric contents. Observe color. ____ ____ ____ _____

Continued

512

	S	U	NP	Comments

E. Measure pH of aspirate with color-coded pH paper that has range of whole numbers from 1 to 11. _____ _____ _____ _____

F. If tube is not in client's stomach, advance it another 2.5 to 5 cm and repeat steps 31C through 31E. _____ _____ _____ _____

31. Anchor the tube:

A. Clamp end of tube or connect it to drainage bag or suction machine after insertion. _____ _____ _____ _____

B. Tape tube to client's nose; avoid putting pressure on nares:

  (1) Apply small amount of tincture of benzoin to lower end of client's nose and allow to dry. Secure tape over client's nose. _____ _____ _____ _____

  (2) Carefully wrap two split ends of tape around tube. _____ _____ _____ _____

  (3) Alternatively, apply tube fixation device using shaped adhesive patch. _____ _____ _____ _____

C. Fasten end of NG tube to client's gown by looping rubber band around tube in slip knot. Pin rubber band to gown. _____ _____ _____ _____

D. Elevate head of bed 30 degrees, unless contraindicated. _____ _____ _____ _____

E. Explain to client that sensation of tube should decrease somewhat with time. _____ _____ _____ _____

F. Remove and dispose of gloves. _____ _____ _____ _____

G. Wash hands. _____ _____ _____ _____

32. Identify tube placement in nose with mark or tape or measure length from nares to connector. _____ _____ _____ _____

33. Irrigate tube:

A. Wash hands. _____ _____ _____ _____

B. Apply disposable gloves. _____ _____ _____ _____

C. Check for tube placement (see step 31). Reconnect NG tube to connecting tube. _____ _____ _____ _____

D. Draw up 30 ml of normal saline into regular or catheter-tipped syringe. _____ _____ _____ _____

E. Clamp NG tube. Disconnect it from connection tubing and lay end of connection tubing on towel. _____ _____ _____ _____

F. Insert tip of irrigating syringe into end of NG tube. Remove clamp. Hold syringe with tip pointed at floor and inject saline slowly and evenly. Do not force solution. _____ _____ _____ _____

G. If resistance occurs, check for kinks in tubing. Turn client onto left side. _____ _____ _____ _____

Continued

	S	U	NP	Comments

H. After instilling saline, immediately aspirate or pull back slowly on syringe to withdraw fluid.

I. Reconnect NG tube to drainage or suction. (If solution does not return, repeat irrigation).

J. Remove and dispose of gloves.

K. Wash hands.

34. Discontinue NG tube:

A. Verify order to discontinue NG tube.

B. Explain procedure to client and reassure client that removal is less distressing than insertion.

C. Wash hands.

D. Apply disposable gloves.

E. Turn off suction and disconnect NG tube from drainage bag or suction. Remove tape from bridge of client's nose and unpin tube from client's gown.

F. Stand on client's right side if you are right-handed and left side if you are left-handed.

G. Hand the client facial tissue. Place clean towel across client's chest. Instruct client to take and hold a deep breath.

H. Clamp or kink tubing securely and then pull tube out steadily and smoothly into towel held in other hand while client holds breath.

I. Measure amount of drainage and note character of content. Dispose of tube and drainage equipment.

J. Clean client's nares and provide mouth care.

K. Assist client to a comfortable position and explain procedure for drinking fluids, if not contraindicated.

35. Clean equipment and return to proper place. Place soiled linen in proper receptacle.

36. Remove and dispose of gloves.

37. Wash hands.

38. Observe amount and character of contents draining from NG tube. Ask if client feels nauseated.

39. Palpate client's abdomen periodically for distention, pain, and rigidity, and auscultate for the presence of bowel sounds. Turn off suction while auscultating.

40. Inspect condition of client's nares and nose.

41. Observe position of tubing.

42. Ask if client's throat feels sore of if there is irritation in the pharynx.

Continued

	S	U	NP	Comments

43. Record time and type of NG tube inserted, client's tolerance of procedure, confirmation of placement, character of client's gastric contents, pH value of contents, and whether tube is clamped or connected to drainage device.
    _____ _____ _____ _____

PROCEDURE PERFORMANCE CHECKLIST
Skill 46-1 Applying Elastic Stockings

	S	U	NP	Comments
Applying Elastic Stockings				
1. Assess client for risk factors to determine need for elastic stockings.	____	____	____	_____
2. Observe for signs, symptoms, and conditions that might contraindicate use of elastic stockings.	____	____	____	_____
3. Obtain prescriber's order.	____	____	____	_____
4. Assess client's or caregiver's understanding of application of elastic stockings.	____	____	____	_____
5. Assess and document condition of client's skin and circulation to legs.	____	____	____	_____
6. Explain procedure and reasons for applying stockings to client or caregiver.	____	____	____	_____
7. Use tape measure to measure client's legs to determine proper stocking size.	____	____	____	_____
8. Wash hands.	____	____	____	_____
9. Position client in supine position. Elevate head of bed to level comfortable for client.	____	____	____	_____
10. Cleanse client's legs. Apply small amount of talcum powder to client's legs and feet if not contraindicated.	____	____	____	_____
11. Apply stockings:				
A. Turn elastic stocking inside out.	____	____	____	_____
B. Place client's toes into foot of elastic stocking, making sure that sock is smooth.	____	____	____	_____
C. Slide remaining portion of stocking over client's foot. Check that toes are covered and that the foot fits into the toe and heel position of the stocking.	____	____	____	
D. Slide stocking up over client's calf until completely extended and smooth.	____	____	____	_____
E. Instruct client to not roll stockings partially down.	____	____	____	_____
12. Assist client to comfortable position.	____	____	____	_____
13. Wash hands.	____	____	____	_____
14. Inspect stocking to make sure there are no wrinkles and no binding at top.	____	____	____	_____
15. Observe client's reactions to stockings.	____	____	____	_____
16. Observe client or caregiver applying stockings.	____	____	____	_____
17. Remove client's stockings at least once per shift and assess skin and circulatory status.	____	____	____	_____

Continued

	S	U	NP	Comments
18. Record date and time of stocking application and stocking length and size.	_____	_____	_____	_____
19. Record and report condition of skin and circulatory assessment.	_____	_____	_____	_____

STUDENT: _____ DATE: _____

INSTRUCTOR: _____ DATE: _____

PROCEDURE PERFORMANCE CHECKLIST
Skill 46-2 Positioning Clients in Bed

	S	U	NP	Comments

Positioning Clients in Bed

1. Assess client's body alignment and comfort level while client is lying down.   _____ _____ _____ _____

2. Assess client for risk factors that may contribute to complications of immobility.   _____ _____ _____ _____

3. Assess client's physical ability to help with moving and positioning.   _____ _____ _____ _____

4. Raise bed to comfortable working height.   _____ _____ _____ _____

5. Remove all pillows and devices used in any previous position.   _____ _____ _____ _____

6. Get extra help as needed.   _____ _____ _____ _____

7. Explain procedure to client.   _____ _____ _____ _____

8. Position client in bed:

   A. Move immobile client up in bed (one nurse):

   (1) Place client on back with head of bed flat. Stand on one side of bed.   _____ _____ _____ _____

   (2) Remove pillow from under client's head and shoulders and place pillow at head of bed.   _____ _____ _____ _____

   (3) Begin at client's feet. Face foot of bed at 45-degree angle. Place feet apart with foot nearest head of bed behind other foot. Flex knees and hips as needed to bring arms level with client's legs. Shift weight from front to back leg, and slide client's legs diagonally toward head of bed.   _____ _____ _____ _____

   (4) Move parallel to client's hips. Flex knees and hips as needed to bring arms level with client's hips.   _____ _____ _____ _____

   (5) Slide client's hips diagonally toward head of bed.   _____ _____ _____ _____

   (6) Move parallel to client's head and shoulders. Flex knees and hips as needed to bring arms level with client's body.   _____ _____ _____ _____

   (7) Slide arm closest to head of bed under client's neck, and reach hand under client to support client's shoulder.   _____ _____ _____ _____

   (8) Place other arm under client's upper back.   _____ _____ _____ _____

Continued

	S	U	NP	Comments

(9) Slide client's trunk, shoulders, head, and neck diagonally toward head of bed. _____ _____ _____ _____

(10) Elevate side rail. Move to other side of bed and lower side rail. _____ _____ _____ _____

(11) Repeat procedure, alternating sides until client reaches desired position in bed. _____ _____ _____ _____

(12) Center client in middle of bed by moving body in same three sections as just described. _____ _____ _____ _____

B. Assist client to move up in bed (one or two nurses):

   (1) Place client on back, with head of bed flat. _____ _____ _____ _____

   (2) Remove pillow from under client's head and shoulders and place pillow at head of bed. _____ _____ _____ _____

   (3) Face head of bed.

     (a) Place one arm under client's shoulders and one arm under client's thighs. _____ _____ _____ _____

     (b) Alternative position: Position one nurse at client's upper body. That nurse will place arm nearest head of bed under client's head and opposite shoulder and other arm under client's closest arm and shoulder. Position other nurse at client's lower torso. That nurse will place arms under client's lower back and torso. _____ _____ _____ _____

   (4) Place feet apart, with foot nearest head of bed behind other foot. _____ _____ _____ _____

   (5) Flex knees and hips. Shift weight from front to back leg, and move client and drawsheet or pullsheet to desired position in bed. _____ _____ _____ _____

C. Position client in supported Fowler's position:

   (1) Elevate head of bed 45 to 60 degrees. _____ _____ _____ _____

   (2) Rest client's head against mattress or on small pillow. _____ _____ _____ _____

   (3) Use pillows to support client's arms and hands if client does not have control of use of them. _____ _____ _____ _____

   (4) Position pillow at client's lower back. _____ _____ _____ _____

Continued

520

	S	U	NP	Comments

(5) Place small pillow or roll under client's thigh. _____ _____ _____ _____

(6) Place small pillow or roll under client's ankles. _____ _____ _____ _____

D. Position hemiplegic client in supported Fowler's position:

  (1) Elevate head of bed 45 to 60 degrees. _____ _____ _____ _____

  (2) Position client in sitting position as straight as possible and support client's affected shoulder. _____ _____ _____ _____

  (3) Position client's head on small pillow with chin slightly forward. Hyperextension of the neck must be avoided. _____ _____ _____ _____

  (4) Provide support for client's involved arm and hand on overbed table in front of client. Place arm away from client's side and support elbow with pillow.

    (a) Position flaccid hand in normal resting position with wrist slightly extended, arches of hand maintained, and fingers partially flexed. Clasp client's hands together. _____ _____ _____ _____

    (b) Position spastic hand with wrist in neutral position or slightly extended and fingers extended with palm down or left in relaxed position with palm up. _____ _____ _____ _____

  (5) Flex client's knees and hips by placing pillow or folded blanket under client's knees. _____ _____ _____ _____

  (6) Support client's feet in dorsiflexion with firm pillow, foot board, or high-top sneakers. _____ _____ _____ _____

E. Position client in supine position:

  (1) Place client on back, with head of bed flat. _____ _____ _____ _____

  (2) Place small rolled towel under lumbar area of client's back. _____ _____ _____ _____

  (3) Place pillow under client's upper shoulders, neck, or head. _____ _____ _____ _____

  (4) Place trochanter rolls or sandbags parallel to lateral surface of client's thighs. _____ _____ _____ _____

  (5) Place small pillow or roll under client's ankles to elevate heels. _____ _____ _____ _____

  (6) Place foot board or firm pillows against bottom of client's feet. _____ _____ _____ _____

  (7) Place high-top sneakers on client's feet. _____ _____ _____ _____

Continued

	S	U	NP	Comments

(8) Place pillows under client's pronated forearms, and keep client's upper arms parallel to client's body. ____ ____ ____ _____

(9) Place hand rolls in client's hands. ____ ____ ____ _____

F. Position hemiplegic client in supine position:

(1) Place client on back, with head of bed flat. ____ ____ ____ _____

(2) Place folded towel or small pillow under client's shoulder or affected side. ____ ____ ____ _____

(3) Keep affected arm away from client's body, with elbow extended and palm up. ____ ____ ____ _____

(4) Place folded towel under client's hip on involved side. ____ ____ ____ _____

(5) Flex client's affected knee 30 degrees by supporting it on a pillow or folded blanket. ____ ____ ____ _____

(6) Support client's feet with soft pillows at right angle to leg. ____ ____ ____ _____

G. Position client in prone position:

(1) Roll client over arm with arm positioned close to client's body, elbow straight, and hand under hip. Position client on abdomen in center of bed. ____ ____ ____ _____

(2) Turn client's head to one side and support head with small pillow. ____ ____ ____ _____

(3) Place small pillow under client's abdomen, below level of diaphragm. ____ ____ ____ _____

(4) Support client's arms in flexed position level at shoulders. ____ ____ ____ _____

(5) Support client's lower legs, and use pillow to elevate toes. ____ ____ ____ _____

H. Position hemiplegic client in prone position:

(1) Move client toward unaffected side. ____ ____ ____ _____

(2) Roll client onto side. ____ ____ ____ _____

(3) Place pillow on client's abdomen. ____ ____ ____ _____

(4) Roll client onto abdomen by positioning involved arm close to client's body with elbow straight and hand under hip. Roll client carefully over arm. ____ ____ ____ _____

(5) Turn client's head toward involved side. ____ ____ ____ _____

(6) Position client's involved arm out to side with elbow bent, hand toward head of bed, and fingers extended (if possible). ____ ____ ____ _____

Continued

522

(7) Flex client's knees slightly by placing pillow under client's legs from knees to ankles.   _____ _____ _____ _____

(8) Keep client's feet at right angles to legs by using pillow high enough to keep toes off mattress.   _____ _____ _____ _____

(9) Place high-top sneakers on client's feet.   _____ _____ _____ _____

I. Position client in lateral position:

(1) Lower head of bed completely or as low as client can tolerate.   _____ _____ _____ _____

(2) Position client to side of bed.   _____ _____ _____ _____

(3) Turn client onto side.   _____ _____ _____ _____

(4) Roll client onto side, toward you.   _____ _____ _____ _____

(5) Place pillow under client's head and neck.   _____ _____ _____ _____

(6) Bring client's shoulder blade forward.   _____ _____ _____ _____

(7) Position both arms in slightly flexed position, with upper arm supported by pillow level and other arm by mattress.   _____ _____ _____ _____

(8) Place tuck-back pillow behind client's back.   _____ _____ _____ _____

(9) Place pillow under semiflexed upper leg for support.   _____ _____ _____ _____

(10) Place sandbag parallel to plantar surface of client's dependent foot. Place high-top sneakers on client's feet.   _____ _____ _____ _____

J. Position client in Sim's position:

(1) Lower head of bed completely.   _____ _____ _____ _____

(2) Place client in supine position.   _____ _____ _____ _____

(3) Position client in lateral position, lying partially on abdomen.   _____ _____ _____ _____

(4) Place small pillow under client's head.   _____ _____ _____ _____

(5) Place pillow under client's flexed upper arm to support arm on level with shoulder.   _____ _____ _____ _____

(6) Place pillow under client's flexed upper legs to support leg on level with hip.   _____ _____ _____ _____

(7) Place sandbags parallel to plantar surface of client's feet.   _____ _____ _____ _____

(8) Place high-top sneakers on client's feet.   _____ _____ _____ _____

(9) Wash hands.   _____ _____ _____ _____

(10) Lower bed and raise side rails.   _____ _____ _____ _____

(11) Observe client's body alignment, position, and level of comfort.   _____ _____ _____ _____

(12) Assess for areas of erythema or skin breakdown.   _____ _____ _____ _____

Continued

	S	U	NP	Comments

9. Record each position change and include amount of assistance needed and client's response and tolerance. _____ _____ _____ _____

10. Record and report any signs of redness (e.g., in areas over bony prominences). _____ _____ _____ _____

PROCEDURE PERFORMANCE CHECKLIST
Skill 46-3 Transfer Techniques

	S	U	NP	Comments
Transfer Techniques				
1. Assess client's status.	____	____	____	_____
2. Identify client's risks for problems with transferring.	____	____	____	_____
3. Explain procedure to client.	____	____	____	_____
4. Provide privacy.	____	____	____	_____
5. Wash hands.	____	____	____	_____
6. Transfer client:				
A. Assist client to sitting position (bed at waist level):				
(1) Place client in supine position.	____	____	____	_____
(2) Face head of bed and remove pillows.	____	____	____	_____
(3) Place feet apart, with foot nearer bed behind other foot.	____	____	____	_____
(4) Place hand farther from client under client's shoulders and support client's head and cervical vertebrae.	____	____	____	_____
(5) Place other hand on bed surface.	____	____	____	_____
(6) Raise client to sitting position by shifting weight from front to back leg.	____	____	____	_____
(7) Push against bed using arm that is placed on bed surface.	____	____	____	_____
B. Assist client to sitting position on side of bed with bed in low position:				
(1) Raise head of bed 30 degrees.	____	____	____	_____
(2) Turn client to side, facing you, on side of bed on which client will be sitting.	____	____	____	_____
(3) Stand opposite client's hips. Turn diagonally so you face client and far corner of foot of bed.	____	____	____	_____
(4) Place feet apart, with foot closer to head of bed in front of other foot.	____	____	____	_____
(5) Place arm nearer head of bed under client's shoulder to support client's head and neck.	____	____	____	_____
(6) Place other arm nearer head and neck.	____	____	____	_____
(7) Move client's lower legs and feet over side of bed. Pivot toward rear leg, allowing client's upper legs to swing downward.	____	____	____	_____
(8) Shift weight to rear leg and elevate client at the same time.	____	____	____	_____

Continued

	S	U	NP	Comments

(9) Remain in front of client until client regains balance. ____ ____ ____ _____

C. Transfer client from bed to chair with bed in low position:

(1) Assist client to sitting position on side of bed. Position chair at 45-degree angle to bed. ____ ____ ____ _____

(2) Apply transfer belt of other transfer aids to client, if needed. ____ ____ ____ _____

(3) Ensure that client has stable, nonskid shoes. Place strong leg forward and weak leg back. ____ ____ ____ _____

(4) Spread feet apart. ____ ____ ____ _____

(5) Flex hips and knees, and align knees with client's knees. ____ ____ ____ _____

(6) Grasp transfer belt from underneath, if used, or reach through client's axillae and place hands on client's scapulas. ____ ____ ____ _____

(7) Rock client up to standing position on count of three while straightening hips and legs and keeping knees slightly flexed. Instruct client to use hands to push up, if able. ____ ____ ____ _____

(8) Maintain stability of client's weak or paralyzed leg with knee. ____ ____ ____ _____

(9) Pivot on foot farther from chair. ____ ____ ____ _____

(10) Instruct client to use armrests on chair for support, and ease client into chair. ____ ____ ____ _____

(11) Flex hips and knees while lowering client into chair. ____ ____ ____ _____

(12) Assess client for proper alignment for sitting position. Provide support for paralyzed extremities. Use lap board or sling to support flaccid arm. Stabilize legs with bath blanket or pillow. ____ ____ ____ _____

(13) Praise client's progress, effort, and performance. ____ ____ ____ _____

D. Perform three-person carry from bed to stretcher (bed at stretcher level):

(1) Stand side by side with two other nurses, facing side of client's bed. ____ ____ ____ _____

(2) Assume responsibility for one of three areas: head and shoulders, hips, or thighs and ankles. ____ ____ ____ _____

(3) Assume wide base of support. ____ ____ ____ _____

Continued

526

	S	U	NP	Comments
(4) Lifters will place arms under client's head and shoulders, hips, and thighs and ankles, with fingers securely around other side of client's body.	_____	_____	_____	_____
(5) Lifters will roll client toward them. On count of three, lift client and hold against chest.	_____	_____	_____	_____
(6) On second count of three, all lifters step back and pivot toward stretcher, moving forward if needed.	_____	_____	_____	_____
(7) Lifters will lower client onto center of stretcher by flexing knees and hips until elbows are level with edge of stretcher.	_____	_____	_____	_____
(8) Assess client's body alignment, place safety straps across client's body, and raise side rails of bed.	_____	_____	_____	_____

E. Use mechanical/hydraulic lift to transfer client from bed to chair:

	S	U	NP	Comments
(1) Bring lift to bedside.	_____	_____	_____	_____
(2) Position chair near bed and allow adequate space to maneuver lift.	_____	_____	_____	_____
(3) Raise bed to high position, with mattress flat. Lower side rail.	_____	_____	_____	_____
(4) Keep bed side rail up on side opposite nurse.	_____	_____	_____	_____
(5) Roll client away from you.	_____	_____	_____	_____
(6) Place hammock or canvas strips under client to form sling; fit lower edge under client's knees and upper edge around client's shoulders.	_____	_____	_____	_____
(7) Raise side rail of bed.	_____	_____	_____	_____
(8) Go to opposite side of bed and lower side rail.	_____	_____	_____	_____
(9) Roll client to opposite side and pull hammock or canvas strips through.	_____	_____	_____	_____
(10) Roll client supine onto canvas seat.	_____	_____	_____	_____
(11) Remove client's glasses, if appropriate. Assess that any tubes remain intact and untangled.	_____	_____	_____	_____
(12) Place lift's horseshoe bar under side of bed (on side with chair).	_____	_____	_____	_____
(13) Lower horizontal bar to sling level by releasing hydraulic valve. Lock valve.	_____	_____	_____	_____
(14) Attach hooks on strap (chain) to holes in sling. Hook short chains or straps to top holes of sling, and hook longer chains to bottom of sling.	_____	_____	_____	_____
(15) Elevate head of bed.	_____	_____	_____	_____

Continued

	S	U	NP	Comments
(16) Fold client's arms over chest.	___	___	___	_____
(17) Pump hydraulic handle using long, slow, even strokes until client is raised off bed.	___	___	___	_____
(18) Use steering handle to pull lift from bed and maneuver to chair.	___	___	___	_____
(19) Roll base around chair.	___	___	___	_____
(20) Release check valve slowly and lower client into chair.	___	___	___	_____
(21) Close check valve as soon as client is down and straps can be released.	___	___	___	_____
(22) Remove straps and mechanical/hydraulic lift.	___	___	___	_____
(23) Check client's sitting alignment.	___	___	___	_____
7. Wash hands.	___	___	___	_____
8. Assess client's tolerance and alignment with each transfer.	___	___	___	_____
9. Record each transfer and position change and client's response and tolerance.	___	___	___	_____
10. Record and report and signs of redness (e.g., over bony prominences).	___	___	___	_____

STUDENT: _____ DATE: _____

INSTRUCTOR: _____ DATE: _____

Skill 47-1 Assessment for Risk of Pressure Ulcer Development

	S	U	NP	Comments
Assessment for Risk of Pressure Ulcer Development				
1. Identify client's general risk for pressure ulcer formation.	_____	_____	_____	_____
2. Assess condition of skin over regions of pressure.	_____	_____	_____	_____
3. Assess client for areas of potential pressure.	_____	_____	_____	_____
4. Observe client for preferred positions when in bed or chair.	_____	_____	_____	_____
5. Observe client's mobility and ability to initiate and assist with position changes.	_____	_____	_____	_____
6. Obtain risk score using Norton or Braden scale.	_____	_____	_____	_____
7. Assist client in changing to one of the following positions: supine, prone, or 30-degree lateral.	_____	_____	_____	_____
8. Palpate any area of client's skin that is discolored or mottled.	_____	_____	_____	_____
9. Monitor length of time any discoloration persists:				
A. Determine appropriate turning interval.	_____	_____	_____	_____
B. Use pressure-relief device, if indicated.	_____	_____	_____	_____
10. Obtain client's nutritional assessment data.	_____	_____	_____	_____
11. Assess client's and family's understanding of risks for pressure ulcers.	_____	_____	_____	_____
12. Observe client's skin for areas at risk for change in color or texture.	_____	_____	_____	_____
13. Observe tolerance of client for position change.	_____	_____	_____	_____
14. Compare client's subsequent risk assessment scores.	_____	_____	_____	_____
15. Record and report client's risk assessment and any preventive measures used.	_____	_____	_____	_____

PROCEDURE PERFORMANCE CHECKLIST
Skill 47-2 Treating Pressure Ulcers

	S	U	NP	Comments

Treating Pressure Ulcers

1. Assess client's level of comfort and need for pain medication. ___ ___ ___ _____

2. Determine if client has allergies to topical agents. ___ ___ ___ _____

3. Review prescriber's order for topical agent or dressing. ___ ___ ___ _____

4. Wash hands. ___ ___ ___ _____

5. Apply disposable gloves. ___ ___ ___ _____

6. Position client to allow dressing removal. ___ ___ ___ _____

7. Assess pressure ulcer and surrounding skin to determine ulcer stage:
   A. Note color, moisture, and appearance of skin around ulcer and of ulcer itself. ___ ___ ___ _____
   B. Measure two maximum perpendicular diameters. ___ ___ ___ _____
   C. Measure depth of pressure ulcer using sterile cotton-tipped applicator or other device. ___ ___ ___ _____
   D. Measure depth of skin undermined by lateral tissue necrosis. Use a cotton-tipped applicator and gently probe under skin edges. ___ ___ ___ _____

8. Wash skin around ulcer gently with warm water and rinse area thoroughly with water. ___ ___ ___ _____

9. Gently and thoroughly dry skin by patting lightly with towel. ___ ___ ___ _____

10. Change to sterile gloves (check agency policy). ___ ___ ___ _____

11. Cleanse ulcer thoroughly with normal saline or cleansing agent:
    A. Use irrigating syringe for deep ulcers. ___ ___ ___ _____
    B. Cleanse ulcer in the shower with hand-held shower head. ___ ___ ___ _____
    C. Use whirlpool treatment to assist with mechanical debridement only. ___ ___ ___ _____

12. Apply topical agents as prescribed:
    A. Enzymes:
       (1) Apply thin, even later of ointment over necrotic areas of ulcer only. ___ ___ ___ _____
       (2) Apply gauze dressing directly over ulcer. ___ ___ ___ _____
       (3) Tape dressing securely in place. ___ ___ ___ _____

Continued

	S	U	NP	Comments

B. Gel agents:
  (1) Cover surface of ulcer with gel agents using applicator or gloved hand. _____ _____ _____ _____
  (2) Apply dry fluffy gauze or hydrocolloid or transparent dressing over gel agent to completely cover ulcer. _____ _____ _____ _____

C. Calcium alginates:
  (1) Pack wound with alginate using applicator or gloved hand. _____ _____ _____ _____
  (2) Apply dry gauze, foam, or hydrocolloid over alginate. _____ _____ _____ _____

13. Reposition client comfortably, off of pressure ulcer. _____ _____ _____ _____

14. Remove and dispose of gloves. _____ _____ _____ _____

15. Discard soiled supplies. _____ _____ _____ _____

16. Wash hands. _____ _____ _____ _____

17. Observe skin surround ulcer for inflammation, edema, and tenderness. _____ _____ _____ _____

18. Inspect dressing and exposed ulcer. Monitor client for signs and symptoms of infection. _____ _____ _____ _____

19. Complete assessment for ulcer healing scale. _____ _____ _____ _____

20. Compare subsequent ulcer measurements. _____ _____ _____ _____

21. Do not use the pressure ulcer staging system to measure pressure ulcer healing. _____ _____ _____ _____

22. Record and report ulcer appearance and treatment. _____ _____ _____ _____

PROCEDURE PERFORMANCE CHECKLIST
Skill 47-3 Applying Dry and Wet-to-Dry Moist Dressings

	S	U	NP	Comments
Applying Dry and Wet-to-Dry Moist Dressings				
1. Assess size and location of wound to be dressed.	___	___	___	_____
2. Assess client's level of comfort. Apply prescribed analgesic, if needed.	___	___	___	_____
3. Review orders for dressing change procedure.	___	___	___	_____
4. Explain procedure to client and instruct client to not touch wound area or sterile supplies.	___	___	___	_____
5. Provide privacy.	___	___	___	_____
6. Assist client to a comfortable position.	___	___	___	_____
7. Drape client with bath blanket to expose only wound site.	___	___	___	_____
8. Place disposable bag within reach of work area. Fold top of bag to make cuff.	___	___	___	_____
9. Apply face mask and protective eyewear, if required.	___	___	___	_____
10. Wash hands.	___	___	___	_____
11. Apply disposable gloves.	___	___	___	_____
12. Remove tape, bandage, or ties from wound site.	___	___	___	_____
13. Remove tape: Pull parallel to skin, toward dressing, and remove remaining adhesive from client's skin.	___	___	___	_____
14. With gloved hand, carefully remove gauze dressings one layer at a time, taking care not to dislodge drains or tubes. Keep soiled undersurface away from client's sight. If dressing sticks on a wet-to-dry dressing, gently free dressing and alert client of potential discomfort.	___	___	___	_____
15. Observe character and amount of drainage on dressing and appearance of wound.	___	___	___	_____
16. Dispose of soiled dressings in disposable bag.	___	___	___	_____
17. Remove and dispose of gloves.	___	___	___	_____
18. Open sterile dressing tray or individually wrapped sterile supplies. Place on bedside table.	___	___	___	_____
19. Apply dressing:				
A. Dry dressing:				
(1) Open bottle of cleansing solution (if ordered) and pour into sterile basin.	___	___	___	_____
(2) Apply sterile gloves.	___	___	___	_____
(3) Inspect wound for appearance, drains, drainage, and integrity. Avoid contact with contaminated material.	___	___	___	_____

Continued

	S	U	NP	Comments

(4) Cleanse wound with solution: ___ ___ ___ _____

    (a) Use separate swab for each cleansing stroke. ___ ___ ___ _____

    (b) Clean from least to most contaminated area. ___ ___ ___ _____

(5) Use dry gauze to swab in same matter as step 19A(4) to dry wound. ___ ___ ___ _____

(6) Apply antiseptic ointment if ordered, using same technique as for cleansing. ___ ___ ___ _____

(7) Apply dry sterile dressings to incision or wound:

    (a) Apply loose, woven gauze as contact layer. ___ ___ ___ _____

    (b) Cut 4 x 4 gauze flat to fit around drain, if present. Precut gauze is also available. ___ ___ ___ _____

    (c) Apply second layer of gauze. ___ ___ ___ _____

    (d) Apply thicker woven pad. ___ ___ ___ _____

B. Wet-to-dry dressing:

(1) Pour prescribed solution into sterile basin and add fine-mesh gauze. ___ ___ ___ _____

(2) Apply sterile gloves. ___ ___ ___ _____

(3) Inspect wound for color, character of drainage, type of sutures, and drains. ___ ___ ___ _____

(4) Cleanse wound with prescribed antiseptic solution or normal saline. ___ ___ ___ _____

(5) Apply moist fine-mesh gauze as a single layer directly onto wound surface. If wound is deep, gently pack gauze into wound with forceps. ___ ___ ___ _____

(6) Apply dry, sterile 4 x 4 gauze over wet gauze. ___ ___ ___ _____

(7) Cover with large dressing pads or gauze. ___ ___ ___ _____

20. Apply tape over dressing, gauze roll, or dressing stabilizing or securing ties. For application of dressing stabilizing or securing ties:

A. Expose adhesive surface of tape on end of each tie. ___ ___ ___ _____

B. Place ties on opposite sides of dressing. ___ ___ ___ _____

C. Place adhesive directly on skin or use skin barrier. ___ ___ ___ _____

D. Secure dressing by lacing ties across it. ___ ___ ___ _____

21. Remove and dispose of gloves. Remove mask and eyewear. ___ ___ ___ _____

22. Assist client to a comfortable position. ___ ___ ___ _____

23. Dispose of supplies. ___ ___ ___ _____

24. Wash hands. ___ ___ ___ _____

Continued

534

	S	U	NP	Comments
25. Report brisk, bright-red bleeding or evidence of wound dehiscence or evisceration to physician immediately.	_____	_____	_____	_____
26. Record and report wound appearance, client's response, and characteristics of drainage at shift change.	_____	_____	_____	_____

PROCEDURE PERFORMANCE CHECKLIST
Skill 47-4 Performing Wound Irrigations

	S	U	NP	Comments

Performing Wound Irrigations
1. Assess client's level of pain.
2. Review client's record for prescription for irrigation of open wound.
3. Assess signs and symptoms related to client's open wound.
4. Explain procedure to client.
5. Administer prescribed analgesic 30 to 45 minutes before starting wound irrigation procedure.
6. Assist client to a comfortable position that will permit gravitational flow of irrigating solution through wound and into collection receptacle.
7. Warm irrigation solution to approximate body temperature.
8. Wash hands.
9. Form cuff on waterproof bag and place it near bed.
10. Provide privacy.
11. Apply gown and goggles, if needed.
12. Apply disposable gloves.
13. Remove soiled dressing and discard in waterproof bag.
14. Remove and dispose of gloves.
15. Prepare equipment and open sterile supplies.
16. Apply sterile gloves.
17. Irrigate wound:
   A. Irrigate wound with wide opening:
      (1) Fill 35-ml syringe with irrigation solution.
      (2) Attach 19-gauge needle or angiocatheter.
      (3) Hold syringe tip 2.5 cm above upper end of wound and over area being cleansed.
      (4) Flush would with continuous pressure.
      (5) Repeat steps 17A(1) through 17A(4) until solution draining into basin is clear.
   B. Irrigate deep wound with very small opening:
      (1) Attach soft angiocatheter to filled irrigating syringe.

Continued

	S	U	NP	Comments

(2) Lubricate tip of catheter with irrigating solution, then gently insert tip of catheter and pull out about 1 cm. ____ ____ ____ _____

(3) Flush wound with slow continuous pressure. ____ ____ ____ _____

(4) Pinch off catheter just below syringe while keeping catheter in place. ____ ____ ____ _____

(5) Remove and refill syringe. Reconnect to catheter and repeat until solution draining into basin is clear. ____ ____ ____ _____

C. Cleanse wound with hand-held shower:

(1) With client seated comfortably in shower chair, adjust spray to gentle flow; warm water temperature. ____ ____ ____ _____

(2) Cover shower head with clean washcloth, if needed. ____ ____ ____ _____

(3) Cleanse wound for 5 to 10 minutes with shower head 30 cm from wound. ____ ____ ____ _____

D. Cleanse wound with whirlpool:

(1) Adjust water level and temperature. Add prescribed cleansing agent. ____ ____ ____ _____

(2) Assist client into whirlpool or place extremity into whirlpool. ____ ____ ____ _____

(3) Allow client to remain in whirlpool for prescribed interval. ____ ____ ____ _____

18. Obtain cultures, if needed, after cleansing wound with nonbacteriostatic saline. ____ ____ ____ _____

19. Dry wound edges with gauze; dry client if shower or whirlpool is used. ____ ____ ____ _____

20. Apply appropriate dressing. ____ ____ ____ _____

21. Remove gloves and, if worn, mask, goggles, and gown. ____ ____ ____ _____

22. Assist client to a comfortable position. ____ ____ ____ _____

23. Dispose of equipment and soiled supplies. ____ ____ ____ _____

24. Wash hands. ____ ____ ____ _____

25. Assess type of tissue in wound bed. ____ ____ ____ _____

26. Inspect dressing periodically. ____ ____ ____ _____

27. Evaluate skin integrity. ____ ____ ____ _____

28. Observe client for signs of discomfort. ____ ____ ____ _____

29. Record wound irrigation and client response on progress notes. ____ ____ ____ _____

30. Immediately report any evidence of fresh bleeding, sharp increase in pain, retention of irrigant, or signs of shock to attending physician. ____ ____ ____ _____

31. Record and report expected and unexpected outcomes. ____ ____ ____ _____

PROCEDURE PERFORMANCE CHECKLIST

Skill 47-5 Applying an Abdominal, T, or Breast Binder

	S	U	NP	Comments
Applying an Abdominal, T, or Breast Binder				
1. Observe client with need for support of thorax or abdomen. Observe client's ability to breathe deeply and cough effectively.	_____	_____	_____	_____
2. Review client's medical record if particular binder is prescribed.	_____	_____	_____	_____
3. Inspect client's skin for actual or potential alterations in integrity.	_____	_____	_____	_____
4. Inspect client's surgical dressings, if any.	_____	_____	_____	_____
5. Assess client's comfort level.	_____	_____	_____	_____
6. Gather necessary data regarding size of client and appropriate binder.	_____	_____	_____	_____
7. Explain procedure to client.	_____	_____	_____	_____
8. Teach procedure to client or caregiver.	_____	_____	_____	_____
9. Wash hands.	_____	_____	_____	_____
10. Apply disposable gloves.	_____	_____	_____	_____
11. Provide privacy.	_____	_____	_____	_____
12. Apply binder:				
A. Abdominal binder:				
(1) Position client in supine position with head slightly elevated and knees slightly flexed.	_____	_____	_____	_____
(2) Fanfold far side of binder toward midline of binder.	_____	_____	_____	_____
(3) Assist client in rolling away from you and toward raised side rail while firmly supporting abdominal incision and dressing with hands.	_____	_____	_____	_____
(4) Place fanfolded ends of binder under client.	_____	_____	_____	_____
(5) Assist client in rolling over onto folded ends.	_____	_____	_____	_____
(6) Unfold and stretch ends out smoothly on far side of bed.	_____	_____	_____	_____
(7) Instruct client to roll back into supine position.	_____	_____	_____	_____
(8) Adjust binder so that supine client is centered over binder using symphysis pubis and costal margins as lower and upper landmarks.	_____	_____	_____	_____

Continued

	S	U	NP	Comments

(9) Close binder. Pull one end over center of client's abdomen. While maintaining tension on that end of binder, pull opposite end over center and secure with Velcro closure tabs, metal fasteners, or horizontally placed safety pins.

(10) Assess client's comfort level.

(11) Adjust binder as necessary.

B. Single-T and double-T binders

(1) Assist client to dorsal recumbent position, with lower extremities slightly flexed and hips rotated slightly outward.

(2) Have client raise hips and place horizontal band around client's waist, with vertical tails extending past client's buttocks. Overlap waistband in front and secure with safety pins.

(3) Complete binder application:

  (a) Single-T binder: Bring remaining vertical strip over perineal dressing and continue up and under center front of horizontal band. Bring ends over waistband and secure all thicknesses with safety pin.

  (b) Double-T binder: Bring remaining vertical strips over perineal or suprapubic dressing with each tail supporting one side of scrotum and proceeding upward on either side of penis. Continue drawing ends behind and then downward in front of horizontal band. Secure all thicknesses with a horizontally placed safety pin.

(4) Assess client's comfort level with client in lying, sitting, and standing positions. Readjust front pins and tails as necessary, ensuring that tails are not too tight. Increase padding if any area rubs against surrounding tissues.

(5) Instruct client regarding removal of binder before defecating or urinating, and inform client of need to replace binder after performing these bodily functions.

Continued

540

	S	U	NP	Comments

C. Breast binder:
    (1) Assist client in placing arms through binder's armholes. _____ _____ _____ _____
    (2) Assist client to supine position in bed. _____ _____ _____ _____
    (3) Pad area under client's breasts, if necessary. _____ _____ _____ _____
    (4) Using Velcro closure tabs or horizontally placed safety pins, secure binder at nipple level first. Continue closure process above and then below nipple line until entire binder is closed. _____ _____ _____ _____
    (5) Make appropriate adjustments, including individualizing fit of shoulder straps and pinning waistline darts to reduce binder size. _____ _____ _____ _____
    (6) Instruct and observe client's skill development in self-care related to reapplying breast binder. _____ _____ _____ _____

13. Remove and dispose of gloves. _____ _____ _____ _____
14. Wash hands. _____ _____ _____ _____
15. Observe wound site for skin integrity, circulation, and characteristics. _____ _____ _____ _____
16. Assess comfort level of client using analog scale of 0 to 10 and noting any objective signs and symptoms. _____ _____ _____ _____
17. Assess client's ability to ventilate properly. _____ _____ _____ _____
18. Identify client's need for assistance with daily activities. _____ _____ _____ _____
19. Record and report application of binder, condition of client's skin, circulation, integrity of dressing, and client's comfort level. _____ _____ _____ _____
20. Report ineffective lung expansion to physician immediately. _____ _____ _____ _____

PROCEDURE PERFORMANCE CHECKLIST
Skill 47-6 Applying an Elastic Bandage

	S	U	NP	Comments
Applying an Elastic Bandage				
1. Inspect client's skin for alterations in integrity.	____	____	____	_____
2. Inspect client's surgical dressing.	____	____	____	_____
3. Observe adequacy of client's circulation distal to bandage.	____	____	____	_____
4. Review client's medical record for specific orders related to application of elastic bandage.	____	____	____	_____
5. Identify client's and primary caregiver's present knowledge level and skill if bandaging will be continued when the client goes home.	____	____	____	_____
6. Explain procedure to client.	____	____	____	_____
7. Teach bandaging skill to client or caregiver.	____	____	____	_____
8. Wash hands.	____	____	____	_____
9. Apply disposable gloves if drainage is present.	____	____	____	_____
10. Provide privacy.	____	____	____	_____
11. Assist client to a comfortable position.	____	____	____	_____
12. Hold roll of elastic bandage in dominant hand and use other hand to lightly hold beginning of bandage at distal body part. Continue transferring roll to dominant hand as bandage is wrapped.	____	____	____	_____
13. Apply bandage from distal point toward proximal boundary using a variety of turns to cover various shapes of body parts.	____	____	____	_____
14. Unroll and very slightly stretch bandage.	____	____	____	_____
15. Overlap turns by one-half to two-thirds width of bandage roll.	____	____	____	_____
16. \Secure first bandage with clip or tape before applying additional rolls. Apply additional rolls without leaving any uncovered skin surface. Secure final bandage applied.	____	____	____	_____
17. Remove and dispose of gloves.	____	____	____	_____
18. Wash hands.	____	____	____	_____
19. Assess client's distal circulation when bandage application is complete and at least twice during each 8-hour period.	____	____	____	_____
20. Have client or caregiver demonstrate bandage application.	____	____	____	_____
21. Record and report condition of client's wound, integrity of dressing, application of bandage, client's circulation, and client's comfort level.	____	____	____	_____

PROCEDURE PERFORMANCE CHECKLIST

Skill 47-7 Applying a Moist Hot Compress to an Open Wound

	S	U	NP	Comments
Applying a Moist Hot Compress to an Open Wound				
1. Refer to client's record for compress order.	____	____	____	_____
2. Inspect condition of client's exposed skin and wound on which compress is to be applied.	____	____	____	_____
3. Assess client's extremities for sensitivity to temperature and pain.	____	____	____	_____
4. Refer to client's medical record to identify any systemic contraindications to heat application.	____	____	____	_____
5. Prepare equipment and supplies.	____	____	____	_____
6. Explain procedure and purpose to client. Describe sensations that will be felt, such as decreasing warmth and wetness. Explain precautions to prevent burning.	____	____	____	_____
7. Provide privacy.	____	____	____	_____
8. Assist client to a comfortable position in proper body alignment. Place waterproof pad under part of client's body that will be treated.	____	____	____	_____
9. Expose client's body part that will be covered with the compress, and drape rest of client with bath blanket.	____	____	____	_____
10. Wash hands.	____	____	____	_____
11. Prepare compress:				
A. Pour solution into sterile container.	____	____	____	_____
B. If using portable heating source, warm solution. Open sterile packages and drop gauze into container to become immersed in solution.	____	____	____	_____
C. Adjust temperature of aquathermia pad.	____	____	____	_____
12. Apply disposable gloves.	____	____	____	_____
13. Remove any existing dressing covering wound.	____	____	____	_____
14. Dispose of gloves and dressings in proper receptacle.	____	____	____	_____
15. Assess condition of wound and surrounding skin.	____	____	____	_____
16. Apply sterile gloves.	____	____	____	_____
17. Pick up one layer of immersed gauze, wring out any excess solution, and apply gauze lightly to open wound.	____	____	____	_____
18. After a few seconds, lift edge of gauze to assess for redness.	____	____	____	_____
19. If client tolerates compress, pack gauze snugly against the wound. Cover all wound surfaces with hot compress.	____	____	____	_____

Continued

	S	U	NP	Comments

20. Cover moist compress with dry sterile dressing and bath towel. If necessary, pin or tie in place. ____ ____ ____ _____

21. Remove sterile gloves. ____ ____ ____ _____

22. Apply aquathermic or waterproof heating pad over towel (optional). Keep in place for desired duration of application. ____ ____ ____ _____

23. If an aquathermic pad is not used to maintain temperature of application, change hot compress using sterile technique every 5 minutes or as ordered during duration of therapy. ____ ____ ____ _____

24. After prescribed time, apply disposable gloves and remove pad, towel, and compress. Reassess wound and condition of skin, and replace dry sterile dressing as ordered. ____ ____ ____ _____

25. Assist client to preferred comfortable position. ____ ____ ____ _____

26. Dispose of equipment and soiled compress. ____ ____ ____ _____

27. Wash hands. ____ ____ ____ _____

28. Inspect area covered by compress and heating pad every 5 to 10 minutes. ____ ____ ____ _____

29. Ask every 5 to 10 minutes if client notices an unusual burning sensation not felt before application of compress. ____ ____ ____ _____

30. Have client explain and demonstrate application of compress. ____ ____ ____ _____

31. Record type, location, and duration of application of compress. Note solution and temperature. ____ ____ ____ _____

32. Record and report condition of wound and skin, treatment, instructions provided, and client's response to compress. ____ ____ ____ _____

PROCEDURE PERFORMANCE CHECKLIST
Skill 49-1 Demonstrating Postoperative Exercises

	S	U	NP	Comments

Demonstrating Postoperative Exercises

1. Assess client for risk of postoperative complications.

2. Explain purpose and importance of exercises.

3. Diaphragmatic breathing:
   A. Ask client to sit or stand upright with hands palm down along lower borders of anterior ribcage with tips of third fingers lightly together.
   B. Instruct client to take slow, deep breaths and inhale through nose.
   C. Tell client that downward movement of diaphragm will be felt during inspiration and to avoid using chest and shoulder muscles while breathing.
   D. Ask client to hold breath to count of three and slowly exhale through mouth.
   E. Tell client to repeat exercise three to five times. Have client practice.
   F. Explain how often exercise should be performed.

4. Incentive spirometry:
   A. Wash hands.
   B. Position client in semi- or high Fowler's position.
   C. Set the spirometer to the volume level to be attained.
   D. Demonstrate correct use of spirometer mouthpiece.
   E. Instruct client on correct techniques for inspiration and expiration while using device.
   F. Instruct client to breathe normally for short period.
   G. Instruct client to repeat maneuver until goals are achieved.
   H. Wash hands.

5. Positive expiratory pressure therapy and "huff" coughing:
   A. Wash hands.
   B. Set positive expiratory pressure device for the positive pressure setting ordered.

Continued

	S	U	NP	Comments

C. Instruct client to assume semi-Fowler's or high Fowler's position and place nose clip on client's nose.   _____ _____ _____ _____

D. Ask client to place lips around mouthpiece of device. Client should take a full breath and then exhale two to three times longer than inhalation.   _____ _____ _____ _____

E. Remove device from client's mouth and have client take a slow, deep breath and hold for 3 seconds.   _____ _____ _____ _____

F. Instruct client to exhale in quick, short, forced inhalations.   _____ _____ _____ _____

6. Controlled coughing:

A. Assist client to an upright position. Explain importance of positioning.   _____ _____ _____ _____

B. Demonstrate coughing: Take two slow diaphragmatic breaths, inhaling through mouth, exhaling through nose.   _____ _____ _____ _____

C. Instruct client to then inhale a third breath deeply, hold breath to count of three, and then cough fully two or three times without inhaling.   _____ _____ _____ _____

D. Caution client against merely clearing throat.   _____ _____ _____ _____

E. If surgical incision is in client's chest or abdominal area, show client how to splint cough with both hands over incision or with pillow. Have client practice technique.   _____ _____ _____ _____

F. Explain how often the patient should cough and splint.   _____ _____ _____ _____

G. Instruct client to examine sputum.   _____ _____ _____ _____

7. Turning:

A. Assist client to supine position on right side of bed.   _____ _____ _____ _____

B. Put side rails up.   _____ _____ _____ _____

C. Ask client to place left hand over incisional area for splinting.   _____ _____ _____ _____

D. Instruct client to keep left leg straight and flex right knee up and over left leg.   _____ _____ _____ _____

E. Ask client to grasp side rail on left side of bed with right hand, pull toward left, and roll onto left side.   _____ _____ _____ _____

F. Teach client when to perform maneuver.   _____ _____ _____ _____

8. Leg exercises:

A. Assist client to supine position.   _____ _____ _____ _____

B. Explain and demonstrate exercises by using passive range of motion exercises.   _____ _____ _____ _____

Continued

	S	U	NP	Comments

C. Rotate each of client's ankles in complete circle. Have client draw imaginary circles with big toe and repeat five times. _____ _____ _____ _____

D. Alternate dorsiflexion and plantar flexion of client's feet. _____ _____ _____ _____

E. Continue exercises by alternately flexing and extending client's knees; repeat five times. _____ _____ _____ _____

F. Have client keep knees straight and alternately raise each leg straight up from bed surface; repeat five times. _____ _____ _____ _____

G. Instruct client when and how often to perform exercises and to coordinate turning and leg exercises with breathing and coughing exercises. _____ _____ _____ _____

9. Observe client's ability to perform all exercises. _____ _____ _____ _____

10. Record procedures performed and observations. _____ _____ _____ _____

Answer Keys to Review Questions

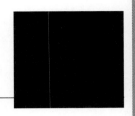

CHAPTER 1
1. c
2. b
3. b
4. d
5. d

CHAPTER 2
1. a
2. d
3. a
4. d
5. c

CHAPTER 3
1. b
2. a
3. a
4. d
5. c

CHAPTER 4
1. a
2. c
3. c
4. d
5. a

CHAPTER 5
1. b
2. d
3. a
4. b
5. a

CHAPTER 6
1. c
2. c
3. d
4. a
5. a

CHAPTER 7
1. a
2. b
3. b
4. b
5. a

CHAPTER 8
1. a
2. c
3. c
4. c
5. a

CHAPTER 9
1. b
2. b
3. a
4. c
5. d

CHAPTER 10
1. c
2. d
3. d
4. a
5. c
6. d

CHAPTER 11
1. b
2. b
3. c
4. b
5. a

CHAPTER 12
1. b
2. a
3. b
4. c
5. b

CHAPTER 13
1. b
2. c
3. a
4. e

CHAPTER 14
1. c
2. a
3. a
4. a
5. b

CHAPTER 15
1. a
2. a
3. b
4. d
5. d

CHAPTER 16
1. d
2. b
3. d
4. d
5. a

CHAPTER 17
1. b
2. d
3. a
4. a
5. c

CHAPTER 18
1. c
2. c
3. b
4. b
5. a

CHAPTER 19
1. a
2. d
3. c
4. a
5. a

CHAPTER 20
1. d
2. d
3. a
4. b
5. c

Answers to Review Questions   551

CHAPTER 21

1. a
2. c
3. d
4. b
5. d

CHAPTER 22

1. b
2. b
3. b
4. a
5. b

CHAPTER 23

1. b
2. c
3. d
4. c
5. b

CHAPTER 24

1. b
2. c
3. c
4. c
5. d

CHAPTER 25

1. b
2. d
3. c
4. b
5. c

CHAPTER 26

1. c
2. c
3. b
4. c
5. d

CHAPTER 27

1. b
2. d
3. c
4. a
5. d

CHAPTER 28

1. a
2. a
3. a
4. a
5. c

CHAPTER 29

1. c
2. c
3. b
4. c
5. d

CHAPTER 30

1. d
2. a
3. a
4. d
5. c
6. d

CHAPTER 31

1. d
2. d
3. b
4. c
5. c

CHAPTER 32

1. d
2. a
3. c
4. c
5. c
6. d

CHAPTER 33

1. d
2. b
3. d
4. a
5. b
6. a

CHAPTER 34

1. b
2. a
3. a
4. a
5. b
6. a

CHAPTER 35

1. c
2. c
3. d
4. a

CHAPTER 36

1. c
2. b
3. a
4. b
5. d

CHAPTER 37

1. d
2. d
3. c
4. d
5. a

CHAPTER 38

1. b
2. a
3. c
4. b
5. c

CHAPTER 39

1. a
2. c
3. b
4. b
5. d
6. b

CHAPTER 40

1. b
2. c
3. a
4. c
5. b
6. d

CHAPTER 41

1. a
2. a
3. c
4. d
5. b

CHAPTER 42

1. b
2. d
3. a
4. b
5. c

CHAPTER 43

1. c
2. d
3. c
4. c
5. b
6. a

CHAPTER 44

1. a
2. b
3. b
4. a
5. d

CHAPTER 45

1. b
2. a
3. c
4. b
5. c

CHAPTER 46

1. a
2. d
3. d
4. a
5. d

CHAPTER 47

1. b
2. b
3. a
4. c
5. b
6. d

CHAPTER 48

1. c
2. a
3. b
4. c
5. a

CHAPTER 49

1. d
2. c
3. c
4. a
5. b

Answers to Synthesis Models

KNOWLEDGE

- Components of self-concept (identity, body image, self-esteem, role performance)
- Self-concept stressors related to identity, body image, self-esteem, role
- Therapeutic communication principles, nonverbal indicators of distress
- Cultural factors that influence self-concept
- Growth and development (middle-age adult)
- Pharmacologic effects of medicine (pain medication)

EXPERIENCE

- Caring for a client who had an alteration in body image, self-esteem, role, or identity
- Jan's own personal experience of threat to self-concept

ASSESSMENT

- Observe the Mr. Johnson's behaviors that suggest an alteration in self-concept
- Assess the Mr. Johnson's cultural background
- Assess the Mr. Johnson's coping skills and resources
- Converse with Mr. Johnson to determine his feelings, perceptions about changes in body image, self-esteem, or role
- Assess the quality of Mr. Johnson's relationships

STANDARDS

- Support Mr. Johnson's autonomy to make choices and express values that support positive self-concept.
- Apply intellectual standards of relevance and plausibility for care to be acceptable to Mr. Johnson
- Jan needs to safeguard Mr. Johnson's right to privacy by judiciously protecting information of a confidential nature

ATTITUDES

- Display curiosity in considering why Mr. Johnson might be behaving or responding in this manner
- Jan needs to display integrity when her beliefs and values differ from Mr. Johnson's; admit to any inconsistencies between her values and his
- Risk taking may be necessary in developing a trusting relationship with Mr. Johnson

Chapter 26   *Synthesis Model for Nursing Care Plan for* **Alterations in Self-Concept (page 141).**

KNOWLEDGE

- A basic understanding of sexual development, sexual orientation, sociocultural dimensions, the impact of self-concept, STDs, safe sex practices.
- Ways to phrase questions regarding sexuality and functioning
- Disease conditions that affect sexual functioning
- How interpersonal relationship factors may affect sexual functioning

EXPERIENCE

- Jack needs to explore his discomfort with discussing topics related to sexuality and develop a plan for addressing these discomforts
- Jack needs to reflect on his personal sexual experiences and how he has responded

ASSESSMENT

- Assess Mr. Clement's developmental stage in regard to sexuality
- Consider self-concept as a factor that will influence sexual satisfaction and functioning
- Physical assessment of urogenital area
- Determine Mr. Clement's sexual concerns
- Assess safe sex practices and the use of contraception
- Assess the severity of his hypertension, which may be affecting his sexual functioning
- Assess the impact of high-risk behaviors on sexual health

STANDARDS

- Jack needs to apply intellectual standards of relevance and plausibility for care to be acceptable to Mr. Clement
- Jack needs to safeguard Mr. Clement's right to privacy by judiciously protecting information of a confidential nature
- Jack needs to apply the principles of ethic of care

ATTITUDES

- Jack needs to display curiosity, consider why Mr. Clement might behave or respond in a particular manner
- Jack needs to display integrity; his beliefs and values may differ from Mr. Clement's
- Jack needs to admit to any inconsistencies in his and Mr. Clement's values
- Risk taking: Jack needs to be willing to explore both personal and Mr. Clement's sexual issues and concerns

Chapter 27 *Synthesis Model for Nursing Care Plan for* **Sexual Dysfunction** **(page 147).**

KNOWLEDGE

- The concepts of faith, hope, spiritual well-being and religion
- Caring practices in the individual approach to a client
- Available services in the community (health care providers and agencies)

EXPERIENCE

- Leah's past experience in selecting interventions that support client's spiritual well-being

PLANNING

- Leah needs to collaborate with James and his family on choice of interventions
- Consult with pastoral care or other clergy, holy leaders as appropriate
- Continue appropriate religious rituals specific to James

STANDARDS

- Standards of autonomy and self determination to support James decisions about the plan

ATTITUDES

- Leah will exhibit confidence in her skills and know to develop a trusting relationship with James

Chapter 28 *Synthesis Model for Nursing Care Plan for Spiritual Well-being* (page 153).

KNOWLEDGE

- Characteristics of a resolution of grief
- Clinical symptoms of an improved level of comfort (applicable for the terminally ill)

EXPERIENCE

- Previous client responses to planned nursing interventions of the loss of a significant other

EVALUATION

- Evaluate signs and symptoms of Mr. Miller's grief and his wife's
- Evaluate his wife's ability to provide supportive care
- Evaluate Mr. Miller's level of comfort

STANDARDS

- Use established expected outcomes to evaluate Mr. Miller's plan of care (participation in life review)
- Evaluate Mr. Miller's role in end-of-life decisions and (or the grieving) process

ATTITUDES

- Persevere in seeking successful comfort measures for Mr. Miller

Chapter 29 *Synthesis Model for Nursing Care Plan for Grief and Loss (page 159).*

KNOWLEDGE

- Characteristics of adaptive behaviors
- Characteristics of continuing stress response

EXPERIENCE

- Previous client responses to planned nursing interventions

EVALUATION

- Reassess Carl for the presence of new or recurring stress related problems/symptoms (fatigue, changes in energy level, weight, or eating habits)
- Determine if change in care promoted Carl's adaptation to stress
- Evaluate if Carl's expectations have been achieved.

STANDARDS

- Use of established expected outcomes to evaluate Carl's plan of care (rest and relaxation, stable weight, positive feelings about wife and their relationship)
- Apply the intellectual standard of relevance; be sure that Carl achieves goals relevant to his needs

ATTITUDES

- Janet needs to demonstrate perseverance in redesigning interventions to promote Carl's adaptation to stress
- Janet needs to display integrity in accurately evaluating nursing interventions

Chapter 30   *Synthesis Model for Nursing Care Plan for* **Care Giver Role Strain (page 166).**

KNOWLEDGE

- The role of physical therapist and exercise trainers in improving Mrs. Swain's CDP program
- Determine Mrs. Swain's ability to increase her level of activity

EXPERIENCE

- Mary needs to consider previous client and personal experiences to therapies designed to improve exercise and activity tolerance
- Mary's personal experience with exercise regimens

PLANNING

- Mary needs to consult and collaborate with members of the health team to increase Mrs. Swain's activity
- Involve Mrs. Swain and her family in designing her activity and exercise plan
- Mary needs to consider Mrs. Swain's ability to increase her activity level and follow a exercise program

STANDARDS

- Therapies need to be individualized to Mrs. Swain's activity tolerance
- Mary needs to apply the goals of the American College of Sports Medicine in the application

ATTITUDES

- Mary needs to be responsible and creative in designing interventions to improve Mrs. Swain's activity tolerance

Chapter 36 *Synthesis Model for Nursing Care Plan for* Activity Intolerance (page 221).

KNOWLEDGE

- Basic human needs
- The potential risks to a client's safety from physical and environmental hazards
- The influence of developmental stage on safety needs (older adult)
- The influence of illness and medications on Ms. Cohen's safety (immobilization and visual impairment)

EXPERIENCE

- Past experiences of Mr. Key in caring for clients with mobility or sensory impairments that threaten safety
- Personal experiences in caring for the older adult

ASSESSMENT

- Identification of actual and potential threats to Ms. Cohen's safety
- Determine the impact of Ms. Cohen's underlying disease on her safety
- The presence of risks for Ms. Cohen's developmental stage

STANDARDS

- Mr. Key needs to apply intellectual standards of accuracy, significance, completeness, and fairness when assessing for threats to Ms. Cohen's safety
- ANA standards of nursing practice
- Fall prevention protocols (Practice Standards)

ATTITUDES

- Perseverance is needed when identifying all threats to Ms. Cohen's safety
- Responsibility for collecting unbiased accurate data regarding Ms. Cohen's threat to safety
- Fairness is appropriate to objectively evaluate the risk to Ms. Cohen's safety with in the home and the community

Chapter 37 *Synthesis Model for Nursing Care Plan for* Risk for Injury (page 227).

KNOWLEDGE

- Principles of comfort and safety
- Adult learning principles to apply when educating the client and family
- Services available through community agencies

EXPERIENCE

- Care of previous clients that required adaptation of hygiene approaches

PLANNING

- Involve Mrs. Wyatt and her family in planning and adapting approaches as well as in hygiene instruction
- Know community resources applicable to Mrs. Wyatt's needs
- Consider the timing of other care activities when choosing the best time for hygienic care

STANDARDS

- Individualize the hygiene care to meet Mrs. Wyatt's preferences
- Apply standards of safety and promotion of client dignity

ATTITUDES

- Jeanette needs to be creative when adapting approaches to any self-care limitations that Mrs. Wyatt might have
- Jeanette needs to take responsibility for following standards of good hygiene practice

Chapter 38 *Synthesis Model for Nursing Care Plan for* Self-Care Deficit, Bathing/Hygiene (page 236).

KNOWLEDGE

- Cardiac and respiratory anatomy and physiology
- Cardiopulmonary pathophysiology
- Clinical signs and symptoms of altered oxygenation
- Developmental factors affecting oxygenation
- Impact on lifestyle
- Environmental impact

EXPERIENCE

- Caring for clients with impaired oxygenation, activity intolerance, and respiratory infections
- Observations of changes in client respiratory patterns made during poor air quality days
- Personal experience with how a change in altitudes or physical conditioning affects respiratory patterns
- Personal experience with respiratory infections or cardiopulmonary alterations

ASSESSMENT

- Identify recurring and present signs and symptoms associated with Mr. Edwards impaired oxygenation
- Determine the presence of risk factors that apply to Mr. Edwards
- Ask Mr. Edwards about the use of medication
- Determine Mr. Edwards activity status
- Determine Mr. Edwards tolerance to activity

STANDARDS

- Apply intellectual standards of clarity, precision, specificity, and accuracy when obtaining a health history for a client with cardiopulmonary alterations

ATTITUDES

- Carry out the responsibility of obtaining correct information about Mr. Edwards and explaining risk factors, health promotion and disease prevention activities, and therapies for disease/symptom management
- Display confidence in assessing Mr. Edwards management of illness

Chapter 39 *Synthesis Model for Nursing Care Plan for* **Ineffective Airway Clearance (page 251).**

Answers to Synthesis Models   563

KNOWLEDGE

- Consider the other health care professionals caring for Mrs. Bottomley
- The impact of specific fluid regimens on the Mrs. Bottomley's fluid balance
- The impact of new medications on Mrs. Bottomley's fluid balance

EXPERIENCE

- Consider the previous clinical assignments you have had and how those clients responded to nursing therapies (what worked and what didn't?)

PLANNING

- Select nursing interventions to promote fluid, electrolyte, and acid-base balance
- Consult with pharmacists and nutritionists
- Involve Mrs. Bottomley and her family in designing the interventions

STANDARDS

- Therapies need to be individualized to Mrs. Bottomley's fluid balance and acid-base requirements

ATTITUDES

- Use creativity to plan interventions that will achieve an effective airway and integrate those into Mrs. Bottomley's activities of daily living
- Be responsible in planning nursing interventions consistent with the client's fluid balance and acid-base requirements

Chapter 40 *Synthesis Model for* Ineffective Airway Clearance/Risk for Fluid Volume Deficit (page 266).

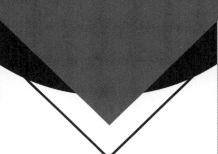

KNOWLEDGE

- The characteristics of a desirable sleep pattern
- Basis for the expected outcomes in the plan of care

EXPERIENCE

- Previous client's responses to planned nursing interventions for promoting sleep
- Previous experience in adapting sleep therapies to personal needs

EVALUATION

- Evaluate signs and symptoms of Julie's sleep disturbance
- Review Julie's sleep pattern
- Have sleep partner report Julie's response to therapies
- The expected outcomes developed during the plan of care serve as the standards to evaluate its success

STANDARDS

- Use established expected outcomes to evaluate Julie's plan of care (improved duration of sleep, fewer awakenings)

ATTITUDES

- Humility may apply if an intervention is unsuccessful; rethink the approach
- In the case of chronic sleep problems, perseverance is needed in staying with the plan of care or in trying new approaches

Chapter 41 *Synthesis Model for Nursing Care Plan for* Sleep Pattern Disturbance (page 276).

KNOWLEDGE

- Physiology of pain
- Factors that potentially increase or decrease responses to pain
- Pathophysiology of conditions causing pain
- Awareness of biases affecting pain assessment and treatment
- Cultural variations in how pain is expressed
- Knowledge of nonverbal communication

EXPERIENCE

- Caring for clients with acute, chronic, and cancer pain
- Caring for clients who experienced pain as a result of a health care therapy
- Personal experience with pain

ASSESSMENT

- Determine Mrs. May's perspective of pain including history of pain, its meaning, and physical emotional and social effects
- Objectively measure the characteristics of Mrs. May's pain
- Review potential factors affecting Mrs. May's pain

STANDARDS

- Refer to AHCPR guidelines for acute pain management
- Apply intellectual standards (clarity, specificity, accuracy, and completeness) when gathering assessment
- Apply relevance when letting Mrs. May's explore the pain experience

ATTITUDES

- Persevere in exploring causes and possible solutions for chronic pain
- Display confidence when assessing pain to relieve Mrs. May's anxiety
- Display integrity and fairness to prevent prejudice from affecting assessment

Chapter 42 *Synthesis Model for Nursing Care Plan for* **Acute Pain (page 287).**

566   Answers to Synthesis Models

KNOWLEDGE

- Roles of dietitians and nutritionists in caring for clients with altered nutrition
- Impact of community support groups and other resources in assisting clients to manage nutrition
- Impact of bad diets on client's overall nutritional status

EXPERIENCE

- Previous client responses to nursing interventions for altered nutrition
- Personal experiences with dietary change strategies (what worked and what didn't)

PLANNING

- Select nursing interventions to promote optimal nutrition
- Select nursing interventions consistent with therapeutic diets
- Consult with other health care professionals (dietitians, nutritionists, physicians, pharmacists, and physical and occupational therapists) to adopt interventions that reflect Mrs. Cooper's needs
- Involve the family when designing interventions

STANDARDS

- Individualize therapy according to Mrs. Cooper's needs
- Therapies consistent with established standards of normal nutrition (e.g., USDA, FDA, WHO, HWC)
- Select therapies consistent with established standards for therapeutic diets (AHA, ADA., ASREP)

ATTITUDES

- Display confidence in selecting interventions
- Creatively adapt interventions for client's physical limitation, culture, personal preferences, budget, and home care needs

Chapter 43 *Synthesis model for Nursing Care Plan for* Altered Nutrition: Less Than Body Requirements (page 299).

KNOWLEDGE

- Physiology of fluid balance
- Anatomy and physiology of normal urine production and urination
- Pathophysiology of selected urinary alterations
- Factors affecting urination
- Principles of communication used to address issues related to self-concept and sexuality

EXPERIENCE

- Caring for clients with alterations in urinary elimination
- Caring for clients at risk for urinary infection
- Personal experience with changes in urinary elimination

ASSESSMENT

- Gather nursing history of the urination pattern, symptoms, and factors affecting urination
- Conduct a physical assessment of body systems potentially affected by urinary change
- Assess the characteristics of urine
- Assess perception of urinary problems as it affects self-concept and sexuality

STANDARDS

- Maintain privacy and dignity
- Apply intellectual standards to ensure history and assessment are complete and in depth
- Apply professional standards of care from professional organizations such as ANA and AHCPR

ATTITUDES

- Display humility in recognizing limitations in knowledge

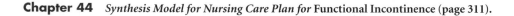

Chapter 44   *Synthesis Model for Nursing Care Plan for* Functional Incontinence (page 311).

KNOWLEDGE

- Role of the other health care professionals in returning the client's bowel elimination pattern to normal
- Impact of specific therapeutic diets and medication on bowel elimination patterns
- Expected results of cathartics, laxatives, and enemas on bowel elimination

EXPERIENCE

- Previous client response to planned nursing therapies for improving bowel elimination (what worked and what didn't)

PLANNING

- Javier needs to select nursing interventions to promote normal bowel elimination
- Consult with nutritionists and enteral stoma therapists
- Involve Larry and his family in designing nursing interventions

STANDARDS

- Individualize therapies to Larry's bowel elimination needs
- Select therapies consistent within wound and ostomy professional practice standards

ATTITUDES

- Javier needs to be creative when planning interventions for Larry to achieve normal bowel elimination patterns
- Display independence when integrating interventions from other disciplines in Larry's plan of care
- Act responsibly by ensuring that interventions are consistent within standards

Chapter 45 *Synthesis Model for Nursing Care Plan for* Constipation *(page 323).*

KNOWLEDGE

- Characteristics of improved mobility status on all physiological systems and the client's psychosocial and developmental status

EXPERIENCE

- Previous client responses to planned mobility interventions.

EVALUATION

- Reassess Miss Adams for signs and symptoms of improved or decreased mobility status
- Ask for Miss Adam's perception of mobility status after intervention
- Evaluate whether or not Miss Adam's expectations of care have been met

STANDARDS

- Use established expected outcomes for the Miss Adam's plan of care (lung fields remain clear) to evaluate her response to care

ATTITUDES

- Display humility when identifying those interventions that were not successful
- Use creativity when redesigning new interventions to improve Miss Adam's mobility status

Chapter 46 *Synthesis Model for Nursing Care Plan for* Impaired Mobility (page 333).

KNOWLEDGE

- Pathogenesis of pressure ulcers
- Factors contributing to pressure ulcer formation or poor wound healing
- Factors contributing to wound healing
- Impact of underlying disease process of skin integrity
- Impact of medication on skin integrity and wound healing

EXPERIENCE

- Caring for clients with impaired skin integrity or wounds
- Observation of normal wound healing

ASSESSMENT

- Identify actual and potential risks to impaired skin integrity
- Identify signs and symptoms associated with impaired skin integrity or poor wound healing
- Determine Mrs. Stein's mobility status

STANDARDS

- Apply intellectual standards of accuracy, relevance, completeness, and precision when obtaining health history regarding skin integrity and wound management
- Knowledge of AHCPR standards for prevention of pressure ulcers

ATTITUDES

- Use discipline to obtain complete and correct assessment data regarding Mrs. Stein's skin and or/wound integrity
- Demonstrate responsibility for collecting appropriate specimens for diagnostic and laboratory tests related to wound management

Chapter 47 *Synthesis Model for Nursing Care Plan for* **Impaired Skin Integrity (page 345).**

KNOWLEDGE

- Understand how a sensory deficit can affect the client's functional status
- Role other health professionals might have in sensory function management
- Services of community resources
- Adult learning principles to apply when educating the client and family

EXPERIENCE

- Previous client responses to planned nursing interventions to promote sensory function

PLANNING

- Select strategies that assist Judy to remain functional in her home
- Adapt therapies based on short- or long-term sensory deficit
- Involve the family in helping Judy adjust to her limitations
- Refer to client to appropriate health care professional and/or community agency

STANDARDS

- Individualize therapies that allow the client to adapt to sensory loss in any setting
- Apply standards of safety

ATTITUDES

- Use creativity to find interventions that help Judy adapt to the home environment

Chapter 48 *Synthesis Model for Nursing Care Plan for* Sensory Perceptual Alterations (page 354).

KNOWLEDGE

- Behaviors that demonstrate learning
- Characteristics of anxiety and/or fear

EXPERIENCE

- Previous client responses to planned preoperative care
- Any personal experience Joe has had with surgery

EVALUATION

- Evaluate Mrs. Cambana's knowledge of surgical procedure and planned postoperative care
- Have Mrs. Cambana demonstrate postoperative exercises
- Observe behaviors or nonverbal expressions of anxiety or fear

STANDARDS

- Use established expected outcomes to evaluate Mrs. Cambana's plan of care (ability to perform postoperative exercises)

ATTITUDES

- Demonstrate perseverance when Mrs. Cambana has difficulty performing postoperative exercises

Chapter 49 *Synthesis Model for Nursing Care Plan for* Knowledge Deficit Regarding Pre and Postoperative Care (page 368).